Lucian Sulica
Andrew Blitzer
Editors

Vocal Fold Paralysis

Lucian Sulica
Andrew Blitzer
Editors

Vocal Fold Paralysis

With 80 Figures, mostly in Color

Springer

Lucian Sulica, MD
Assistant Professor
Department of Otorhinolaryngology
Weill Medical College of Cornell University
New York, New York

Andrew Blitzer, MD, DDS
Professor of Clinical Otolaryngology
Department of Otolaryngology
Columbia University College
of Physicians and Surgeons
Director, NY Center for Voice
and Swallowing Disorders
New York, New York

ISBN   3-540-23765-8
Springer Berlin Heidelberg New York

ISBN   978-3-540-23765-5
Springer Berlin Heidelberg New York

Library of Congress Control Number: 2005930275

This work is subject to copyright. All rights are reserved, whether the whole or part of the material is concerned, specifically the rights of translation, reprinting, reuse of illustrations, recitation, broadcasting, reproduction on microfilms or in any other way, and storage in data banks. Duplication of this publication or parts thereof is permitted only under the provisions of the German Copyright Law of September 9, 1965, in its current version, and permission for use must always be obtained from Springer-Verlag. Violations are liable for prosecution under the German Copyright Law.

Springer is a part of Springer Science+Business Media
springer.com

© Springer-Verlag Berlin Heidelberg 2006
Printed in Germany

The use of general descriptive names, registered names, trademarks, etc. in this publication does not imply, even in the absence of a specific statement, that such names are exempt from the relevant protective laws and regulations and therefore free for general use.

Product liability: The publishers cannot guarantee the accuracy of any information about dosage and application contained in this book. In every individual case the user must check such information by consulting the relevant literature.

Editor: Marion Philipp, Heidelberg, Germany
Desk Editor: Irmela Bohn, Heidelberg, Germany
Production: LE-TeX Jelonek, Schmidt & Vöckler GbR, Leipzig, Germany
Cover: Frido Steinen-Broo, eStudio Calamar, Spain
Typsetting and reproduction of the figures:
Satz-Druck-Service, Leimen, Germany
Printed on acid-free paper   24/3100YL/Di

Dedication

This volume is dedicated with love and the most profound gratitude to my first two clinical professors, Lucian O. Sulica, MD and Virginia I. Sulica, MD, who taught me (among other things) that medicine requires equal measures of logic and intuition, skepticism and faith, perseverance and enthusiasm, doggedness and curiosity, and compassion above all.

Lucian Sulica, MD

Preface

Vocal fold paralysis is not a rare clinical entity. The length and path of the laryngeal nerves makes them vulnerable to compromise from a variety of sources, and many physicians – surgeons, oncologists, endocrinologists, neurologists – encounter the consequences. Yet for all of its clinical familiarity, vocal fold paralysis has preserved its mysteries to a remarkable extent. When faced with straightforward questions from patients – What are the chances that I will recover my voice? What are the chances the vocal fold will move again? When is either of these likely to happen? – we are able to offer only the most approximate answers, based on a consensus that is rarely supported by unequivocal clinical evidence. Basic treatment considerations, such as when to intervene and what kind of intervention to make, are founded as much on dogma and physician preference as on information regarding outcomes and efficacy. Comparison with facial nerve palsy, another cranial mononeuropathy familiar to most otolaryngologists, reveals the gaps in knowledge regarding vocal fold paralysis rather starkly.

Under these circumstances, it seemed appropriate to attempt to collect the available information between two covers, not necessarily to close these lacunae, for much clinical investigation remains to be done before that can happen, but to offer an integrated reference and sourcebook on the subject of vocal fold paralysis. The resulting volume is divided into three sections. The first summarizes current knowledge regarding the relevant neuroanatomy, aberrant reinnervation, natural history and clinical evaluation. The second addresses treatment considerations, both as part of an integrated treatment algorithm, and also with respect to each principal medialization option. All commonly used injection medialization substances and available laryngoplasty techniques are presented in turn, and authors have included not only a detailed discussion of surgical technique enriched by observations from personal experience, but also available efficacy data. Finally, the third section addresses dynamic rehabilitation of vocal fold paralysis in the form of pacing and reinnervation, where the future must necessarily lie, and special topics like pediatric vocal fold paralysis and bilateral vocal fold paralysis.

We intended to make this book useful on several levels: as a grounding in relevant basic science, as a guide to informed clinical decision-making, as a practical "how-to" in the operating room or office, and as a springboard for further thought and investigation. Most of all, though, we hope that the clinical questions that remain to be answered concerning vocal fold paralysis are better framed, and perhaps posed more strongly and with a greater sense of urgency.

To the extent that we have succeeded in these aims, it is entirely due to our contributors. We are in their debt for their expertise and their commitment to sharing it, and their good grace in the face of our editorial demands. Most of all, we are grateful for their investment of time and effort in support of scholarship and education, in a medical environment that encourages it less and less.

We also wish to acknowledge the professionalism of Marion Philipp, Irmela Bohn and Martina Himberger at Springer, and we thank them for their patience and equanimity in the face of the difficulties that inevitably arise in the course of such a project.

Finally, we wish to thank our colleagues and our students with whom we have discussed these topics, and most of all our patients, who are not cowed by our white coats and push us for better answers every day.

Lucian Sulica, MD
Andrew Blitzer, MD, DDS
New York, NY

Contents

Part I
Basic Science and Clinical Evaluation

Chapter 1
Neuroanatomy of the Larynx
Ajay E. Chitkara

Introduction	3
CNS	4
Superior Laryngeal Nerve	4
Cervical Segment of SLN	5
Internal Branch of SLN	5
External Branch of SLN	5
Recurrent Laryngeal Nerve	6
Cervical Segment of RLN	6
RLN Branching Patterns	7
Relationship of RLN with Inferior Thyroid Artery	8
Retrothyroid Segment of RLN	10
Laryngeal Segment of RLN	10
Neuromuscular Junctions	12
RLN Communication with SLN	12
Conclusion	14

Chapter 2
Synkinesis and Dysfunctional Reinnervation of the Larynx
David L. Zealear, Cheryl R. Billante

Introduction	17
Innervation and Functional Anatomy of Laryngeal Muscles	17
Consequence of RLN Injury	21
Conventional Treatment for Laryngeal Paralysis	24
Studies in Selective Reinnervation	25

Chapter 3
Vocal Fold Paralysis: Causes, Outcomes, and Clinical Aspects
Lucian Sulica, Anthony Cultrara, Andrew Blitzer

Introduction	33
Sources of Nerve Damage	33
Overview	33
Surgery/Trauma	38
Surgery in the Neck	38
Surgery in the Chest	44
Surgery at the Skull Base	45
Other Procedures and Interventions	45
Medical Disease	46
Malignancy	46
Nonmalignant Disease	46
Stroke	47
Other Neurologic Disease	47
Idiopathic Vocal Fold Paralysis	47
Conclusion	48

Chapter 4
Evaluation of Vocal Fold Paralysis
C. Blake Simpson, Esther J. Cheung

History	55
Vocal Quality and Swallowing	55
Vocal Inventory	55
Airway	56
Medical History: Establishing an Etiology	56
Physical Examination	57
General	57
Laryngeal	57
Work-up	59
Serology	59
Imaging Studies	59
Conclusion	61

Chapter 5
Diagnostic Electromyography for Unilateral Vocal Fold Dysmotility
Al Hillel, Lawrence Robinson

Introduction 63
Definition of Immobility 63
Definition of Electromyography 63
Techniques of Electromyography 64
EMG Waveforms: How They Are Derived, and What They Mean 64
How LEMG Defines Dysmotility and Refines the Diagnosis 66
How LEMG Can Guide Treatment. 69
   Philosophy of LEMG. 70
Case Examples. 70
   Case 1 70
   Case 2 70

Part II
Treatment

Chapter 6
Decision Points in the Management of Vocal Fold Paralysis
Lucian Sulica, Andrew Blitzer

Introduction 77
Dysphagia and Aspiration 77
Prognosis 78
Laryngeal Electromyography 80
Adjusting the Treatment Algorithm 81
Conclusion 83

Chapter 7
Voice Therapy for Unilateral Vocal Fold Paralysis
Celia F. Stewart, Elizabeth Allen

Introduction 87
Assessment. 87
   Perceptual Assessment. 87
   Self-Ratings 87
   Objective Measurements 88
   Compensations 89
Guidelines for Planning Voice Therapy ... 89
   Patterns of Vocal Symptoms 90
   Rehabilitation Hypotheses 90
Therapy Procedures 90

Indirect Rehabilitation 90
Direct Rehabilitation 91
Transfer of Skills 92
Vocal Practice. 92
Communicating in Noisy Environments 92
Results 93
Conclusion 93

Chapter 8
Injection Augmentation
Karen A. Cooper, Charles N. Ford

Introduction 97
Indications 97
Historical Note. 97
Timing of Intervention 98
Technique 99
Office-Based Procedure. 99
Results 102
Complications. 102
Current Status and Future Goals 102

Chapter 8.1
Autologous Fat for Vocal Fold Injection
Clark A. Rosen

Introduction 105
Rationale for Vocal Fold Lipoinjection ... 105
Patient Selection 105
Technical Aspects of Vocal Fold Lipoinjection. 106
   Fat Harvest 106
   Lipoinjection 108
   Post-operative Care Following Lipoinjection 108
Duration of Benefit. 109
Complications of Lipoinjection of the Vocal Folds. 109
   Airway 109
   Suboptimal Voice Improvement 109
   Overinjection. 110

Chapter 8.2
Collagen in Vocal Fold Injection
Mark S. Courey

Physiologic Considerations 111
Historical Considerations. 111
Technical Considerations. 112

Clinical Applications 114
Conclusion 114

Chapter 8.3
Treatment of Glottal Insufficiency Using Micronized Human Acellular Dermis (Cymetra)
Albert L. Merati

Introduction 117
Background 117
Advantages and Disadvantages
   of Micronized Acellular Dermis
     for Clinical Use 118
Micronized Human Acellular Dermis
   in Clinical Laryngology 119
   Complications 119
   Technical Aspects
     for Using Micronized Acellular
       Human Dermis 120
Conclusion 120

Chapter 8.4
Vocal Fold Augmentation with Calcium Hydroxylapatite
Peter C. Belafsky, Gregory N. Postma

Introduction 123
   Indications for Vocal Fold Augmentation
     with CaHA 123
Technique of Injection Augmentation
   with CaHA 123
   In-Office Injection of CaHA 124
   Injection of CaHA
     in the Operating Room 124
Conclusion 126

Chapter 8.5
Treatment of Glottal Insufficiency Using Hyaluronan
Stellan Hertegård, Åke Dahlqvist, Lars Hallén, Claude Laurent

Introduction and Core Messages 127
Rationale 128
Indications 128
   Indication Under Investigation 129
Patient Selection 129
Advantages 130
Disadvantages 131

Complications 131
Technique 131

Chapter 9
Principles of Medialization Laryngoplasty
C. Blake Simpson, Lucian Sulica

Introduction 135
Indications for Surgery 135
Arytenoid Adduction 137
Procedure Selection:
   Framework Surgery vs Injection
     Augmentation 137
Patient Selection 137
Timing of Medialization Laryngoplasty . . . 138
Technical Notes and Pertinent
   Anatomic Landmarks 138
Complications 140
Suboptimal Results / Surgical Errors 141
Revision Surgery 142
Long-Term Surgical Issues 142
Conclusion 142

Chapter 9.1
Silastic Medialization Laryngoplasty
C. Blake Simpson

Introduction 145
Procedure 145
   Preparation 145
   Surgical Approach 145
   Endolaryngeal/
     Paraglottic Manipulation 146
   Carving the Silastic Implant 147
   Implant Insertion 148
   Closure 150
   Postoperative Care 150
   Postoperative Issues
     and Expected Vocal Recovery 150

Chapter 9.2
Medialization Thyroplasty Using the Montgomery Thyroplasty System
Mark A. Varvares, Rebecca M. Brandsted

Introduction 153
Design of Thyroplasty Prosthesis 153
Patient Selection 154
Anesthesia 154
Surgical Technique 154

Window Measurement 155
Window Outline 155
Method for Cutting Window 156
Implant Measurement. 156
Insertion of Implant 157
Closure 157
Postoperative Care. 157
Complications. 157
Results 157
Conclusion 158

Chapter 9.3
Medialization Thyroplasty Using the VoCoM Vocal Cord Medialization System
Tanya K. Meyer, Andrew Blitzer

Introduction 159
Surgical Technique. 160
Revision. 163
Complications. 163
Results 163
Conclusion 163

Chapter 9.4
Titanium Medialization Implant
Berit Schneider

Titanium as a Biomaterial 165
Titanium Vocal Medialization Implant . . . 165
Preoperative Medication 166
Anesthesia 166
Surgical Technique. 166
Objective Outcome Measures. 167
Advantages 167
Complications. 167
Other Titanium Implant Devices 168

Chapter 9.5
Medialization Laryngoplasty with Gore-Tex (Expanded Polytetrafluoroethylene)
Timothy M. McCulloch, Henry T. Hoffman

Introduction 169
Technique of Gore-Tex Thyroplasty 170
   Patient Preparation Steps 171
   Operative Steps 171
Complications. 174
Conclusion 175

Chapter 10
Arytenoid Repositioning Surgery
Gayle E. Woodson

Introduction 177
Indications 177
Vocal Fold Motion 178
What Is a Posterior Gap? 178
History of Arytenoid Surgery 179
Mechanics of Arytenoid Surgery. 180
Technique of Arytenoid Adduction 181
Conclusion 184

Part III
Special Topics

Chapter 11
Laryngeal Reinnervation
Randal C. Paniello

Introduction 189
Rationale for Reinnervation in UVFP. 189
Choice of Donor Nerve 190
Choice of Anesthesia /
   Contingency Plans 191
Technique of Ansa Cervicalis
   to RLN Anastomosis 192
Technique of Hypoglossal Nerve
   to RLN Anastomosis 193
Postoperative Care. 194
Results of Animal Studies 194
Clinical Results 195
   Ansa-RLN 195
   Ansa-RLN and Medialization 195
   Hypoglossal Nerve 196
   Original RLN. 196
Reinnervation or Medialization? 197
Cricothyroid Reinnervation 197
Abductor Reinnervation 198
   Phrenic Nerve 198
   Ansa Cervicalis 199
Combined Adductor and Abductor
   Reinnervation 199
Bidirectional Motion: Animal Models 199
Reinnervation for Laryngeal
   Transplantation 199
Conclusion 200

Chapter 12
Electrical Stimulation for Vocal Fold Paralysis
Michael Broniatowski

Introduction 203
Background and Justification 203
    The Problem 203
    Critique of Traditional Management
      of Laryngeal Paralyses 204
    Physiological Bases
      for Laryngeal Stimulation 204
    Challenges in Approaches
      to Laryngeal Stimulation 205
    Laryngeal Stimulating Strategies 207
    Issues of Long-Term Stimulation
      and Biocompatibility of Implanted
      Circuits 207
Current Human Applications 207
    Dynamic Laryngotracheal Closure
      for Aspiration 208
    Dynamic Restoration of Laryngeal Patency
      After Bilateral Vocal Fold Paralysis 209
Potential Future Human Applications 212
    Integrated Swallowing Rehabilitation . . . 213
    Laryngeal Transplantation 213
    Artificial Control of Voice
      and Spasm 213
Conclusion 215

Chapter 13
Bilateral Medialization Laryngoplasty
Gregory N. Postma, Peter C. Belafsky

Introduction 219
Surgical Indications 219
Surgical Technique 219
Results 222
Complications 222
Discussion 222
Approach to Surgical Treatment 223
Conclusion 223

Chapter 14
Vocal Fold Paralysis in Children
Marshall E. Smith

Introduction 225
Spectrum of Presentation 225
The Newborn and Infant: Airway
    and Swallowing Assessment
    and Management 226
Management of Airway, Voice,
    and Swallowing in Vocal Fold Paralysis
    in Infants 227
Bilateral Vocal Fold Paralysis:
    Long-Term Management Options 228
Voice Concerns in the Older Child
    and Adolescent 229
Unilateral Laryngeal Paralysis:
    Management Options 230
Laryngeal EMG in Children 231
Familial Vocal Fold Paralysis 232
Conclusion 232

Chapter 15
Bilateral Vocal Fold Immobility
George Goding

Introduction 237
History 237
Etiology 238
Evaluation 239
Adjunctive Measures
    and Nonsurgical Management 240
Surgical Management 241
Posterior Glottic Stenosis 241
Direct Muscle Reinnervation 242
Lateralization 243
Tissue Removal 244
Research 245
Conclusion 246

Subject Index 249

List of Contributors

Elizabeth Allen
Department of Speech-
Language Pathology and Audiology
Steinhardt School of Education
New York University
New York, New York
USA

Peter C. Belafsky, MD, PhD
Associate Professor
Center for Voice and Swallowing
Department of Otolaryngology
UC Davis Medical Center
Sacramento, California
USA

Cheryl R. Billante, PhD
Assistant Professor
Department of Otolaryngology –
Head and Neck Surgery
Vanderbilt University Medical School
Nashville, Tennessee
USA

Andrew Blitzer, MD, DDS
Professor of Clinical Otolaryngology
Department of Otolaryngology
Columbia University College of Physicians and
Surgeons
Director, NY Center for Voice and Swallowing
Disorders
New York, New York
USA

Rebecca M. Brandsted
Department of Otolaryngology
St. Louis University School of Medicine
St. Louis, Missouri
USA

Michael Broniatowski, MD
Professor
Department of Otolaryngology –
Head and Neck Surgery
Case Western Reserve University
Cleveland, Ohio
USA

Esther J. Cheung, MD
Resident Physician
Division of Otolaryngology –
Head and Neck Surgery
Pennsylvania State College of Medicine
Hershey, Pennsylvania
USA

Ajay E. Chitkara, MD
Clinical Assistant Professor
Division of Otolaryngology
State University of New York at Stony Brook
Smithtown, New York
USA

Karen Cooper, MD
Attending Physician
Division of Otolaryngology –
Head and Neck Surgery
Manhattan Eye, Ear and Throat Hospital
New York, New York
USA

Mark S. Courey, MD
Professor
Director, The UCSF Voice and Swallowing Center
Department of Otolaryngology –
Head and Neck Surgery
UCSF School of Medicine
San Francisco, California
USA

List of Contributors

Anthony Cultrara, MD
Attending Physician
Private Practice
Vorhees, NJ
USA

Åke Dahlqvist, MD, PhD †
Department of Clinical Sciences –
Otorhinolaryngology
Umeå University Hospital
Umeå
Sweden
(deceased in the tsunami catastrophe,
Thailand, December 26, 2004)

Charles N. Ford, MD
Professor
Department of Otolaryngology –
Head and Neck Surgery
University of Wisconsin Hospitals and Clinics
Madison, Wisconsin
USA

George Goding, MD
Associate Professor
Department of Otolaryngology
University of Minnesota
Hennepin County Medical Center
Minneapolis, Minnesota
USA

Lars Hallén, MD, PhD
Department of Otorhinolaryngology
Central Hospital Falun
Falun
Sweden

Stellan Hertegård, MD, PhD
Department of Logopedics and Phoniatrics
Karolinska Institute
Huddinge University Hospital
Stockholm
Sweden

Allen Hillel, MD
Professor
Department of Otolaryngology –
Head and Neck Surgery
University of Washington School of Medicine
Seattle, Washington
USA

Henry T. Hoffman, MD
Professor
Department of Otolaryngology –
Head and Neck Surgery
University of Iowa
Iowa City, Iowa
USA

Claude Laurent, MD, PhD
Department of Otorhinolaryngology
Rikshospitalet University Hospital
Oslo
Norway

Timothy M. McCulloch, MD
Professor
Department of Otolaryngology –
Head and Neck Surgery
University of Washington School of Medicine
Seattle, Washington
USA

Albert L. Merati, MD
Associate Professor
Chief, Division of Laryngology
Department of Otolaryngology and
Communication Sciences
Medical College of Wisconsin
Milwaukee, Wisconsin
USA

Tanya K. Meyer, MD
Assistant Professor
Department of Otolaryngology
University of Maryland School of Medicine
Baltimore, Maryland
USA

List of Contributors

Randall C. Paniello, MD
Associate Professor
Department of Otolaryngology
Washington University School of Medicine
St. Louis, Missouri
USA

Gregory N. Postma, MD
Professor
Director, Center for Voice
and Swallowing Disorders
Department of Otolaryngology
Medical College of Georgia
Augusta, Georgia
USA

Lawrence Robinson, MD
Professor
Department of Rehabilitation Medicine
University of Washington School of Medicine
Seattle, Washington
USA

Clark A. Rosen, MD
Associate Professor
Department of Otolaryngology
University of Pittsburgh School of Medicine
Pittsburgh, Pennsylvania
USA

Berit Schneider, MD
Universitäts HNO-Klinik
Klinische Abteilung Phoniatrie-Logopädie
AKH der Stadt Wien
Vienna
Austria

C. Blake Simpson, MD
Associate Professor
Department of Otolaryngology –
Head and Neck Surgery
The University of Texas Health Science Center
San Antonio, Texas
USA

Marshall E. Smith, MD
Associate Professor
Division of Otolaryngology –
Head and Neck Surgery
University of Utah School of Medicine
Salt Lake City, Utah
USA

Celia F. Stewart, PhD
Professor
Department of Speech – Language
Pathology and Audiology
Steinhardt School of Education
New York University
New York, New York
USA

Lucian Sulica, MD
Assistant Professor
Department of Otorhinolaryngology
Weill Medical College of Cornell University
New York, New York
USA

Mark Varvares, MD
Professor and Chairman
Department of Otolaryngology
St. Louis University School of Medicine
St. Louis, Missouri
USA

Gayle E. Woodson, MD
Professor
Division of Otolaryngology
Southern Illinois School of Medicine
Springfield, Illinois
USA

David L. Zealear, PhD
Associate Professor
Department of Otolaryngology –
Head and Neck Surgery
Vanderbilt University Medical School
Nashville, Tennessee
USA

Part I
Basic Science and Clinical Evaluation

Chapter 1
Neuroanatomy of the Larynx 3
Ajay E. Chitkara

Chapter 2
Synkinesis and Dysfunctional Reinnervation of the Larynx 17
David L. Zealear, Cheryl R. Billante

Chapter 3
Vocal Fold Paralysis: Causes, Outcomes, and Clinical Aspects 33
Lucian Sulica, Anthony Cultrara, Andrew Blitzer

Chapter 4
Evaluation of Vocal Fold Paralysis 55
C. Blake Simpson, Esther J. Cheung

Chapter 5
Diagnostic Electromyography for Unilateral Vocal Fold Dysmotility 63
Al Hillel, Lawrence Robinson

Chapter 1

Neuroanatomy of the Larynx

Ajay E. Chitkara

Introduction

The course of the recurrent laryngeal and superior laryngeal nerves has been studied throughout the modern era of surgery, most often in the context of thyroidectomy and cadaver dissection. Classical anatomy of the larynx has maintained that the recurrent laryngeal nerve (RLN) innervates intrinsic muscles of the larynx except for cricothyroid and sensation at and below the glottis, whereas superior laryngeal nerve (SLN) innervates cricothyroid muscle and sensation above the level of the true vocal folds [1–3]. This traditional understanding of the nerve supply to the larynx has been evolving into a more contemporary model as a result investigations using fine microscopic dissection and neurospecific staining techniques, and attention to neural relationships during thyroid surgery. These studies have revealed a complex relationship among the four main nerves which innervate the larynx (Fig. 1.1). It now seems that there is a less clear line of separation between inferior and superior laryngeal afferent innervation in the glottic and subglottic region. The superior and inferior laryngeal nerves appear to have more connections than the well-known anastomosis of Galen. There is anatomical evidence that raises the possibility that the superior laryngeal nerve may contribute motor innervation to muscles other than the cricothyroid. Some intrinsic muscles of the larynx are comprised of more than one anatomic belly, each with separate nerve supply suggesting distinct neural control of these distinct units. The vast majority of our current understanding of the innervation of the larynx comes from anatomical or surgical dissection, with occasional histological evidence. Physi-

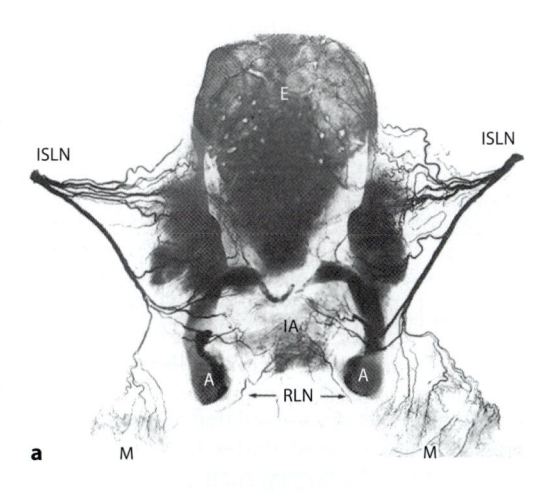

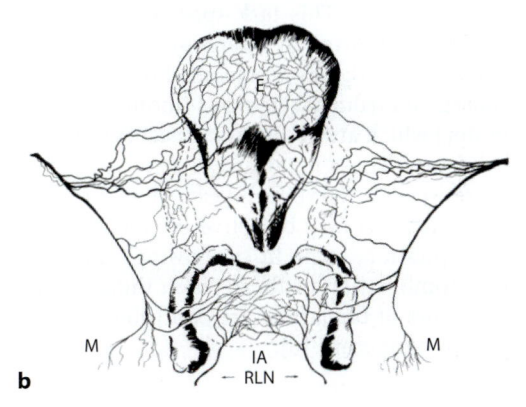

Fig. 1.1. Top: Sihler's neurospecific staining technique. The larynx has been dissected and configured into two dimensions. This specimen depicts complex anastomoses among branches of the internal branch of the superior laryngeal nerve (*ISLN*) and between *ISLN* and the recurrent laryngeal nerve (*RLN*) in the interarytenoid plexus. Bottom: schematic of figure above. *E* epiglottis cartilage *IA* interarytenoid muscle, *A* arytenoid, *M* mucosa. (Adapted with permisson from [18])

ological evidence is rare. As a result, there is still a large amount of information about the functional neuroanatomy of the larynx which remains to be uncovered.

CNS

The central pathways which control the various laryngeal functions are numerous and complex. These communications have been investigated in various animal models. In the region of the upper medulla and lower pons, the nucleus ambiguus and the nucleus tractus solitarius are the primary ganglia for the efferent and afferent pathways to the larynx, respectively.

Yoshida et al. [4] studied the motoneuron distribution in the monkey brainstem. Motoneurons to the recurrent laryngeal nerve were distributed in the rostral part of the ipsilateral nucleus ambiguus with a more compact distribution laterally, and a more scattered array in the dorsomedial region. The motoneurons to the cricothyroid muscle originate in the ipsilateral nucleus ambiguus and retrofacial nucleus and are scattered around the outer, compact cell group. Yajima and Hayashi [5] described physiological evidence of branching of motoneurons originating in the nucleus ambiguus. They demonstrated that a single motoneuron could have one axonal branch coursing with the SLN and another branch coursing with the RLN. This simultaneous innervation of two distinct muscles supports the idea that central control of coordinated movements of distinct muscles contributes to specific tasks performed by the larynx, such as respiration or swallowing [5]. This task-specific motor control was supported by later work from Yajima and Larson [6]. They concluded that there are subsets of medullary neurons (motor and nonmotor) which are involved in specific laryngeal behaviors. These neurons are active in one or more specific laryngeal tasks. For example, some neurons may be active in voicing, some in respiration, some in swallowing, and some in a combination of these tasks; thus, specific behaviors of the larynx are controlled by subgroups of neurons [6].

The afferent pathway of SLN and RLN were studied in the rat by Patrickson et al. [7]. The SLN had terminal fields bilaterally in the interstitial and medial subnuclei of the nucleus tractus solitarius, with greater density in the ipsilateral projections compared with the contralateral projections. The RLN distribution was similar except it was only ipsilateral, and there were significantly less dense terminal projections [7]. The convergence of these afferents to the interstitial and dorsomedial subnuclei support these areas as sensory integrators of the larynx [7].

Sympathetic innervation to the larynx arises from the superior cervical ganglion and travels among the laryngeal nerve fibers to the laryngeal submucosa [8]. The parasympathetics that travel with the vagus nerve originate in the dorsal motor nucleus of the vagus. These preganglionic axons travel through the pharyngeal plexus, the cardiac plexus, and the esophageal plexus, then synapse in their respective ganglia in the walls of the end organs. The secretomotor fibers which supply the larynx travel through the recurrent laryngeal and the superior laryngeal nerves [2].

Superior Laryngeal Nerve

The superior laryngeal nerve (SLN) provides the main sensory innervation to the larynx in the glottic and supraglottic regions with some contribution to the posterior subglottis. Motor innervation supplies the cricothyroid muscle. There is also some evidence for motor contribution to the interarytenoid and thyroarytenoid muscles. Traditional nosology has maintained that injury to the external branch of the superior laryngeal nerve (exSLN) results in bowing and flaccidity of the true vocal fold, decreased vocal range, and laryngeal rotation [9–12]. Sulica has brought to light that these perceptions of the effect of exSLN paralysis upon the function of the larynx may not be completely accurate [9]. When placed in the context of the human larynx and SLN's functional interrelationship with the recurrent laryngeal nerve, the role of injury and compensation of either nerve is one of significant complexity.

Cervical Segment of SLN

The SLN is the second major branch of the tenth cranial nerve [2]. The SLN branches from the vagus at or below the inferior cervical (nodose) ganglion. The SLN travels from the medial aspect of the vagus nerve, superficial to the superior sympathetic cervical ganglion from which it receives sympathetic contribution [13]. The SLN courses deep to the internal carotid artery as it emerges in an anteromedial direction towards the larynx. In this region it supplies branches posteriorly to the carotid body [14]. The average length of the SLN trunk is 1.9 cm in males and 1.4 cm in females [15]. The main trunk of SLN divides into the internal branch (inSLN) and external branch (exSLN) prior to supplying the larynx.

Internal Branch of SLN

The internal branch of the SLN is predominantly a sensory nerve, though there may be a small degree of motor input [15–17]. After dividing from the SLN trunk, the internal branch of SLN runs parallel and medial to the superior laryngeal artery [15]. As it passes the greater cornu of the hyoid it turns medially, passing deep to thyrohyoid muscle [10, 15]. The inSLN then enters the larynx through the thyrohyoid membrane just superior to the superior border of the inferior pharyngeal constrictor muscle [10]. Prior to entering the larynx, this branch runs deep or superior to the superior laryngeal artery which ramifies from the superior thyroid artery [10, 13]. After entrance into the larynx, the inSLN branches into three main divisions: superior; middle; and inferior. Sanders and Mu [16] studied the course of these branches using the Sihler neurospecific staining technique to demonstrate the fine terminal branches of the nerves which are often too delicate for anatomical dissection [18]. Occasionally, after the inSLN enters the larynx it will anastomose with the exSLN through the thyroid foramen in the superoposterior aspect of the thyroid cartilage [17].

The superior division of inSLN ramifies into two to three secondary branches. The most superior branch innervates the lingual aspect of epiglottis. The next branch provides sensory input to the lateral aspect of the glossoepiglottic fold. The caudal branch of the superior division courses through the aryepiglottic fold to innervate the laryngeal aspect of the epiglottis. The laryngeal mucosa of the epiglottis has a richer nerve supply than the lingual aspect [16].

The middle division of the inSLN divides into four to six branches; these innervate the aryepiglottic fold, the mucosa superior to the true vocal fold, the vestibule, and the posterior aspect of the arytenoid. The most dense sensory supply of the middle division is to the true and false vocal folds, and the aryepiglottic folds [16].

The descending division of inSLN is the largest branch of the three. This divides into eight to ten secondary branches. The main trunk of this inferior division courses inferiorly along the medial aspect of the piriform sinus supplying branches medially. The first branch travels to the posterior aryepiglottic fold and the outer aspect of the tip of arytenoid [16]. The next few branches pass to the posterior surface of the arytenoid and to the interarytenoid muscle. These interarytenoid branches divide further to supply the interarytenoid muscle, posterior glottic mucosa, medial aspect of arytenoid, and posterior subglottic mucosa. The terminal branches of the inSLN continue inferiorly as they pass over the posterior aspect of posterior cricoarytenoid (PCA) muscle to provide sensation to the anterior hypopharyngeal mucosa. The inSLN also provides the branch which communicates with RLN via Galen's anastomosis [16, 17, 19]. Communication between the inferior and superior laryngeal nerves is discussed in greater detail below.

External Branch of SLN

The external branch of SLN is of much smaller caliber than the internal branch, measuring approximately 0.2 mm in diameter [20]. The exSLN provides motor supply to the cricothyroid (CT) muscle. It may occasionally supply motor innervation to the thyroarytenoid muscle, and perhaps sensation to the glottis [17, 18, 21]. After the external branch separates from the main trunk of SLN, in the region of the greater cornu of the hyoid bone, it courses posterior to the superior thyroid artery (STA) in 96% of cases [10]. Kierner et al. [22] examined the SLNs of 31 cadavers and classified the course of the SLN into four types. In type-1 nerves (42%), the exSLN crossed the STA greater than 1 cm cephalad to the superior pole of the thyroid gland. Type-2 nerves (30%) crossed the STA within 1 cm of the superior pole of the thyroid gland. Type-3 nerves (14%) crossed the STA under cover of the superior pole of the thyroid gland. Type-4 nerves (14%) descended dorsal to the STA and crossed branches of the STA immediately above the superior pole of the thyroid gland. The nerve generally travels from posterior to anterior passing beneath the superior thyroid vessels on its way to the CT muscle. Prior to entering the CT muscle, the exSLN usually pierces the inferior pharyngeal constrictor muscle. In 17–22% of cases, however, nerves pass directly to the CT muscle, remaining superficial to the inferior constrictor muscle [10, 23]. Lennquist et al. studied 50 cadaver nerves and noted the exSLN entered the inferior constrictor muscle within 5 mm of the CT muscle 38% of the time, and entered between 5 and 10 mm in 20% of cases. They also found the exSLN covered by inferior constrictor fibers and not visible in this region in 20% of cases [23]. Friedman et al. [24] reviewed 1057 thyroid lobectomies in which they attempted to identify the exSLN. They classified the exSLN relationship with inferior constrictor muscle into three categories: type-1 nerves course entirely superficial to the inferior constrictor; type-2 nerves enter the inferior constrictor muscle within 1 cm of this muscle's junction with the CT muscle; and type-3 nerves enter the inferior constrictor muscle in its superior fibers. The type-I nerves were usually associated with the exSLN crossing the STA at or below the superior thyroid lobe; thus placing the nerve at greater risk of injury when dividing the superior vascular supply during thyroidectomy [24]. The variability of relations of exSLN with the STA and the inferior constrictor muscle mandate a thorough understanding of these variations on the part of the head and neck surgeon in order to identify and preserve this structure in the operating room.

The exSLN then ramifies into two divisions to supply the oblique and rectus bellies of the CT muscle [18]. Occasionally, branches of the exSLN pass through the CT muscle into the larynx and anastomose with the RLN in the body of the thyroarytenoid muscle [17, 18].

Recurrent Laryngeal Nerve

The recurrent laryngeal nerve supplies motor input to all of the intrinsic muscles of the larynx, except for the CT. This nerve also supplies sensory innervation to the glottis, subglottis, proximal trachea and esophagus. Other branches from RLN contribute to the motor function of the cricopharyngeus muscle, and supply parasympathetics to the cardiac and esophageal plexus and to the larynx. The nerve's course has been extensively studied and follows some general rules; however, upon close inspection, the details of the course of this nerve are quite varied and rarely abide by anatomical criteria which can safely be applied in all cases.

Cervical Segment of RLN

The axons which comprise the RLN are situated anteriorly in the vagus as this nerve exits the brain stem. The vagus nerve courses inferiorly in the neck after passing through the jugular foramen. During the cervical segment the RLN axons congregate at the ventromedial aspect of the vagus nerve 40 mm prior to branching from the main trunk [25]. The vagus travels in the carotid sheath posterior to the internal and common carotid arteries. On the right side of the neck the vagus passes over the subclavian artery. In this region the recurrent laryngeal nerve branches from the main trunk of the vagus and loops around the subclavian artery from anterior to posterior and travels cephalad in the neck towards the larynx [26]. In less than 1% of cases the right inferior laryngeal nerve branches directly from the vagus to the larynx at approximately the level of the cricoid cartilage. The so-called non-recurrent inferior laryngeal nerve crosses posterior to the common carotid artery and enters the larynx posterior to the CT joint [13]. This aberrant pathway is explained by abnormal embryological development. Normally, the recurrent laryngeal nerves are pulled caudad in the neck and chest around the sixth arches of the aorta. The left sixth arch remains as the ductus arteriosus, and later the ligamentum arteriosum. The right sixth arch normally resorbs, allowing the right RLN to pass inferior to the right fourth aortic arch, which becomes the subclavian artery. In rare cases, the right fourth aortic arch also resorbs during embryonic development. The consequence is that the right subclavian artery arises from the descending aorta and the right inferior laryngeal nerve tracks from the vagus directly to the larynx without looping around a vascular structure [26–28].

As the RLN ascends in the neck it courses from lateral to medial until it reaches the tracheoesophageal (TE) groove prior to entering the larynx. Ardito et al. [29] studied 2626 RLNs during 1543 thyroidectomies over 10 years and found that 61.4% of right RLNs reach the TE groove and ascend in this sulcus, 37.8% remain lateral to the TE groove then enter the larynx, and 0.6% course anterolateral to the TE groove prior to entering the larynx. This variability, especially when the nerve travels anterolateral to the TE groove, may pose significant risk for iatrogenic injury.

The left recurrent laryngeal nerve branches from the main trunk of the vagus at the level of the aortic arch as it passes anterior to the branching points of the left common carotid and subclavian arteries [13]. The RLN loops beneath the aorta lateral to the ligamentum arteriosum which is a sixth aortic arch derivative [28]. The nerve then courses cranially and medially towards the larynx. As the RLN ascends in the left side of the neck it courses toward the TE groove. Ardito et al. found that 67.3% of nerves reach the TE groove, 31% remain lateral to the TE groove, and 1.6% course anterolateral to the TE groove [29]. There are only a few reports of non-recurrent left inferior laryngeal nerves in the literature; these have been associated with a right aortic arch with anomalous left subclavian artery, essentially the mirror image of the anomaly present with a right non-recurrent nerve [25, 30].

In the majority of necks the RLN courses from the mediastinum as a single nerve trunk on each side until it approaches the cricoid cartilage. Rarely is there more than one main trunk on a side of the neck. Ardito et al. found 4 cases out of 2626 RLNs which had two ipsilateral, parallel trunks ascending from the mediastinum, and 4 cases with a fan-shaped arrangement in the nerve's proximal course through the neck [29]. Sun et al. examined 100 cadaver RLNs and found two double RLNs ascending from the mediastinum [31].

RLN Branching Patterns

The recurrent laryngeal nerve provides multiple branches along its course from the main trunk of the vagus. As the right RLN recurs around the subclavian artery and the left RLN recurs around the aorta, each supplies branches to the deep cardiac plexus [13]. During the ascent through the neck each nerve also supplies the trachea and esophagus with sensory and motor branches [30, 31]. Finally, it supplies the cricopharyngeus muscle prior to entering the larynx where it provides motor function to the intrinsic laryngeal muscles except for CT and sensation to the glottis, subglottis, and proximal trachea. By the time the inferior laryngeal nerve courses around the CT joint and enters the larynx, it is often already divided into anterior and posterior branches.

Nemiroff and Katz [32] reviewed the extralaryngeal branching patterns of 153 RLNs in patients undergoing thyroid or parathyroid surgery. They found that 41.2% of the nerves branched prior to entering the larynx. There was no difference in incidence among right and left sides; in 14.5% of patients bilateral branching was present. The branching occurred between 0.6 and 4.0 cm from the inferior border of the cricoid cartilage, although 73% of the nerves which branched did so between 1.2 and 2.3 cm from the cricoid cartilage. A later series by the same authors [33] reviewed 1177 RLNs in surgical patients. They found 63% of nerves bifurcated or trifurcated (11 nerves trifurcated) more than 0.5 cm from the inferior border of the cricoid cartilage, and 23.6% of all patients had bilateral bifurcation. Page et al. [34] had a lower incidence of branching in their series of 251 thyroidectomies (403 nerves) with 23.41% of right nerves branching and 15.15% of left nerves branching prior to entering the larynx. Moreau et al. [35] found 10 bifurcating RLNs in 34 dissected cadavers. Other investigators report RLN branching ranging from 30 to 100% of nerves [34–40]. It is not always clear in these reports whether branches to extralaryngeal structures are considered when labeling a nerve as branching.

Most of the RLN branching prior to the larynx results in bifurcation. There are patients in whom there are more than two branches of RLN prior to entering the larynx. Nemiroff and Katz had only 4 nerves out of 153 which trifurcated [32]. Sun et al. [31] examined 50 cadaver larynges and found between two and five cervical branches of the RLN. There were two branches in 17%, 3 branches in 48%, 4 branches in 25%, and 5 branches in 10% of the nerves examined. It is important to note that the foregoing numbers refer to branches which terminate both within and outside of the larynx. Regarding branches of the RLN entering the larynx, Sun et al. [31] found 94 nerves with two or more branches (two nerves with four branches), and only six nerves with one trunk entering the larynx. Of the 100 nerves studied by Sun et al. [31], the branching pattern in 87 was of tree-branching type, and the remaining 13 nerves demonstrated anastomoses of multiple branches and/or anastomoses with branches from the cervical sympathetic chain to form a loop-type configuration. In Ardito et al.'s review of 2626 RLNs, 1891 nerves branched, 1856 of the nerves bifurcated, 23 nerves trifurcated, and 14 nerves had multiple small branches before entering the larynx [29]. The discrepancy among these reports may be related to cadaver [31] vs intraoperative [29, 32] studies, although this is unlikely to fully account for the vast disparity among the multiple studies.

Previous investigators noted a predominance of anterior and posterior branching of the laryngeal portion of the RLN. These branches were designated motor and sensory, respectively, based purely on anatomical location [25]. Contemporary RLN anatomists prefer to classify the anterior and posterior branches as adductor and abductor branches; both likely contain sensory and motor fibers [17, 18, 41].

In light of the variation in incidence and type of extralaryngeal branching patterns, the surgeon's best approach to prevent inadvertent trauma to this crucial structure is to assume there is greater than one branch of the nerve. The pattern of branching may also play a role in the configuration of the true vocal fold in the setting of paresis or paralysis [32, 33]. Whether one or more branches are injured would result in selective denervation with or without synkinesis of specific intrinsic muscles of the larynx. Whatever the case, it is certain that variability in neural anatomy and compensatory laryngeal adjustments make the relationship of vocal fold position to pattern of neural injury virtually impossible to decipher clinically. The Wagner-Grossman hypothesis, which related vocal fold position to the integrity of cricothyroid innervation, and Semon's law, which related it to different vulnerability of abductor and adductor innervation, dominated the clinical discourse on this subject for decades. Careful work has shown that both are invalid [42, 43].

Relationship of RLN with Inferior Thyroid Artery

The recurrent laryngeal nerve's intimate course with the inferior thyroid artery has long been the subject of anatomists endeavors in an effort to simplify the surgical approach and technique. Unfortunately, the course of the RLN as it relates to the inferior thyroid artery does not lend itself to broad and safe generalizations.

Historically, the left RLN is described coursing deep to the inferior thyroid artery (ITA) in the majority of cases, and the right RLN passing deep to, superficial to, or between branches of the ITA in approximately equal proportions [1]. There is clear variability in these findings among investigators, and all variations have been documented on both sides including a spiraloid relationship of the artery around the nerve encountered by Ardito et al. [29]. Most published reports classify the relationship between these structures into three categories: RLN coursing superficial to ITA; RLN coursing deep to ITA; and RLN coursing between branches of ITA (Tables 1.1, 1.2). Lore and others [26, 30, 35] report no consistent relationship between these structures citing Reed [44] who described 28 variations of the branching patterns of the ITA and RLN. As many of these investigators have shown, and based upon the variability of the branching patterns of both the RLN and the ITA, there are few reliable generalizations in the relationship of these two structures.

The proximity of the RLN and the ITA is also of physiological importance. The ITA provides the main blood supply for the RLN. Proximally the RLN is fed by TE branches of the ITA. On the left the proximal thoracic RLN is supplied by the anterior bronchoesophageal artery [45].

As the RLN ascends in the neck the blood supply is via the inferior laryngeal artery which is a branch of the ITA. As the RLN courses through the neck, the supplying vessel can often be found immediately superficial and anterior to the nerve [13]. There is often a branch of the ITA accompanying the anterior and posterior branches of the RLN as they enter the larynx. This close anatomic association can place the nerve at significant surgical risk when bleeding is present from one of these vessels [31].

Retrothyroid Segment of RLN

As the RLN courses towards the larynx it travels posterior to the thyroid gland. This is a segment of the nerve which is susceptible to surgical trauma. Classically the nerve was thought to run posterior to the thyroid

Table 1.1. Relationship of right recurrent laryngeal nerve (RLN) to inferior thyroid artery (ITA)

Reference	RLN superficial	RLN deep	RLN between branches of ITA (%)	Number	Study type
Skandalakis [26]	31	20	48	204	Cadaver
Sun [31]	50	22	28[b]	100	Cadaver
Monfared [13]	21	28	50	21	Cadaver
Ardito [29]	12	61	27	1342	Surgical
Page [34][a]	67	33	–	205	Surgical

[a] Percentages in this study represent initial site of RLN crossing ITA
[b] Includes RLN passing between branches of ITA, ITA passing among branches of RLN, and branches of the RLN and ITA interrelated

Table 1.2. Relationship of left recurrent laryngeal nerve (RLN) to inferior thyroid artery (ITA)

Reference	RLN superficial to ITA (%)	RLN deep to ITA (%)	RLN between branches of ITA (%)	Number	Study type
Skandalakis [26]	10	64	27	204	Cadaver
Sun [31]	14	56	30[b]	100	Cadaver
Monfared [13]	21	50	28	21	Cadaver
Ardito [29]	2	77	21	1284	Surgical
Page [34][a]	11	89	–	205	Surgical

[a] Percentages in this study represent initial site of RLN crossing ITA
[b] Includes RLN passing between branches of ITA, ITA passing among branches of RLN, and branches of the RLN and ITA interrelated

gland, occasionally penetrating through some thyroid tissue [25, 46]. It was also thought to have a variable relationship with the posterior suspensory ligament of Berry, traveling lateral, medial, or through this structure [25, 30, 46, 47]. Berlin [46] reported the nerve traveling in the tracheoesophageal groove in 65% of cases, piercing the suspensory ligament in 25%, and traveling through the gland in 10% of cases. Hunt [47] reported the RLN is embedded within the posterior suspensory ligament in 50% of patients. Lore et al. [30] stated that the RLN consistently runs posterior and lateral to the ligament of Berry. Later investigators supported Lore et al., including Sasou et al. [48], who reported on 689 RLNs encountered during thyroid surgery and an additional 46 RLNs examined in cadavers. The RLN consistently passed dorsolaterally to the ligament of Berry without evidence of penetration through this dense connective tissue. The authors did note in one cadaver a small area of connective tissue overlying the RLN in the region of the posterior suspensory ligament. This was reportedly less dense and histologically distinct from Berry's ligament. An apparent variation may present during surgery with medial traction of the thyroid lobe bringing the RLN more anteriorly such that it appears to course over the ligament of Berry [30, 47].

Another anatomical variation in the retrothyroid region of the RLN is the tubercle of Zuckerkandl, a posterolateral protuberance of thyroid tissue found in up to 63% of patients [49]. This prominence represents the embryological fusion of the ultimobranchial body and the principal median thyroid process, and is usually located just caudal to the superior parathyroid gland. Gauger found the tubercle to be larger than 1 cm in 41 of 63 patients who demonstrated this variation (100 patients studied overall) [49]. Other authors have found this to be true in 15–55% of patients [50, 51]. In 93% of people with a 1-cm or greater tubercle the nerve coursed medial to this tissue in a narrow fissure between the tubercle of Zuckerkandl and the main thyroid parenchyma [49]; the remaining 7% had the nerve lateral to the tubercle in a more vulnerable location. In this series of 161 thyroid lobectomies there were no instances of the RLN passing through the thyroid tissue. This finding of the RLN coursing between these two portions of the thyroid gland led Gauger et al. to surmise that prior reports of the nerve penetrating the gland may instead be referring to the course of the nerve through this anatomical fissure [49].

The penultimate landmark before the RLN enters the larynx is the cricothyroid (CT) articulation. This is also the most constant landmark for identification of the nerve. As the nerve courses toward its entry into the larynx, it passes posterior to the CT joint [13, 14, 26]. This relationship holds true even when the nerve ramifies proximal to this juncture; others use the inferior cornu of the thyroid cartilage as the constant reference point for the RLN [25, 30, 31, 52]. Sun et al. [31] examined this relationship in 100 cadaver RLNs and found the anterior and posterior branches of RLN enter the larynx at 7.30 mm and 7.13 mm inferior to the inferior cornu of the thyroid cartilage, respectively. In addition, approximately 72% of the anterior branches pass anteroinferior to the inferior cornu and 93% of the posterior branches pass posteroinferior to the inferior cornu of the thyroid cartilage [31]. This reliable anatomic association can be useful when attempts at locating the RLN in other areas are unsuccessful. The main caution is the likely presence of more than one branch in the region of the CT joint.

Laryngeal Segment of RLN

When the RLN reaches the inferior cornu of the thyroid cartilage it begins its intralaryngeal course. At this point the branching, although still variable, is more predictable. The RLN ramifies into a posterior or abductor division, and an anterior or adductor division. The abductor portion supplies the posterior cricoarytenoid (PCA) muscle and the adductor division supplies the interarytenoid (IA) muscle, lateral cricoarytenoid (LCA) muscle, and thyroarytenoid (TA) muscle. In addition to the efferent axons there are sensory branches providing sensation, temperature, and pressure signals to the brainstem [53, 54].

The first intralaryngeal branch ramifies posteriorly to the PCA muscle. This nerve branches from the main trunk of RLN inferior to the inferior cricothyroid ligament [55]. Most frequently there is one main trunk from the RLN to PCA, some larynges have two trunks to PCA, and rarely there are three [55, 56]. There may be further secondary branching after the trunks separate from the main division of RLN. Sanders et al. noted two main PCA trunks in one-half to two-thirds of laryngeal specimens [18, 57]. Regardless, prior to termination in the PCA muscle all specimens ended in two main divisions which supply its two bellies [18]. Nguyen et al. [56] examined 30 cadavers and found one PCA trunk in 67% of larynges, two trunks in 27%, and three trunks in 7%. Damrose et al. [55] noted 8 of 10 cadavers with a single trunk to PCA and 2 of 10 with two trunks. The first division to PCA innervates the lateral PCA belly and the second division innervates the medial belly [18, 57]. This difference is significant in light of the distinct biomechanical action the two bellies of the PCA affect upon the arytenoid cartilage: the medial belly rotates the cartilage about a vertical axis, and the lateral belly moves the cartilage along an anterior/posterior axis [58].

Distal to the PCA branches, the remainder of the RLN is the adductor division. The next branch, which ramifies from the RLN superior to the inferior CT ligament, supplies the interarytenoid muscle [55]. This nerve passes medially around the cricoarytenoid joint, ascends beneath the PCA, and enters at the inferior aspect of the IA muscle [18]. There are often anastomoses with the PCA nerve, and more significantly with the contralateral RLN and also the inSLN [18, 56]. The majority of inSLN input in this region is sensory. There is anatomical (but not physiological) evidence that motor input to IA may also be supplied from inSLN via this intricate plexus [59]. The IA nerve plexus is a variable, complex, and dense anastomotic network which is the only site in the larynx which exhibits bilateral RLN communication [18].

The next division of the RLN is to the lateral cricoarytenoid muscle. Sanders et al. [18] found this to be a consistent single branch which ends in a dense anastomotic plexus at the center of the muscle. Nguyen et al. [54] reported greater variability. They found one branch to the LCA muscle in 70%, two branches in 25%, and three branches in 5% of cadaver larynges. Nguyen et al. also described variability in the location of the pedicles as they enter the LCA muscle. Of the 42 unipedicular nerves, 38 entered via a middle pedicle, 4 via an inferior pedicle, and none entered from superiorly. The LCA is comprised of a single muscle belly.

The terminal motor branch of the RLN innervates the thyroarytenoid muscle. This nerve branch courses along the external surface of the LCA as it travels toward the TA muscle [56]. The terminal branch then ramifies into multiple fascicles prior to entering the body of the TA muscle [18, 56]. The terminal branches of the TA nerve supply the true vocal fold and the ventricular fold. These branches form the most dense anastomotic network of neural tissue in the larynx and are especially dense along the medial edge of the TA muscle [18]. Complementary to these findings is the distinction of a superior and inferior muscle compartment of the TA muscle [60]. The superior compartment, which lies along the medial aspect of the true vocal fold vibratory edge, is composed of numerous, small muscle fascicles containing loosely packed muscle fibers. The inferior compartment is comprised of a large single muscle fascicle with tightly packed muscle fibers [60]. Furthermore, 85% of the muscle spindles are densely located in the superomedial compartment of the TA muscle. These muscle spindles provide afferent information from the larynx to the brainstem regarding length and change of length of the adjacent muscle fibers [61]. This fine neuromotor development along the superomedial edge of the vocal fold is unique to humans and primates [61]. The superior compartment appears to have motor input independent from the remaining TA muscle. These anatomic findings suggest selective neurological control likely related to fine-tuning of the voice. This phenomenon is demonstrated in the falsetto voice, with increasing pitch there is selective dampening of vibration at the superomedial vocal fold edge [61, 62].

It is important to keep the findings of these investigators in perspective. Our understanding of the variable and complex course of the RLN, especially its intralaryngeal course, is based upon fine anatomical dissection and inspection of thin nerves coursing around and through small structures that comprise the larynx. Despite their elegance, these dissections do not provide physiological information to definitively differentiate the efferent supply from the afferent supply.

Neuromuscular Junctions

Once the branches of the RLN and SLN enter the appropriate muscles, they interface at the neuromuscular junctions (NMJ). The morphology of the NMJs have been classified as plate-like, grape-like, or complex, all of which have been identified in the PCA, IA, TA, and CT muscles [63]. The TA muscle is principally comprised of the complex motor end plates. In addition, the TA muscle has a higher incidence of double NMJs on a given muscle fiber. These dual NMJs are always innervated by the same nerve. In older larynges there is evidence of neurons innervating adjacent NMJs which have lost there native innervation [63]. Initial studies of the TA distribution of NMJs found a relatively scattered distribution within the thyroarytenoid muscle [63, 64]. Sheppert et al. [65] looked at the NMJs in the TA muscle using immunolabeled anti-synaptophysin antibody. They found 75% of the NMJs distributed among the middle one-third of the TA in an anterior/posterior dimension with relative even distribution in the superior/inferior dimension. Examination of the LCA found consistent distribution of NMJs in the mid portion of the muscle [66, 67]. The NMJs in the PCA muscle form an arc-like distribution [68] which is less consistent than in the other muscles, and appears to be related to the distribution among the two bellies of the PCA muscle. Staining of the cricothyroid muscle revealed a propensity of the NMJs for the medial two-thirds of the muscle with minimal staining at the extreme ends [21].

RLN Communication with SLN

The interrelationship of the RLN with the SLN has been noted since the first century A.D. when Galen described his eponymous anastomosis [19]. The present controversy over these anastomoses is not whether they exist, but whether they contain motor fibers, sensory fibers, or both. During the twentieth century various authors supported and disputed the motor communication based upon anatomical and physiological studies. Contemporary research convincingly shows that there is more than one site of anastomosis between the SLN and RLN, and that some of these communications may relay motor control (Fig. 1.2).

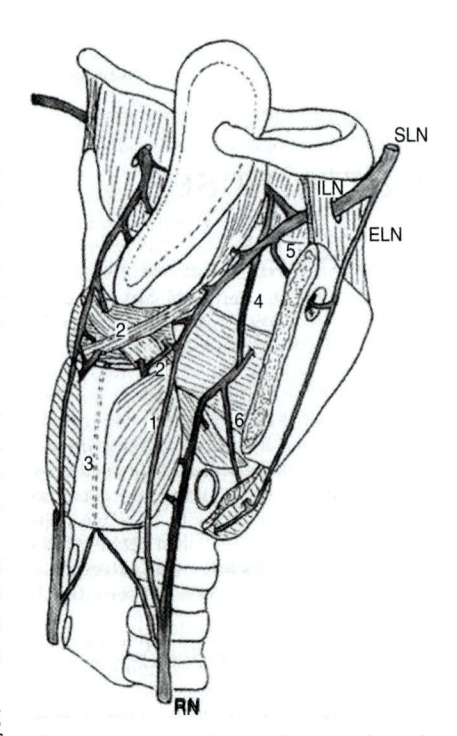

Fig. 1.2. Anastomotic sites between branches of superior and recurrent laryngeal nerves. *SLN* superior laryngeal nerve, *ILN* internal branch superior laryngeal nerve, *ELN* external branch superior laryngeal nerve, *RN* recurrent laryngeal nerve, *1* Galen's anastomosis, *2* deep arytenoid plexus, *2'* superficial arytenoid plexus, *3* cricoid anastomosis, *4* thyroarytenoid anastomosis, *5* thyroid foramen, *6* cricothyroid anastomosis. (Adapted from [17])

Galen's anastomosis is the most well-known communication among the laryngeal nerves. This occurs between the dorsal branch of inSLN and the posterior branch of the RLN. This communicating nerve passes from RLN along the posterior aspect of the PCA and interarytenoid muscles, deep to the hypopharyngeal mucosa as it travels cephalad. Galen's anastomosis is present in the majority of human larynges. In reviewing prior reports of 30 or more dissections of human larynges, Furlan found this anastomosis present in 75–100% of cases in 6 of 7 studies [17, 19, 69–72]. Sanders et al., using Sihler's staining technique, found this communication between the inSLN and the RLN in the region of the interarytenoid neural plexus in most of their ten specimens [18]. Galen's anastomosis is often described as a single nerve branch, although from a study of 90 larynges, Sanudo et al. [17] reported a double trunk in 3% and a plexiform communication in 2% of cases. This anastomotic branch also supplies small branches of sensory innervation to the pharynx and may supply motor input to the interarytenoid muscles [17].

The interarytenoid plexus is a second site of consistent anastomosis between the inferior and superior laryngeal nerves [17, 18]. The RLN contribution comes from the anterior branch supplying the interarytenoid muscles which courses cephalad beneath the PCA muscles to the interarytenoideus. The SLN contribution arises from the dorsal branch of the inSLN which ends in one to three branches supplying the interarytenoid and arytenoid region. The interarytenoid plexus is comprised of both superficial and deep anastomotic networks. The superficial communication, present in 86% of larynges, occurs between the arytenoid branches of the RLN and the lower arytenoid branches of the inSLN which communicate over the dorsal aspect of the interarytenoid muscles [17]. The deep plexus, present in all larynges, is situated within the interarytenoid muscles between RLN and SLN and provides both motor input to the interarytenoideus and sensory innervation to the posterior commissure mucosa [17]. The interarytenoid plexus is not only significant for the communication between superior and inferior laryngeal nerves, it also provides the only peripheral neurological communication between the right and left sides of the larynx [17, 18].

The communicating nerve as described by Sanders et al. [18] and Wu et al. [41] links the exSLN with the RLN in 44% of the laryngeal dissections. Sanudo [17] and Wu et al. [41] noted this in 68% of the hemilarynges studied. The exSLN enters the superolateral aspect of the CT muscle where it divides into several branches. Some of these branches exit the medial aspect of the CT muscle, pass between the thyroid and cricoid cartilages, traverse the LCA muscle, and enter the thyroarytenoid muscle. Some of these branches, presumably motor neurons based upon anatomical and histological evidence, anastomose with RLN and terminate in the TA muscle as intramuscular branches [41]. Sensory branches of the communicating nerve pass through the TA muscle and terminate in either the subglottic mucosa or at the CT joint. The communicating nerve infrequently bypasses the TA to anastomose directly with the inSLN [41].

The cricoid anastomosis has been described by Sanudo et al. [17]. They found this communication in 6 of 10 larynges. This anastomotic network is formed by the deep arytenoid plexus (RLN and SLN) and small branches of the RLN before this nerve enters the larynx. This cricoid anastomosis is situated anterior to the posterior cricoid lamina and supplies mucosal branches to the lateral and posterior subglottis [17]. Sanudo also found a small percentage of larynges with communication at the level of the TA between inSLN and RLN. This occurred at the superficial aspect of the TA muscle via the ventral branch of inSLN and an anterior branch of RLN in 14% of nerves studied [17].

The physiological relationship of the anastomoses of the superior and inferior laryngeal nerves was investigated in dogs by Dedo and Ogura [73]. They sectioned RLNs and found persistent EMG activity in the thyroarytenoid muscle. This activity was unrelated to CT muscle activity, and was dissociated from contralateral RLN input. Only after sectioning the SLN, or dissecting the CT muscle from the cricoid or thyroid cartilage, did the electrical activity cease [18, 73].

These multiple communications between RLN and SLN are undoubtedly significant in the overall function of the larynx. Their role will be elucidated as we better understand the physiology behind these neural anastomoses.

Conclusion

The numerous sites of branching and communication among the laryngeal nerves help us to view the innervation of the larynx in a more complex light. The laryngeal organ does not appear to be supplied by four individual nerves. Instead, it is controlled by a complex, interrelated nerve plexus with varying motor and sensory contributions provided by two superior and two inferior laryngeal nerves. According to Sanudo et al.'s dissection of 90 specimens, 98% of human larynges have between two and four sites of anastomoses between laryngeal nerves, with the remaining 2% having five anastomotic points [17].

The presence of these numerous anastomoses among the RLN and SLN, as well as the right and left sides, have contributed to our contemporary understanding of the larynx in the setting of vocal fold paralysis and have the potential to shed light on issues of compensation, reinnervation and recovery, and the variability of the clinical presentation of vocal fold paralysis from patient to patient. As we further investigate the function of these varied anastomoses we can begin to better understand the complexity that innervates the human larynx. A comprehensive understanding of the pathway of these nerves is paramount to better understanding the nature of vocal fold paralysis, vocal fold immobility, and the rehabilitation of the immobile vocal fold.

References

1. Hollinshead WH (1982) The pharynx and larynx. In: Anatomy for surgeons: the head and neck, 3rd edn. Lippincott, Philadelphia, pp 389–441
2. Wilson-Pauwels L, Akesson EJ, Stewart PA (1988) Vagus nerve. In: Cranial nerves: anatomy and clinical comments. BC Decker, Philadelphia, pp 125–138
3. Meller SM (1984) Functional anatomy of the larynx. Otolaryngol Clin North Am 17:3–12
4. Yoshida Y, Mitsumasu T, Miyazaki T, Hirano M, Kaneseki T (1984) Distribution of motoneurons in the brain stem of monkeys, innervating the larynx. Brain Res Bull 13:413–419
5. Yajima Y, Hayashi Y (1989) Electrophysiological evidence for axonal branching of ambiguous laryngeal motoneurons. Brain Res 478:309–314
6. Yajima Y, Larson CR (1993) Multifunctional properties of ambiguous neurons identified electrophysiologically during vocalization in the awake monkey. J Neurophysiol 70:529–540
7. Patrickson JW, Smith TE, Zhou S-S (1991) Afferent projections of the superior and recurrent laryngeal nerves. Brain Res 539:169–174
8. Graney DO, Flint PW (1998) Anatomy of the larynx/hypopharynx/trachea/bronchus/esophagus. In: Cummings CW, Fredrickson JM, Harker LA, Krause CJ, Schuller DE, Richardson MA (eds) Otolaryngology: head and neck surgery, 3rd edn. Mosby, St. Louis, pp 1823–1833
9. Sulica L (2004) The superior laryngeal nerve: function and dysfunction. Otolaryngol Clin North Am 37:183
10. Durham CF, Harrison TS (1964) The surgical anatomy of the superior laryngeal nerve. Surg Gynecol Obstet 118:38–44
11. Droulias C, Tzinas S, Harlaftis N, Akin JT, Gray SW, Skandalakis JE (1976) The superior laryngeal nerve. Am Surg 42:635–638
12. Moosman DA, DeWeese MS (1968) The external laryngeal nerve as related to thyroidectomy. Surg Gynecol Obstet 127:1011–1016
13. Monfared A, Gorti G, Kim D (2002) Microsurgical anatomy of the laryngeal nerves as related to thyroid surgery. Laryngoscope 112:386–392
14. Monfared A, Kim D, Jaikumar S, Gorti G, Kam A (2001) Microsurgical anatomy of the superior and recurrent laryngeal nerves. Neurosurgery 49:925–933
15. Furlan JC, Brandao LG, Ferraz AR, Rodrigues AJ Jr (2003) Surgical anatomy of the extralaryngeal aspect of the superior laryngeal nerve. Arch Otolaryngol Head Neck Surg 129:79–82
16. Sanders I, Mu L (1998) Anatomy of the human internal superior laryngeal nerve. Anat Rec 252:646–656
17. Sanudo J-R, Maranillo E, Leon X, Mirapeix R-M, Orus C, Quer M (1999) An anatomical study of anastomoses between laryngeal nerves. Laryngoscope 109:983–987
18. Sanders I, Wu B-L, Mu L, Li Y, Biller HF (1993) The innervation of the human larynx. Arch Otolaryngol Head Neck Surg 119:934–939

19. Furlan JC, Brandao LG, Ferraz AR (2002) Prevalence of Galen's anastomosis: an anatomical and comparative study. J Laryngol Otol 116:823–825
20. Kambic V, Zargi M, Radsel Z (1984) The topographical anatomy of the external branch of the superior laryngeal nerve: its importance in head and neck surgery. J Laryngol Otol 98:1121–1124
21. DeVito MA, Malmgren LT, Gacek RR (1985) Three-dimensional distribution of neuromuscular junctions in human cricothyroid. Arch Otolaryngol 111:11–113
22. Kierner AC, Aigner M, Burian M (1998) The external branch of the superior laryngeal nerve: its topographical anatomy as related to surgery of the neck. Arch Otolaryngol Head Neck Surg 124:301–303
23. Lennquist S, Cahlin C, Smeds S (1987) The superior laryngeal nerve in thyroid surgery. Surgery 102:999–1008
24. Friedman M, LoSavio P, Ibrahim H (2002) Superior laryngeal nerve identification and preservation in thyroidectomy. Arch Otolaryngol Head Neck Surg 128:296–303
25. Sepulveda A, Sastre N, Chousleb A (1996) Topographic anatomy of the recurrent laryngeal nerve. J Reconstruct Microsurg 12:5–10
26. Skandalakis JE, Droulias C, Harlaftis N, Tzinas S, Gray SW, Akin JT (1976) The recurrent laryngeal nerve. Am Surg 42:629–634
27. Steinberg JL, Khane GJ, Fernandes CMC, Nel JP (1986) Anatomy of the recurrent laryngeal nerve: a redescription. J Laryngol Otol 100:919–927
28. Gray SW, Skandalakis JE, Akin JT (1976) Embryological considerations of thyroid surgery: developmental anatomy of the thyroid, parathyroids and the recurrent laryngeal nerve. Am Surg 42:621–628
29. Ardito G, Revelli L, D'Alatri L, Lerro V, Guidi ML, Ardito F (2004) Revisited anatomy of the recurrent laryngeal nerves. Am J Surg 187:249–253
30. Lore JM, Kim DJ, Elias S (1977) Preservation of the laryngeal nerves during total thyroid lobectomy. Ann Otol 86:777–788
31. Sun SQ, Zhao J, Lu H et al. (2001) An anatomical study of the recurrent laryngeal nerve: its branching patterns and relationship to the inferior thyroid artery. Surg Radiol Anat 23:363–369
32. Nemiroff PM, Katz AD (1982) Extralaryngeal divisions of the recurrent laryngeal nerve: surgical and clinical significance. Am J Surg 114:466–469
33. Katz AD, Nemiroff P (1993) Anastamoses and bifurcations of the recurrent laryngeal nerve: report of 1177 nerves visualized. Am Surg 59:188–191
34. Page C, Foulon P, Strunski V (2003) The inferior laryngeal nerve: Surgical and anatomic considerations. Report of 251 thyroidectomies. Surg Radiol Anat 25:188–191
35. Moreau S, de Rougy MG, Babin E et al. (1998) The recurrent laryngeal nerve: related vascular anatomy. Laryngoscope 108:1351–1353
36. Riddell VH (1956) Injury to the recurrent laryngeal nerves during thyroidectomy. Lancet 271:638–641
37. Armstrong WG, Hinton JW (1951) Multiple divisions of the recurrent laryngeal nerve: an anatomic study. Arch Surg 62:532–539
38. Bowden REM (1955) The surgical anatomy of the recurrent laryngeal nerve. Br J Surg 43:153–163
39. Clader DN, Luter PW, Daniels BT (1957) A photographic study of the superior and inferior laryngeal nerves and the superior and inferior thyroid arteries. Am J Surg 23:608–618
40. Weeks C, Hinton JW (1942) Extralaryngeal divisions of the recurrent laryngeal nerve: its significance to vocal cord paralysis. Am J Surg 16:251–258
41. Wu B, Sanders I, Mu L, Biller HF (1994) The human communicating nerve: an extension of the external superior laryngeal nerve that innervates the vocal fold. Arch Otolaryngol Head Neck Surg 120:1321–1328
42. Woodson GE (1993) Configuration of the glottis in laryngeal paralysis. I: Clinical study. Laryngoscope 103:1227–1234
43. Koufman JA, Walker FO, Joharji GM (1995) The cricothyroid muscle does not influence vocal fold position in laryngeal paralysis. Laryngoscope 105:369–272
44. Reed AF (1943) The relation of the inferior laryngeal nerve to the inferior thyroid artery. Anat Rec 85:17
45. Filaire M, Garcier JM, Harouna Y, Laurent S, Mom T, Naamee A, et al. (2001) Intrathoracic blood supply of the vagus and recurrent laryngeal nerves. Surg Radiol Anat 23:249–252
46. Berlin DD (1935) The recurrent laryngeal nerves in total ablation of the normal thyroid gland. An anatomical and surgical study. Surg Gynecol Obstet 60:19–26
47. Hunt PS (1968) A reappraisal of the surgical anatomy of the thyroid and parathyroid glands. Br J Surg 55:63
48. Sasou S, Nakamura S, Kurihara H (1998) Suspensory ligament of Berry: its relationship to recurrent laryngeal nerve and examination in 24 autopsies. Head Neck 20:695–698
49. Gauger PG, Delbridge LW, Thompson NW, Crummer P, Reeve TS (2001) Incidence and importance of the tubercle of Zuckerkandl in thyroid surgery. Eur J Surg 167:249–254
50. Pelizzo MR, Toniato A, Gemo G (1998) Zuckerkandl's tuberculum: an arrow pointing to the recurrent laryngeal nerve (constant anatomical landmark). J Am Coll Surg 187:333–336

51. Hisham AN, Aina EN (2000) Zuckerkandl's tubercle of the thyroid gland in association with thyroid symptoms: a coincidence or consequence? Aust N Z J Surg 70:251–253
52. Wang CA (1975) The use of the inferior horn of the thyroid cartilage in identifying the recurrent laryngeal nerve. Surg Gynecol Obstet 140:91–94
53. Sant'Ambrogio G, Mathew OP, Fisher JT, Sant'Ambrogio FB (1983) Laryngeal receptors responding to transmural pressure, airflow and local muscle activity. Respir Physiol 54:317–330
54. Sant'Ambrogio G, Mathew OP (1986) Laryngeal receptors and their reflex responses. Clin Chest Med 7:211–222
55. Damrose EJ, Huang RY, Ye M, Berke GS, Sercarz JA (2003) Surgical anatomy of the recurrent laryngeal nerve: implications for laryngeal reinnervation. Ann Otol Rhinol Laryngol 112:434–438
56. Nguyen M, Junien-Lavillauroy C, Faure C (1989) Anatomical intra-laryngeal anterior branch study of the recurrent (inferior) laryngeal nerve. Surg Radiol Anat 11:123–127
57. Sanders I, Li Y, Biller H (1995) Axons enter the human posterior cricoarytenoid muscle from the superior direction. Arch Otolaryngol Head Neck Surg 121:754–757
58. Bryant NJ, Woodson GE, Kaufman K et al. (1996) Human posterior cricoarytenoid muscle compartments. Anatomy and mechanics. Arch Otolaryngol 122:1331–1336
59. Mu L, Sanders I, Wu B-L, Biller HF (1994) The intramuscular innervation of the human interarytenoid muscle. Laryngoscope 104:33–39
60. Sanders I, Rai S, Han Y, Biller HF (1998) Human vocalis contains distinct superior and inferior subcompartments: possible candidates for the two masses of vocal fold vibration. Ann Otol Rhinol Laryngol 107:826–833
61. Sanders I, Han Y, Wang J, Biller H (1998) Muscle spindles are concentrated in the superior vocalis subcompartment of the human thyroarytenoid muscle. J Voice 12:7–16
62. Pressman JJ (1942) Physiology of the vocal cords in phonation and respiration. Arch Otolaryngol 35:355–398
63. Perie S, St. Guily JL, Callard P, Sebille A (1997) Innervation of adult human laryngeal muscle fibers. J Neurol Sci 149:81–86
64. Rosen M, Malmgren LT, Gacek RR (1983) Three dimensional computer reconstruction of the distribution of neuromuscular junctions in the thyroarytenoid muscle. Ann Otol Rhinol Laryngol 92:424–429
65. Sheppert AD, Spirou GA, Berrebi AS, Garnett JD (2003) Three-dimensional reconstruction of immunolabeled neuromuscular junctions in the human thyroarytenoid muscle. Laryngoscope 113:1973–1976
66. Freije J, Malmgren LT, Gacek RR (1986) Motor endplate distribution in the human lateral cricoarytenoid muscle. Arch Otolaryngol 112:176–179
67. Gambino DR, Malmgren LT, Gacek RR (1985) Three-dimensional computer reconstruction of the neuromuscular junction distribution in the human posterior cricoarytenoid muscle. Laryngoscope 95:556–560
68. Sanders I, Mu L, Wu B-L, Biller HF (1993) The intramuscular nerve supply of the human lateral cricoarytenoid muscle. Acta Otolaryngol (Stockh) 113:679–682
69. Williams AF (1951) The nerve supply of the laryngeal muscles. J Laryngol Otol 65:343–348
70. Pichler H, Gisel A (1953) The clinical significance of the ramification of the recurrent laryngeal nerves: a critical anatomic study. Laryngoscope 67:105–117
71. Rueger RS (1972) The superior laryngeal nerve and the interarytenoid muscle in humans: an anatomic study. Laryngoscope 82:2008–2031
72. Schweizer V, Dorfl J (1997) The anatomy of the inferior laryngeal nerve. Clin Otolaryngol 22:362–369
73. Dedo HH, Ogura JH (1965) Vocal cord electromyography in the dog. Laryngoscope 75:201–211

Chapter 2

Synkinesis and Dysfunctional Reinnervation of the Larynx

David L. Zealear, Cheryl R. Billante

Introduction

While a tremendous volume of energy and literature has been devoted to laryngeal paralysis in the past decade, there are still substantial gaps in our understanding of fundamental issues. Controversy remains regarding the actual innervation pathways of the larynx, and whether the paralyzed larynx is truly denervated or dysfunctionally reinnervated. An appreciation of these basic issues is prerequisite to making prudent decisions regarding the most appropriate type of intervention. The purpose of this chapter is to provide a brief overview of basic laryngeal anatomy and neurophysiology in order to prepare the reader for a subsequent discussion of future research for treatment of laryngeal paralysis. A novel approach is described which can induce selective reinnervation of individual laryngeal muscles by their original motor fibers within the recurrent laryngeal nerve; thus, synkinetic reinnervation following nerve injury can be avoided. The possible mechanisms underlying selective reinnervation are proposed, and the potential for translating this technology into clinical medicine utilizing electrotherapy and gene therapy is considered.

Innervation and Functional Anatomy of Laryngeal Muscles

As a matter of basic orientation, a conventional view of laryngeal anatomy is briefly presented. The intrinsic laryngeal muscles have both their origin and insertion on the cricoid, thyroid, or arytenoid cartilage. In concert, they orchestrate the motion of the vocal folds during respiration, vocalization, and airway protection. The paired posterior cricoarytenoid (PCA) muscles are situated on the posterior larynx (Fig. 2.1A). When the PCA contracts, it rocks the arytenoid cartilage in a posteromedial direction to swing open the vocal process and fold (Fig. 2.1B). The articular facets of the cricoarytenoid joint are contoured to also permit a sliding motion along the mediolateral axis. The PCA is the sole abductor of the vocal folds during inspiration and acts as a co-contractor antagonist to the adductors during phonation. The thyroarytenoid (TA) muscle is the principal adductor and intrinsic tensor of the vocal fold (Fig. 2.1C). In synergy with the lateral cricoarytenoid (LCA) and interarytenoid (IA) muscles, it acts to close the glottic airway during vocalization and airway protection. The cricothyroid (CT) does not insert on the arytenoid, and therefore affects vocal fold motion indirectly. It tilts the thyroid cartilage toward the cricoid ring ventrally in a visor-like action, effectively stretching the vocal folds. It is known to have a dual role: it is active in both adduction and abduction. With the exception of the CT, the abductor and adductor muscles are supplied by motor fibers in the recurrent laryngeal nerve (RLN). The CT, on the other hand, receives its innervation from the external branch of the superior laryngeal nerve (SLN). Sensory information from the larynx is carried in both the RLN and SLN. For the most part, sensory fibers in the RLN originate from receptors below the level of the vocal folds, while those in the internal branch of the SLN originate at the glottal level and above; however, some sensory fibers in the internal SLN or RLN originate remotely and cross over via Galen's anastomosis.

Recent reports provide a radical departure from this conventional view of anatomy and suggest an anatomical complexity not previously appreciated. Careful dissection and analysis has revealed that each laryngeal muscle is not a single entity but rather an assembly of anatomically distinct compartments potentially adapted for different functions. While this notion can be traced back as far as the seventeenth century, in the past decade Sanders et al. have published a series of articles providing strong evidence for the existence of functional compartments [1–4]. Based on the presence of fascial barriers, differences in fiber direction and site of insertion, the PCA, TA, and CT

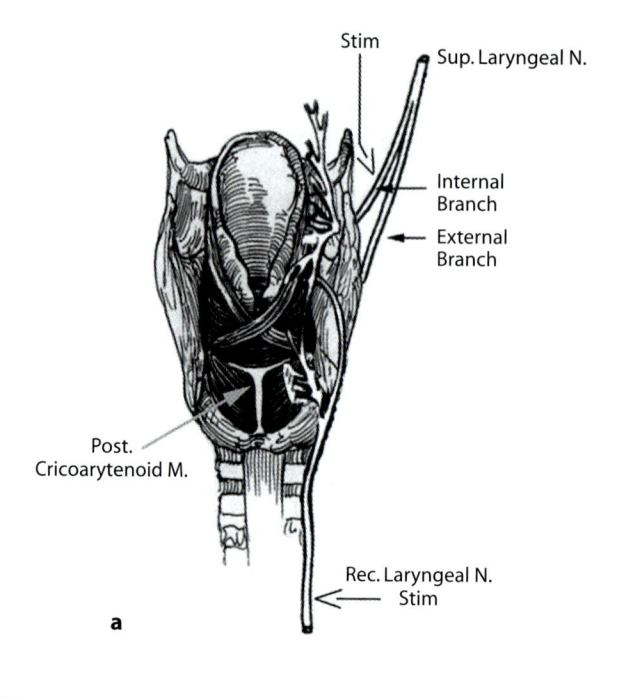

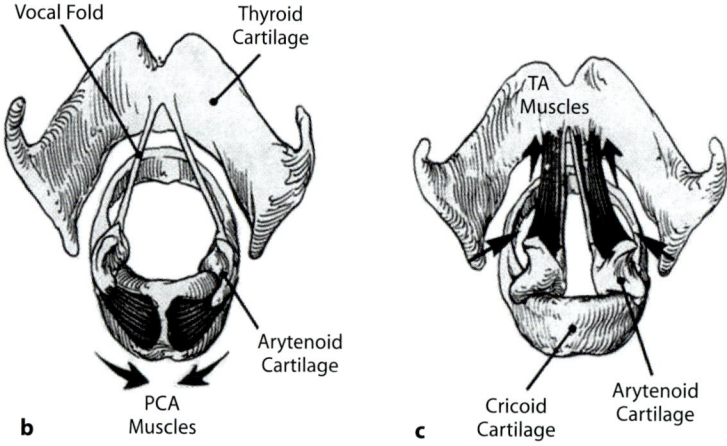

Fig. 2.1. a–c Laryngeal anatomy and muscle actions. For the normally innervated larynx, stimulation of afferents in the superior laryngeal nerve (internal branch) reflexly activate reflex glottic closure motor units in the recurrent laryngeal nerve and thyroarytenoid (*TA*) muscle to adduct the vocal fold and close the airway (*arrows*, c). Inspiratory motor units in the recurrent laryngeal nerve and posterior cricoarytenoid (*PCA*) muscle are recruited during hypercapnia to abduct the vocal fold and open the airway (*arrows*, b).

muscles have been found to comprise two to three distinct compartments (Fig. 2.2). Muscle biochemistry may lend support for the theory of functional compartmentalization. For example, the horizontal division of the PCA has a greater percentage of slow-twitch type-I fibers than the vertical or oblique compartments. Likewise, the superior medial division of the thyroarytenoid muscle, known as the vocalis, contains a highly specialized slow-twitch fiber that is multiply innervated and fatigue resistant [5]. In general, these slow contracting fibers are optimally adapted for tonic functions such as vocalization or quiet respiration. A high density of muscle spindles in these two compartments suggests that they are engaged in a motor behavior requiring fine control with feedback [6]. In contrast, the vertical and oblique divisions of the PCA and the lateral division of the TA have a higher concentration of fast-twitch type-II fibers, which likely reflects their specialization for rapid breathing and airway protection, respectively.

The theory of compartmentalization is further strengthened by recent studies of the innervation pattern of laryngeal muscles. Although the branching pattern is quite variable among individuals and even between the two sides of the larynx, the compartments of a muscle often receive innervation by separate nerve branches. There is inference from work by Maranillo et al. [7] and Sanders et al. [8] that the horizontal and vertical-oblique divisions of the human PCA muscle are innervated independently, most commonly by two different branches off the RLN (Fig. 2.3). In some cases, it

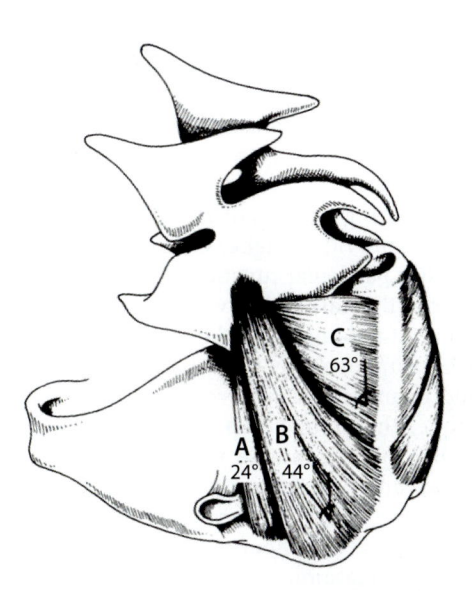

Fig. 2.2. Compartments of the canine PCA muscle. Dissection reveals three discrete anatomical compartments, each with a distinctive origin and angle of insertion on the muscular process of the arytenoids: *A* vertical compartment; *B* oblique compartment; *C* horizontal compartment. In the human PCA muscle, the vertical and oblique compartments are combined. (From Sanders et al. [81])

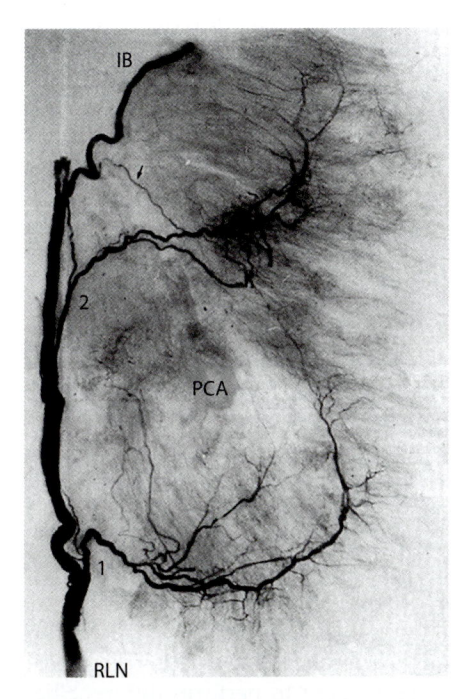

Fig. 2.3. Innervation of the human posterior cricoarytenoid (*PCA*) muscle. The initial branch of the recurrent laryngeal nerve (*RLN*) is to this muscle. On entering the larynx, the RLN passes superiorly along the lateral edge of the PCA. In half of the specimens, two branches came off separately from the RLN to innervate two different areas of the muscle. The first branch innervates the vertical–oblique compartment of the muscle (*1*), while the second branch innervates the horizontal compartment (*2*). The arrow points to one of the communicating nerve branches that connect the nerves to the PCA and the interarytenoid muscles. *IB* indicates the nerve branch to the interarytenoid muscle. (From Sanders et al. [8])

appears that the vocalis may receive additional motor innervation from the external branch of the SLN in addition to its normal source, the RLN [9].

The laryngeal muscles engage in a great diversity of motor behaviors from ballistic-type phasic movements during coughing to finely graded more tonic motor acts such as singing a scale. Presented with functions of such a range of complexity, it is tempting to postulate that a muscle may have become compartmentalized with specialization of its muscle fiber contraction properties and organization. Certainly, the vocalis with its slow twitch fiber composition, multilobar construction, and muscle spindle density is most suited for the accurate generation of sound used in communication; however, there is no direct evidence that compartments are actually involved in different laryngeal behaviors. Furthermore, the variation in fiber type between compartments is apparently no greater than regional differences within a compartment. In general, slow contracting type-I fibers tend to be located deep within a muscle in apposition to the bone or cartilage and nearest the midline for axial muscles. This is true for the CT and PCA muscles and is simply an adaptation of nature to conserve heat loss since these fibers are more dependent upon a circulatory supply than type-II fibers. Teleologically, type-II fibers may have also been reserved a more peripheral location in a muscle to give them a greater mechanical advantage in generating high levels of torque across a joint. High levels of torque are not required in the maintenance of tonus by type-I fibers.

Although it is uncertain whether laryngeal muscles are adapted to perform different behaviors through compartmentalization, there is direct evidence that the motor units that compose them are specialized. In 1979, Zealear performed a study of single motor units of the TA muscle in the cat [10]. Two types of motor units were discovered; of these, 85% were fast-twitch fatigue-resistant motor units. They had faster conducting axons, had a greater range in the number of muscle fibers innervated, and could generate larger tension. The remaining motor units were slow-twitch fatigue-resistant. They had slower conducting axons and tended to be smaller in size. The fiber type composition of the muscle, as revealed histochemically, was found to correlate with its motor unit makeup. Approximately 80% of the fibers were type IIA and 20% type I. Differences in the muscle fiber characteristics of these two types of motor units appeared to make them suited for different functions: the fast type for gagging and the slow type for vocalization. Recordings from their axons confirmed this hypothesis. During arousal in light anesthesia, only slow motor units were recruited for tonic firing during expiration as a prelude to vocalization. This finding was not unexpected since slow motor units have smaller motoneuron cell bodies and are recruited first by synaptic activity for any motor behavior, according to Henneman's size principle [11]; however, fast motor units appeared to be recruited preferentially for airway protection, counter to the size principle. Although gag activity from slow motoneurons could be recorded with stimulation of the internal branch of the SLN, fast motor units exhibited a greater number of spikes at any stimulus level. It can be concluded from this study that fast and slow motor units that comprise each laryngeal muscle have special adaptations and may be preferentially recruited for phasic and tonic functions irrespective of the particular motor behavior performed. Coordination of the participating muscles or their subdivisions would then provide a higher level of control in mediating a particular function.

The idea that fast and slow motor unit adaptations are fundamental to laryngeal behavior is further supported by the report of Hinrichsen and Ryan [12]. Using a retrograde labeling technique, they found that the motoneurons projecting to each muscle were grouped into large and small neurons, presumably providing the source for dual innervation of muscles by fast and slow motoneurons.

The new anatomical reports confirm Dilworth's early description of laryngeal innervation as being complex, composed of many branches with anastomotic channels, and terminating in plexus formations [13]. There is even speculation that some laryngeal muscles may be innervated by both the SLN and RLN. Using the Sihler's stain technique, the interarytenoid muscle has been shown to have innervation from the internal branch of the SLN as well as the RLN [8]. Apparently, some of these fibers may terminate in the PCA muscle as well, providing it innervation by two different pathways. Unfortunately, Sihler's stain cannot differentiate motor from sensory fibers. Until physiological proof is provided, these secondary pathways of innervation must be viewed as strictly sensory, likely representing a more complicated version of Galen's anastomosis. With regard to this, there has been no report that stimulation of the internal branch of the SLN will cause a direct, non-reflexive response of any laryngeal muscle. Furthermore, injury of the RLN in both animal and patient subjects results in paralysis of all laryngeal muscles, with the exception of the CT. There is no indication of secondary innervation that contributes to vocal fold movement.

Consequence of RLN Injury

Acute temporary laryngeal paralysis known as neurapraxia may be more common than indicated by patient numbers, as it resolves quickly within days or weeks. The paralysis stems from loss of signal conduction due to demyelinization without disruption of axons. Full recovery follows remyelinization by Schwann cells. Rehabilitation may take longer in case of axonotmesis (e.g., nerve crush), where the injury is severe enough to anatomically disrupt axons. Recovery ensues because regenerating axons enter their native endoneurial tubes leading back to original target muscles. If the structural integrity of the nerve is disrupted, as occurs in neurotmesis, reinnervation may be inappropriate, inadequate, or non-existent. Reinnervation may be inappropriate if regenerating axons randomly enter endoneurial conduits to the wrong muscle. This dysfunctional or synkinetic reinnervation results in chronic paralysis due to simultaneous contraction of antagonistic muscles. In case of a more extensive injury, an inadequate number of regenerating neurons successfully reach their endoneurial conduits. Even if muscle reconnection is appropriate, paralysis results because of partial muscle denervation and abnormalities in the type, size, and number of reinnervating motor units. Neurotmesis may be so severe that axon regeneration is completely impeded by neuroma formation at the severed RLN stump, or scarred endoneurial tubes and matrix in case of stretch injury. In these instances, reinnervation may fail completely, leaving a muscle chronically denervated.

By virtue of the name synkinesis, contraction of abductor and adductor antagonists produces no net vocal fold motion during vocalization, inspiration, or airway protection. Siribodhi et al. were the first to propose that aberrant regeneration of nerve fibers was responsible for vocal fold paralysis following RLN injury [14]. In a canine study, Boles and Frizell cut and anastomosed the RLN and demonstrated successful regeneration histologically and muscle reinnervation electromyographically, but poor functional recovery "likely due to random reinnervation" [15]. Murakami and Kirchner observed synkinetic paralysis of the vocal folds following end-to-end anastomosis of the RLN in canines. They reported that synkinesis could be relieved and vocal fold abduction restored only when the nerves to the adductors were divided [16]. Almost two decades later, Crumley confirmed laryngeal synkinesis in the human. The EMG recordings from the TA and LCA demonstrated motor unit firing throughout both the inspiratory and expiratory phases of respiration [17]. In 2000, he further described the varied vocal fold positions that are observed in the balance of reinnervation between abductors and adductors, and proposed a clinical classification scheme reflecting the severity of synkinesis [18].

There are numerous reports in the literature attesting to the prevalence of synkinetic reinnervation in both experimental animals and patients with vocal fold paralysis. These studies have provided indirect verification of crossed reinnervation using vocal fold movement, position and electromyography as an index. Flint et al. provided direct evidence of the random nature in which motoneurons project from the brainstem to their target laryngeal muscles after RLN neurorrhaphy [19]. Using different fluorescent retrograde tracers injected into the TA and PCA muscles of the rat, quantitative vector analysis of the cell body locations of motoneurons for each muscle confirmed their segregation into a dorsolateral and ventromedial group, as suggested by previous reports in other species (Fig. 2.4) [20–23]. Following section and repair of the RLN, the motoneurons were no longer segregated; PCA motoneurons became co-localized with TA motoneurons in the dorsolateral pool. This finding corroborates that of Nahm et al., who reported loss of functional organization of the nucleus ambiguus after reinnervation in the guinea pig [24]. In Flint et al.'s study, regeneration of adductor motoneurons may have been favored during synkinetic reinnervation, as noted by the overall shift of motoneurons' locations into that pool [19].

Loss of vocal fold motion from synkinesis is clearly problematic; however, laryngeal paralysis can also arise when reinnervation of a muscle is appropriate but inadequate. Some muscle fibers may be left denervated and eventually atrophy, compromising the muscle's force generating capacity. The reinnervation that does occur may also be dysfunctional because of the limited number of motoneurons that have successfully regenerated to target muscles. In the absence of healthy competition, single motoneurons may elaborate too many terminals synapsing onto many muscle fibers within a limited region of the muscle. Poor interdigitation of motor unit territories is reflected histochemically by replacement of the normal mosaic pattern with that of fiber type clustering. Lack of interdigitation may result in regional muscle twitching without overall tetanic fusion that allows a coordinated contraction of units and proper force development. Abnormally large motor units may be susceptible to

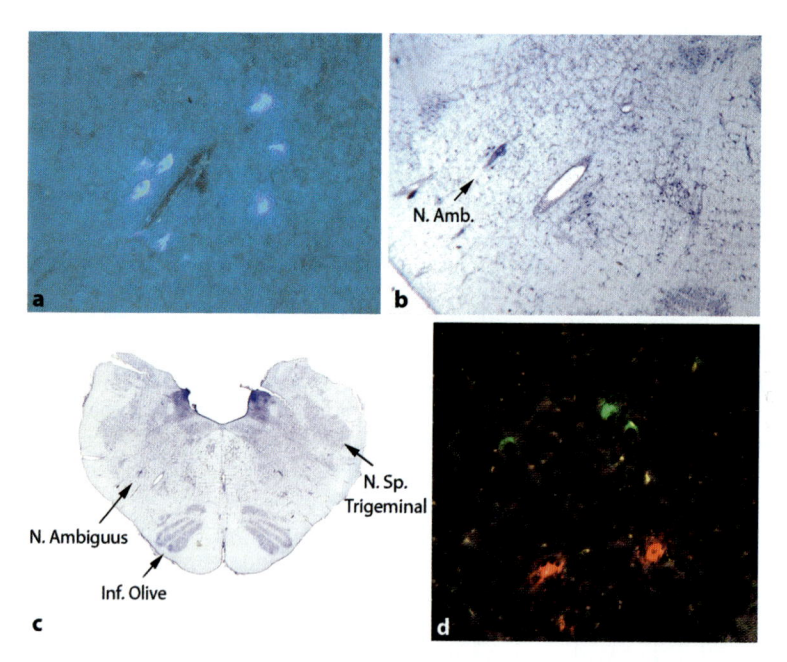

Fig. 2.4. Labeling of canine laryngeal motoneurons with the fluorescent tracer Fast Blue. a Brainstem cross-section shows PCA motoneurons fluorescing blue following injection into the abductor muscle. b, c After counterstaining the section with Cresyl Violet, low-magnification photomicrographs localized the fluorescent neurons to the nucleus ambiguus. In a second canine experiment, Fluoro-Emerald tracer was injected into the TA muscle and Fluoro-Ruby into the PCA muscle. d The TA and PCA motoneurons were segregated along the dorsal–ventral axis, with green fluorescing TA motoneurons located in a more dorsal region and red fluorescing PCA motoneurons located more ventrally. There was no segregation along the medial–lateral axis in the dog, as observed for the rat.

synaptic fatigue and conduction block, since the cell body's reserve of neurotransmitter and axoplasm cannot support so many terminals. The normal sequence of motor unit recruitment for a particular laryngeal behavior may be disturbed because of a change in the relative number of phasic and tonic motoneurons.

In summary, paralysis may arise from reinnervation inadequacy due to lack of neuromuscular reconnection or motor unit pathophysiology as proposed by many authors [17, 25]. In this regard, much of the literature does not distinguish the dysfunction of inadequate reinnervation from that of synkinesis, even though they represent different phenomena.

It is a common misconception that vocal fold paralysis is the result of complete muscle denervation. Animal experiments demonstrate that synkinetic reinnervation accounts for 66–88% of all paralysis, which is thought to be comparable to that in humans [14, 19, 26, 27]. In our own clinic, EMG recordings from the paralyzed TA muscle surface during thyroplasty found evidence of reinnervation in 17 of 20 (85%) patients at least 6 months post-injury. These findings suggest that many, if not most, vocal folds reinnervate, although it is uncertain as to whether synkinetic or inadequate reinnervation predominates. It is remarkable that reinnervation of laryngeal muscles can occur in the face of a severe RLN injury. In an RLN stimulation study in the canine, Crumley and McCabe reported regeneration and laryngeal muscle reinnervation following 2.5-cm nerve resection with stump ligation [28]. In a denervation study in our own laboratory, we were surprised to find that reinnervation of the PCA muscle could not be entirely prevented even when 10 cm of RLN was resected and the stumps ligated. It was interesting that in the three of seven cases where reinnervation occurred, the source of regeneration was the proximal stump of the RLN. Regenerated axon filaments were observed to stream from the proximal stump; vocal fold movement was produced by stimulation of these filaments [29]. The impression that laryngeal muscles are extraordinarily resistant to chronic atrophy following nerve injury is likely an illusion and better explained by the relentless nature of the peripheral nervous system to regenerate and reconnect. But not all reports are consistent with this perspective. In a study of 15 patients undergoing a reinnervation procedure for laryngeal paralysis, Damrose et al. failed to record an evoked potential from the laryngeal mucosa during RLN stimulation in all but one patient. They concluded from these findings that laryngeal paralysis stemmed from complete muscle denervation [30]; however, there is concern regarding their interpretation. In order to definitively rule out the presence of any dysfunctional reinnervation, needle electromyography in the awake patient should have been performed. Furthermore, the methodology employed was not optimally suited for measuring evoked potentials from paralyzed laryngeal muscles. Near-field recording from the laryngeal mucosa surface may not have had sufficient sensitivity to detect subnormal EMGs of the paralyzed fold. More importantly, stimulation was applied to regenerated axon filaments distal to the site of injury, rather than to the more proximally located parent axons. Regenerated filaments are small in diameter with thin myelinization. They typically require longer pulse durations and higher amplitude than the 0.1-ms to 3-mA stimuli used in this study (D.L Zealear, unpublished observations). Despite these criticisms, complete denervation may have been the cause of paralysis in some of these patients. In this regard, Blitzer et al. [31] examined 14 patients with vocal fold paralysis, half of which had good voice and half with poor voice. The patients with reasonable voice had evidence of synkinetic reinnervation and a relatively normal position of the arytenoid cartilage. In contrast, those patients with poor voice were largely silent electromyographically, with an anteriorly displaced arytenoid, suggesting flaccidity and atrophy of laryngeal muscles. This study points out that while spontaneous dysfunctional reinnervation does not restore motion, it may yield a better voice than complete denervation because it maintains vocal fold bulk and tonus [31].

The clinical reality is that paralysis is individual and may involve some degree of inappropriate or inadequate reinnervation as well as denervation atrophy.

Conventional Treatment for Laryngeal Paralysis

Decisions regarding intervention in cases of vocal fold paralysis are made on the basis of the laryngeal function that is most compromised. In the case of unilateral paralysis, the voice is breathy and the patient is at risk for aspiration due to compromised adduction. Inspiratory capacity is minimally impaired, as abduction of the opposite vocal fold provides adequate ventilation. In bilateral paralysis, the gravest concern is total loss of abduction. Because the vocal folds are paralyzed in proximity to one another, voice tends to be functional but airway embarrassment is often severe enough to warrant emergency intubation or tracheotomy to relieve inspiratory stridor and dyspnea [25, 32].

In unilateral paralysis, the objective of treatment is to medialize the paralyzed vocal fold to improve glottal closure. Despite the improvement in voice and aspiration that thyroplasty or injectable materials provide, the static nature of these types of implants ignore the long-term effects of atrophy on vocal fold mass and position. In some patients, voice undergoes a gradual deterioration over time, such that a larger implant or repeat injection is required.

The aim of treatment for bilateral paralysis is to restore adequate ventilation. Tracheotomy is a simple procedure for establishing an emergency airway in case of acute bilateral paralysis. Unfortunately, permanent tracheostomy is known to have the complications of tracheal stenosis, chronic infection, and psychosocial impairment. Procedures such as arytenoidectomy and cordotomy, while regarded as the standard of care for enlarging the glottis, also have inherent complications. Specifically, these procedures irreversibly destroy voice and may compromise airway protection during swallowing.

The limitations associated with current therapy for both unilateral and bilateral paralysis have prompted investigation into more physiological, dynamic approaches to rehabilitation: reanimation of laryngeal muscles by functional electrical stimulation or selective reinnervation. Electrical stimulation of the PCA muscle, when paced with inspiration, offers an innovative method for restored ventilation in case of bilateral vocal fold paralysis, with none of the disadvantages associated with conventional surgical treatment. Paced muscle stimulation has been studied in animals and explored more recently in preliminary clinical trials using an implantable commercial stimulator [33, 34]. Of six patients successfully implanted, five demonstrated stimulated abduction sufficient to restore mouth breathing. Three patients were subsequently decannulated. Unlike conventional treatment, pacing had no negative effect on voice quality [35]. Laryngeal pacing is covered in depth elsewhere in this text.

While electrical reanimation of the paralyzed larynx appears promising, the more natural approach to treatment would be to manipulate the process of nerve regeneration and muscle reinnervation. Since Horseley's original report of successful restoration of vocal fold mobility following RLN anastomosis [36], many investigators have attempted to reinnervate the paralyzed larynx using a variety of approaches in both animal experiments and limited clinical trials. Despite early favorable reports, the present consensus is that end-to-end RLN anastomosis results in crossed innervation of abductor and adductor muscles [15, 17, 25, 37]. Attempts to prevent synkinesis have looked to extrinsic sources for reinnervation of the larynx.

With respect to bilateral paralysis, phrenic nerve to RLN anastomosis has been performed to restore abduction, but with poor results [38–41]. Other approaches have focused on reinnervation of individual muscles. Tucker transposed a nerve–muscle pedicle, composed of a branch of the ansa hypoglossi and a pedicle of the omohyoid muscle, into the denervated PCA of dogs and humans, and reported return of vocal fold abduction [42–44]; however, failure of reinnervation with this procedure has been observed histochemically and electromyographically [37, 45]. Furthermore, other investigators have been unable to replicate good return of abduction. In animal experiments and limited clinical trials, Crumley et al. attempted to reinnervate the PCA by grafting the phrenic nerve to the abductor branch of the RLN and cutting the adductor branch [46]. Although this approach remains experimental, fair results were obtained in his study.

At present, it would appear that there has been more progress made toward reinnervation of adductor muscles in case of unilateral laryngeal paralysis. Despite failure to restore unilateral mobility, a new generation of reinnervation experiments has found success in using an extrinsic nerve to give the muscles bulk and tonus. One of the most pursued approaches, introduced in 1924 by Fraser [47], is an ansa cervicalis to RLN transfer. A purported advantage of the approach is that the nerve subserves only tonic, postural function, and therefore causes no extraneous twitching of the vocal fold or voice disturbance after transfer [48–50]; however, failure to restore adduction during vocalization requires that a medialization procedure still be used in combination with reinnervation [51]. Another promising new approach is that introduced by Paniello [52] and Paniello et al. [53], a hypoglossal nerve to RLN transfer. In animal and human experiments, they showed strong indication that the CXII can serve as a suitable donor for not only maintenance of vocal fold bulk, but also reanimation for deglutition and voice. In the animal studies, all animals showed strong return of adduction, particularly during swallowing. In the preliminary clinical study, 5 patients were reported to have excellent voice quality with no aspiration 1 year after surgery. The return of motion with this strategy could supersede ansa cervicalis transfer, as it obviates the need for a primary thyroplasty; however, this approach has its own inherent disadvantages: a longer distal RLN segment is needed for anastomosis, and the procedure creates a lingual deficit.

These novel trends in clinical research attempt to address laryngeal paralysis through reinnervation of individual muscles using an extrinsic, non-native source. There are two fundamental problems with this strategy. Firstly, stealing another muscle's nerve supply compromises that muscle's function. In case of bilateral paralysis, splitting the phrenic nerve for PCA reinnervation will result in hemidiaphragm paresis. The second problem arises from the differences between the host and donor muscle functions. Clearly, all complex voluntary and involuntary functions cannot be accommodated by the external nerve source. Indeed, because of this problem, the strategy for reinnervating the adductor muscles in case of unilateral paralysis is to identify a nerve source that performs minimal, only tonic function such as the ansa cervicalis. The goal is to maintain or restore bulk to the vocal fold without inducing extraneous motion. Ideally, a means could be found to selectively control reinnervation of laryngeal muscles by their original motoneurons in the RLN.

Studies in Selective Reinnervation

In a study of denervated canine laryngeal muscles following RLN neurorrhaphy, Zealear et al. found that the basic nature of reinnervation could be manipulated by electrical stimulation of the target muscle. Specifically, stimulation of the denervated posterior cricoarytenoid (PCA) muscle promoted selective reinnervation by native inspiratory motoneurons over foreign adductor motoneurons [54]. Eight animals were implanted with a planar array of 36 electrodes for chronic stimulation and recording of spontaneous and evoked electromyographic (EMG) potentials across the entire muscle surface. The PCA muscle in four experimental animals was stimulated during the 11-month experiment, using a 1-s, 30-pps, biphasic pulse train composed of 1-ms pulses 2–6 mA in amplitude and repeated every 10 s. The remaining four animals served as non-stimulated controls. Appropriate reinnervation by native inspiratory motoneurons was indexed behaviorally by the magnitude of vocal fold opening, and electromyographically by the averaged potential across all electrode sites (Fig. 2.5A). Inappropriate reinnervation by foreign reflex glottic closure motoneurons was quantitated by recording EMG potentials following stimulation of the internal branch of the SLN (Fig. 2.5D). All four experimental animals showed a greater level of correct ($p<0.0064$) and a lesser level of incorrect reinnervation ($p<0.0084$) than controls. These findings are consistent with a previous report [55] and suggest that stimulation of a mammalian muscle may profoundly affect its receptivity to reinnervation by a particular motoneuron type.

Although induction of specificity in motoneuron–muscle reconnection by electrical stimulation has not been described by other investigators, there are reports that regenerating motoneurons are influenced by trophic factors in distal nerve stumps. In the invertebrate, Wigston and Donahue described selective reinnervation of surgically exchanged axolotl muscles by their native motoneurons [56]. In the mammal, Brushart et al. observed that collaterals of single motor axons often regenerate down both sensory and motor pathways at a nerve bifurcation. Subsequently, the collaterals in the sensory pathway are pruned, while those in the motor pathway are maintained [57]. This process, termed "preferential motor reinnervation," is believed to be triggered by Schwann cell tube neurotropins and directed by motoneuron cell bodies. In particular, brief electrical stimulation of motoneurons has been found to accelerate the speed and accuracy of regeneration [58]. Politis reported preferential regeneration of peroneal and tibial components of the sciatic nerve down their native branches [59]. These branches each contain motor fibers; however, preferential regeneration down individual muscle pathways in the mammal cannot be inferred from these studies. Indeed, although target muscle recognition may occur in the invertebrate, reinnervation in the adult mammal is believed to be random, with high probability of a synkinetic outcome. With regard to laryngeal muscles, any neurotrophic effect on regeneration is inadequate to prevent misdirected regeneration of adductor fibers in the RLN and inappropriate reinnervation of the PCA muscle. Apparently, reinnervation specificity may be conferred only when muscle fibers or their reconnecting motoneurons are electrically activated [54].

Two postulates are offered as to how electrical stimulation could confer neuromuscular specificity. The first idea holds that muscle stimulation maintains the motoneuron-muscle fiber specificity that was established during development [60] and prevents its loss upon denervation. The second idea assumes that the

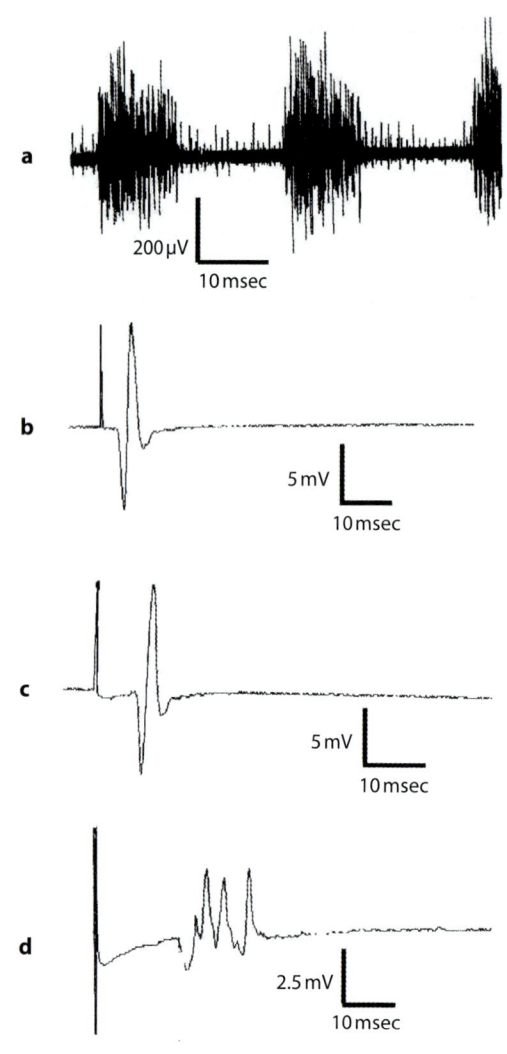

Fig. 2.5. Recordings from same PCA muscle electrode site. **a** Inspiratory activity at beginning of CO_2/air delivery. **b** EEMG following RLN stimulation. **c** EEMG following inadvertent stimulation of RLN motor fibers within vagus nerve just posterior to the superior laryngeal nerve. **d** The reflex glottic closure motor units activated polysynaptically via superior laryngeal nerve stimulation. Note latency increased from **b** to **c**, and **c** to **d**, due to increased conduction path. Response due to direct activation of PCA motor fibers in **c** could be distinguished from indirect response evoked in **d** on the basis of latency and waveform differences, as illustrated.

concept of muscle plasticity extends to the synapse, and that electrical stimulation can modulate not only contractile protein synthesis and muscle fiber properties, but receptivity of the endplate for a particular motoneuron type.

Evidence in support of the first hypothesis comes from basic studies in neurophysiology. The specificity between a single neuron and its endplate is established during development with the competitive elimination of redundant innervation [60, 61]. Following denervation in the adult, motoneurons revert to a more embryonic or dedifferentiated state but retain some specificity for their original muscle target [57, 62]. Denervation induces formation of extrajunctional (de novo) receptors on each muscle fiber; however, the original endplate may be distinguished from these de novo receptors by its recognition and affinity for the original motoneuron [63]. Stimulation of a muscle represses the formation of extrajunctional receptors without making the original endplate refractory to reinnervation [64]; thus, stimulation may favor reconnection between an original endplate and its nerve fiber, and foster restoration of the synapse which was competitively selected in development.

The second hypothesis, that electrical stimulation can modulate endplate receptivity, originated from basic studies in neuromuscular plasticity. In an early landmark study by Buller et al., it was discovered that fast and slow muscles cross-reinnervated by each others nerves switched their contraction speeds [65, 66]. This led to the dogma that the trophic influence of a nerve is needed in order to maintain the integrity and characteristic contractile properties of a muscle; however, in a later study, Salmons and Sreter opposed the putative chemotrophic effects of a nerve on its muscle's contraction speed with patterned electrical stimulation of the nerve [67]. Whether a muscle was innervated by its intrinsic nerve or cross-reinnervated by a nerve of opposite type, the contraction speed was determined by the pattern of electrical stimulation. Finally, Lomo and Westgaard demonstrated that denervated muscles, chronically stimulated with different electrical patterns, varied their contraction speeds in accordance with the pattern with which they were stimulated [68]. Apparently, the activity induced by electrical stimulation can maintain a muscle's characteristics in the absence of nerve supply. More recent studies have supported the idea that there is some feature of electrically induced activity which influences both the synthesis of contractile proteins (myosin heavy chain, MHC) and the contractile properties of muscle [69–71].

Regardless of which hypothesis is responsible for induction of selective reinnervation, it is probable that this event is genetically controlled. If the second hypothesis is true, some of the genes that control muscle transformation may also regulate receptivity to regrowing motor axons. The PCA muscle is distinguished from the adductor antagonists in having a slower contraction speed and higher abundance of type-I (slow-twitch) muscle fibers [10]. Following PCA denervation and reinnervation by the RLN, there is a change in muscle composition to favor type-II (fast-twitch) fibers and a corresponding acceleration of muscle contraction speed. Transformation of the muscle from slow to fast fibers can be prevented or reversed in the presence of electrical stimulation using the paradigm found to induce selective reinnervation [72]. These findings are consistent with reports of activity-dependent changes on muscle contraction in other motor systems [73, 74]. Apparently, the muscle transformation is controlled at a transcriptional level. Recent reports have identified specific genes and their promoters responsible for changes in MHC expression, paralleled by changes in muscle contraction speed induced by alteration in muscle activity [75, 76].

A recent report provides strong evidence that the MHC composition of a laryngeal muscle is correlated with the appropriateness of reinnervation [70]. In case of a nerve-crush injury, there was observed a transient shift in MHC expression characteristic of a denervated muscle. In particular, there was a consistent increase in type-IIA/IIX MHC and a decrease in type-IIB MHC, with a tendency toward a decrease in type-I MHC. Some weeks later upon appropriate reinnervation, the MHC composition reverted to that of the normally innervated control muscle of the same type (i.e., PCA vs

Table 2.1. Normal myosin heavy chain composition in rat laryngeal muscles (%). PCA posterior cricoarytenoid, TA thyroarytenoid, VOC vocalis, CT cricothyroid, LCA lateral cricoarytenoid, MHC myosin heavy chain. (From Shiotani and Flint [71])

	Type I	Type IIA	Type IIX	Type IIB	Type IIL
PCA	6.5 ± 0.7	12.0 ± 2.0	28.8 ± 2.2	46.3 ± 2.3	8.3 ± 1.2
TA	–	–	–	67.0 ± 1.2	33.0 ± 1.2
	Type I	Type IIA + IIX		Type IIB	Type IIL
VOC	–	81.0 ± 3.3		10.7 ± 2.3	8.4 ± 1.6
CT	8.6 ± 1.4	76.3 ± 3.1		15.0 ± 2.5	–
LCA	4.4 ± 0.7	51.3 ± 4.8		37.0 ± 3.9	7.4 ± 1.5

TA; Table 2.1). In case of nerve transection and repair, the course of MHC expression was dramatically different. The MHC profiles characteristic of denervation were expressed initially, but there was no normalization of the MHC pattern over time despite the presence of reinnervation. Apparently, reinnervation must be functional and appropriate in order for MHC profiles to normalize. Synkinetic reinnervation failed to restore normal gene expression characteristic of the particular muscle. The state of no activity associated with denervation was not distinguished from the state of random or nonspecific activity consequent to synkinesis.

While manipulation of nerve activity can influence muscle expression, it is less certain whether the reverse is true. Is the influence across the neuromuscular junction bidirectional? The strong effect of electrical stimulation in promoting selective reinnervation suggests that the pattern of induced activity in muscle can influence the type of nerve fibers that reconnect. As such, it may be possible to alter MHC composition through gene manipulation and thereby direct specificity in reinnervation. Recently, human insulin-like growth factor (hIGF-1) gene therapy has been explored as a potential treatment for peripheral nerve injury [77–80]. When applied to a rat model of laryngeal denervation, injection of hIGF-1 demonstrated both myotrophic and neurotrophic protective effects on the muscle. Specifically, the myotrophic effect of hIGF-1 gene transfer prevented the denervation profile from appearing; it normalized MHC composition with suppression of type-IIA/IIX MHC and promotion of type-IIB/IIL [79]. Coincidentally, the gene transfer produced a significant increase in motor endplate–nerve contact and a reduction in motor endplate length, as shown with acetylcholinesterase and silver staining techniques (Fig. 2.6). Although promising, it remains to be determined whether hIGF-1 gene therapy can promote specificity in reinnervation and become a future clinical tool for preventing synkinesis.

Conventional treatments for laryngeal paralysis fail to correct the inherent problem caused by nerve injury: denervation or dysfunctional reinnervation. New directions in research could for the first time provide a cure for laryngeal paralysis. Remarkably, electrical stimulation of a muscle has been shown to attract the return of its original innervation. Furthermore, gene expression could be regulated by pharmacological agents designed to encourage appropriate reinnervation of muscle denervated by disease or injury. Ultimately, electrical stimulation and gene therapy may prevent muscle atrophy and muscle transformation to a foreign type. Regenerating nerve fibers would recognize their native receptors on a healthy target muscle and enable normal laryngeal function to be restored.

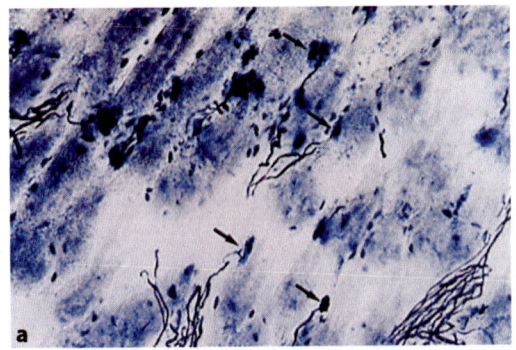

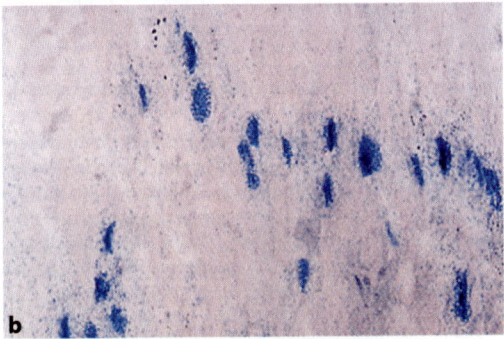

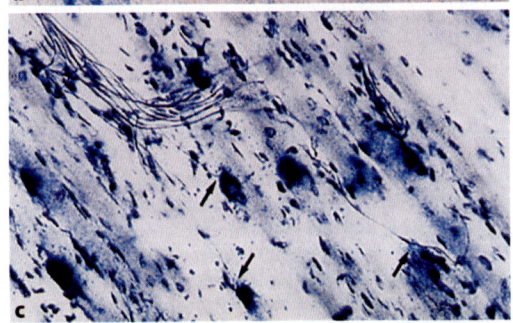

Fig. 2.6. a Photomicrograph of normal laryngeal muscle demonstrating motor endplates and nerve terminals (*arrows*) using cholinesterase or silver–gold staining technique. **b** Untreated denervated muscle 4 weeks after nerve section demonstrates elongation of motor endplates and the absence of neural filaments. **c** Photomicrograph of laryngeal muscle transfected with hIGF-1 plasmid demonstrates nerve sprouting and motor endplate contact (*arrows*) 4 weeks after nerve section and injection with plasmid formulation (magnification ×400). (From Flint et al. [79])

Acknowledgements

This work was supported by the National Institutes of Health grant no. 2RO1 DCO1149.

References

1. Zaretsky L, Sanders I (1992) The three bellies of the canine cricothyroid muscle. Ann Otol Rhinol Laryngol (Suppl) 156:3–16
2. Sanders I, Jacobs I, Wu, Biller HF (1993) The three bellies of the canine posterior cricoarytenoid muscle: implications for understanding laryngeal function. Laryngoscope 103:171–177
3. Sanders I, Bei-Lian W, Liancai M, Biller HF (1994) The innervation of the human posterior cricoarytenoid muscle: evidence for at least two neuromuscular compartments. Laryngoscope 104:880–884
4. Sanders I, Han Y, Surinder R, Biller HF (1998) Human vocalis contains distinct superior and inferior subcompartments: possible candidates for the two masses of vocal fold vibration. Ann Otol Rhinol Laryngol 107:826–833
5. Han Y, Wang J, Fischman DA, Biller HF, Sanders I (1999) Slow tonic muscle fibers in the thyroarytenoid muscles of human vocal folds; a possible specialization for speech. Anat Rec 256:146–157
6. Sanders I, Han Y, Wang J, Biller H (1998) Muscle spindles are concentrated in the superior vocalis subcompartment of the human thyroarytenoid muscle. J Voice 12:7–16
7. Maranillo E, Leon X, Ibanez M, Orus C, Quer M, Sanudo JR (2003) Variability of the nerve supply patterns of the human posterior cricoarytenoid muscle. Laryngoscope 113:602–606
8. Sanders I, Bei-Lian W, Liancai M, Youzhu L, Biller HF (1993) The innervation of the human larynx. Arch Otolaryngol Head Neck Surg 19:934–939
9. Bei-Lian W, Sanders I, Liancai M, Biller HF (1994) The human communicating nerve. Arch Otolaryngol Head Neck Surg 120:1321–1328
10. Zealear DL (1983) The contractile properties and functions of single laryngeal motor units. In: Bless DM, Abbs JH (eds) Vocal fold physiology: temporary research and clinical issues. College-Hill Press, San Diego, pp 96–106
11. Henneman E, Somjen G, Carpenter DO (1965) The functional significance of cell size in spinal motoneurons. J Neurophys 28:560–580
12. Hinrichsen CF, Ryan AT (1981) Localization of laryngeal motoneurons in the rat: morphologic evidence for dual innervation? Exp Neurol 74:341–355
13. Dilworth TFM (1921) The nerves of the human larynx. J Anat 56:48–52
14. Siribodhi C, Sundmaker W, Atkins JP, Bonner FJ (1963) Electromyographic studies of laryngeal paralysis and regeneration of laryngeal motor nerves in dogs. Laryngoscope 73:148–164

15. Boles R, Fritzell B (1969) Injury and repair of the recurrent laryngeal nerves in dogs. Laryngoscope 70:1405–1418
16. Murakami Y, Kirchner JA (1971) Vocal cord abduction by regenerated recurrent laryngeal nerve. An experimental study in the dog. Arch Otolaryngol 94:64–68
17. Crumley RL (1989) Laryngeal synkinesis: its significance to the laryngologist. Ann Otol Rhinol Laryngol 98:87–92
18. Crumley RL (2000) Laryngeal synkinesis revisited. Ann Otol Rhinol Laryngol 109:365–371
19. Flint PW, Downs DH, Coltrera MD (1991) Laryngeal synkinesis following reinnervation in the rat. Neuroanatomic and physiologic study using retrograde fluorescent tracers and electromyography. Ann Otol Rhinol Laryngol 100:797–806
20. Davis PJ, Nail BS (1984) On the location and size of laryngeal motoneurons in the cat and rabbit. J Comp Neurol 230:13–32
21. Hisa Y, Sato F, Fukui K, Ibata Y, Mizuokoshi O (1984) Nucleus ambiguus motoneurons innervating the canine intrinsic laryngeal muscles by the fluorescent labeling technique. Exp Neurol 84:441–449
22. Yoshida Y, Miyazaki T, Hirano M, Shin T, Kanaseki T (1982) Arrangement of motoneurons innervating the intrinsic laryngeal muscles of cats as demonstrated by horseradish peroxidase. Acta Otolaryngol (Stockh) 94:329–334
23. Gacek RR, Malmgren LT, Lyon MJ (1977) Localization of adductor and abductor motor nerve fibers to the larynx. Ann Otol Rhinol Laryngol 86:771–776
24. Nahm I, Shin T, Chiba T (1990) Regeneration of the recurrent laryngeal nerve in the guinea pig. Reorganization of motoneurons after freezing injury. Am J Otolaryngol 11:90–98
25. Dedo H (1970) The paralyzed larynx: an electromyographic study in dogs and humans. Laryngoscope 80:1455–1514
26. Tashiro T (1972) Experimental studies of the reinnervation of the larynx after accurate neurorrhaphy. Laryngoscope 82:225–236
27. Dedo HH (1971) Electromyographic and visual evaluation of recurrent laryngeal nerve anastomosis in dogs. Ann Otol Rhinol Laryngol 80:664–668
28. Crumley RL, McCabe BF (1982) Regeneration of the recurrent laryngeal nerve. Otolaryngol Head Neck Surg 90:442–447
29. Zealear DL, Hamdan AL, Rainey CL (1994) The effects of denervation on posterior cricoarytenoid muscle physiology and histochemistry. Ann Otol Rhinol Laryngol 103:780–788
30. Damrose EJ, Huang RY, Blumin JH, Blackwell KE, Sercarz JA, Berke GS (2001) Lack of evoked laryngeal electromyography response in patients with a clinical diagnosis of vocal cord paralysis. Ann Otol Rhinol Laryngol 110:815–819
31. Blitzer A, Jahn AF, Keidar A (1996) Semon's law revisited: an electromyographic analysis of laryngeal synkinesis. Ann Otol Rhinol Laryngol 105:764–769
32. Holinger L, Holinger PC, Holinger PH (1976) Etiology of the bilateral abductor vocal cord paralysis. Ann Otol 85:428–436
33. Zealear DL, Billante CR, Courey MS, Netterville JL, Paniello R, Sanders I, Herzon, GD, Goding GS, Mann W, Ejnell H, Van de Heyning P (2003) Reanimation of the paralyzed human larynx with an implantable stimulation device. Laryngoscope 113:1149–1156
34. Zealear DL, Billante CR, Courey MS, Sant'anna GD, Netterville JL (2002) Electrically stimulated glottal opening combined with adductor muscle botox blockade restores both ventilation and voice in a patient with bilateral laryngeal paralysis. Ann Otol Rhinol Laryngology 111:500–506
35. Billante CR, Zealear DL, Courey MS, Netterville JL (2002) Effect of chronic electrical stimulation of laryngeal muscle on voice. Ann Otol Rhinol Laryngol 111:328–332
36. Horseley JS (1909) Suture of the recurrent laryngeal nerve with report of a case. Trans South Surg Gynecol Assoc 22:161
37. Crumley RL (1979) Mechanisms of synkinesis. Laryngoscope 89:1847–1854
38. Crumley RL (1982) Experiments in reinnervation. Laryngoscope 92:1–27
39. Fex S (1970) Functioning remobilization of vocal colds in cats with permanent recurrent laryngeal nerve paralysis. Acta Otolaryngol 69:294–301
40. Morledge D, Lauvstad WA, Calcaterra T (1973) Delayed reinnervation of the paralyzed larynx. Arch Otol 97:291–293
41. Taggart JP (1971) Laryngeal reinnervation by phrenic nerve implantation in dogs. Laryngoscope 81:1330–1336
42. Tucker HM (1978) Human laryngeal reinnervation: long-term experience with the nerve muscle pedicle technique. Laryngoscope 88:598–604
43. Tucker HM (1982) Nerve–muscle pedicle reinnervation of the larynx: avoiding pitfalls and complications. Ann Otol Rhinol Laryngol 91:440–444
44. Tucker HM (1989) Long-term results of nerve-muscle pedicle reinnervation for laryngeal paralysis. Ann Otol Rhinol Laryngol 98:674–676
45. Rice DH, Owens O, Burstein F, Verity A (1983) The nerve–muscle pedicle: a visual, electromyographic and histochemical study. Arch Otolaryngol 109:233–234
46. Crumley RL, Horn K, Slendenning D (1980) Laryngeal reinnervation using the split-phrenic

47. Fraser CH (1924) The treatment of paralysis of the recurrent laryngeal nerve by nerve anastomosis. Ann Surg 79:161–166
48. rumley RL (1991) Update: ansa cervicalis to recurrent laryngeal nerve anastomosis for unilateral laryngeal paralysis. Laryngoscope 101:384–388
49. Zheng H, Li Z, Zhou S, Cuan Y, Wen W, Lan J (1996) Experimental study on reinnervation of vocal cord adductors with the ansa cervicalis. Laryngoscope 106:1516–1521
50. Zheng H, Li Z, Zhou S, Cuan Y, Wen W (1996) Update: laryngeal reinnervation for unilateral vocal cord paralysis with the ansa cervicalis. Laryngoscope 106:1522–1527
51. Olson DEL, Goding GS, Michael DD (1998) Acoustic and perceptual evaluation of laryngeal reinnervation by ansa cervicalis transfer. Laryngoscope 108:1767–1772
52. Paniello RC (2000) Laryngeal reinnervation with the hypoglossal nerve. II: Clinical evaluation and early patient experience. Laryngoscope 110:739–747
53. Paniello RC, Lee P, Dahm JD (1999) Hypoglossal nerve transfer for laryngeal reinnervation: a preliminary study. Ann Otol Rhinol Laryngol 108:239–244
54. Zealear DL, Rodriguez RJ, Kenny T, Billante MJ, Cho Y, Billante CR, Garren KC (2002) Electrical stimulation of a denervated muscle promotes selective reinnervation by native over foreign motoneurons. J Neurophys 87:2195–2199
55. Zealear DL, Billante CR, Chongkolwatana C, Herzon GD (2000) The effects of chronic electrical stimulation on laryngeal muscle reinnervation. ORL J Otorhinolaryngol Relat Spec 62:87–95
56. Wigston DJ, Donahue SP (1988) The location of cues promoting selective reinnervation of axolotl muscles. J Neurosci 8:3451–3458
57. Brushart TM, Gerber J, Lessens P, Shen YG, Royall RM (1998) Contributions of pathway and neuron to preferential motor reinnervation. J Neurosci 18:8674–8681
58. Al-Majed A, Neumann CM, Brushart TM, Gordon T. Brief electrical stimulation promotes the speed and accuracy of motor axonal regeneration. J Neurosci 2000; 20(7):2602–08.
59. Politis MJ. Specificity in mammalian peripheral nerve regeneration at the level of the nerve trunk. Brain Res 1985;328:271.
60. Thompson W. Synapse elimination in neonatal rat muscle is sensitive to pattern of muscle use. Nature 1983;302:614–6.
61. Bennett MR, Robinson J (1989) Growth and elimination of nerve terminals at synaptic sites during polyneuronal innervation of muscle cells: a trophic hypothesis. Proc R Soc Lond B 235:299–320
62. Gordon T, Bambrick L, Orozco R (1988) Comparison of injury and development in the neuromuscular system. Ciba Found Symp 138:210–226
63. Lomo T, Waerhaug O (1985) Motor endplates in fast and slow muscles of the rat: What determines their difference? J Physiol (Paris) 80:290–297
64. Kallo JR, Steinhardt FA (1983) The regulation of extrajunctional acetylcholine receptors in the denervated rat diaphragm muscle in culture. J Physiol (Lond) 344:433–453
65. Buller AJ, Eccles JC, Eccles RM (1960) Differentiation of fast and slow muscles in the cat hind limb. J Physiol 150:399–416
66. Buller AJ, Eccles JC, Eccles RM (1960) Interactions between motoneurons and muscles in respect of the characteristic speeds of their muscle responses. J Physiol 150:417–439
67. Salmons S, Sreter FA (1976) Significance of impulse activity in the transformation of skeletal muscle type. Nature 263:30
68. Lomo T, Westgaard RH, Dahl HA (1974) Contractile properties of muscle: control by pattern of muscle activity in the rat. Proc Royal Soc Lond (B) 187:99
69. Windisch A, Gundersen K, Szabolcs H, Gruber H, Lomo T (1998) Fast to slow transformation of denervated and electrically stimulated rat muscle. J Physiol 510:623–632
70. Shiotani A, Nakagawa H, Flint PW (2001) Modulation of myosin heavy chains in rat laryngeal muscle. Laryngoscope 111:472–477
71. Shiotani A, Flint PW (1998) Myosin heavy chain composition in rat laryngeal muscles after denervation. Laryngoscope 108:1225–1229
72. Zealear DL, Billante CL, Chongkolwatana C, Rho YS, Hamdan AL, Herzon GD (2000) The effects of chronic electrical stimulation on laryngeal muscle physiology and histochemistry. ORL J Otorhinolaryngol Relat Spec 62:81–86
73. Vrbova G, Pette D (1999) What does chronic electrical stimulation teach us about muscle plasticity? Muscle Nerve 22(6):666–677
74. Gundersen K (1998) Determination of muscle contractile properties: the importance of the nerve. Acta Physiol Scand 162:333–341
75. Murgia M, Serrano AL, Calabria E, Pallafacchina G, Lomo T, Schiaffino S (2000) Ras is involved in nerve-activity-dependent regulation of muscle genes. Nat Cell Biol 2:142–147
76. Wittwer M, Fluck M, Hoppeler H, Muller S, Desplanches D, Billeter R (2002) Prolonged unloading of rat soleus muscle causes distinct adaptations of the gene profile. FASEB J 16:884–886
77. Flint PW, Nakagawa H, Shiotani A, Coleman ME, O'Malley BW Jr (2004) Effects of insulin-like

growth factor-1 gene transfer on myosin heavy chains in denervated rat laryngeal muscle. Laryngoscope 114:368–371

78. Shiotani A, O'Malley BW Jr, Coleman ME, Flint PW (1999) Human insulinlike growth factor 1 gene transfer into paralyzed rat larynx: single vs multiple injection. Arch Otolaryngol Head Neck Surg 125:555–560

79. Flint PW, Shiotani A, O'Malley BW Jr (1999) IGF-1 gene transfer into denervated rat laryngeal muscle. Arch Otolaryngol Head Neck Surg 125:274–279

80. Shiotani A, O'Malley BW Jr, Coleman ME, Alila HW, Flint PW (1998) Reinnervation of motor endplates and increased muscle fiber size after human insulin-like growth factor I gene transfer into the paralyzed larynx. Hum Gene Ther 20:2039–2047

81. Sanders I, Jacobs I, Wu BL, Biller HF (1993) The three bellies of the canine posterior cricoarytenoid muscle: implications for understanding laryngeal function. Laryngoscope 103:171–177

Chapter 3

Vocal Fold Paralysis: Causes, Outcomes, and Clinical Aspects

Lucian Sulica, Anthony Cultrara, Andrew Blitzer

Introduction

The paths of the recurrent nerves from the central nervous system largely determine the causes of vocal fold paralysis. While the superior laryngeal nerve alone may be dysfunctional, recurrent nerve injury, either alone or in combination with the superior nerve, is necessary for gross vocal fold immobility.

The recurrent nerve may be subjected to a variety of mechanical trauma. It may be sectioned during surgery. It may be stretched or compressed acutely during surgical manipulation, or chronically by a mass growing adjacent to the nerve. It may be invaded by malignancy, and it may be devascularized as a result of nearby surgical dissection. Radiation produces fibrosis in and around nerves that may result in neuropathy as well.

Mild pressure to a peripheral nerve produces segmental demyelinization and impairs axonal transport, the degree and severity of the conduction block being proportional to the severity of the injury [1]. Remyelinization over the preserved axon usually restores conduction and function. Injuries which interrupt the axon, such as nerve section or severe crush, produce complete wallerian degeneration along the entire length of the nerve distal to the injury beginning within 24 h of injury. Functional recovery depends on preservation of the neural conduits for axonal regeneration. The basal lamina of the original nerve fibers is usually preserved in severe crush (axonotmesis), and proximal axonal sprouts may reach the appropriate muscle. If the nerve is transected (neurotmesis), the proportion of fibers that find their way to the original target is low and generally inversely proportional to the size of the gap between proximal and distal segments.

Regeneration of the recurrent nerve is more problematic than most peripheral nerves, because it carries mixed adductor and abductor fibers to a population of highly specialized muscles whose function must be precisely graded and tightly integrated for breathing, swallowing and phonation. The problems of synkinesis and misdirected reinnervation are detailed elsewhere in this volume.

Sources of Nerve Damage

Overview

Most sources of nerve injury fall into three broad categories: damage from surgery or other trauma; compromise from a range of medical conditions; and dysfunction due to factors yet to be completely identified and characterized, designated "idiopathic." The roster of surgeries during which the laryngeal nerves are at risk, once limited to thyroidectomy, now includes a variety of base of skull, cervical and thoracic procedures, and continues to expand (Table 3.1). In modern series, mediastinal tumors, usually metastases from primary lung malignancies, account for the majority of vocal fold paralyses from medical causes. This was not always so, because historically other disease processes occurred with greater frequency and accounted for a much larger proportion of cases. Certain cases have always defied diagnosis. Early speculation regarding their etiology focused on toxins and inflammatory or infectious conditions, even before the notion of viral pathogens existed. It is interesting to note that, on the whole, the incidence of idiopathic paralysis has not changed dramatically since the introduction of advanced imaging techniques.

Table 3.1. Surgeries and procedures which place laryngeal nerves at risk

Cervical surgery
— Thyroidectomy/parathyroidectomy
— Anterior approach to the cervical spine
— Carotid endarterectomy
— Implantation of vagal nerve stimulator
— Cricopharyngeal myotomy/repair of Zenker's diverticulum
Thoracic procedures
— Pneumonectomy and pulmonary lobectomy
— Repair of thoracic aortic aneurysm
— Coronary artery bypass graft
— Aortic valve replacement
— Esophageal surgery
— Tracheal surgery
— Mediastinoscopy
— Thymectomy
— Ligation of persistent ductus arteriosus
— Cardiac and pulmonary transplant
Other surgery
— Skull base surgery
— Brainstem surgery, or neurosurgery which required brainstem retraction
Other medical procedures
— Central venous catheterization
— Endotracheal intubation

The frequency of etiologies of vocal fold paralysis varies considerably, both between and within these broad categories. Table 3.2 presents a summary of series of unilateral vocal fold paralysis since 1932, and reveals the extent of such variation. Cases of bilateral paralysis included in some of the reports have been discarded, and the many series which do not distinguish between unilateral and bilateral paralysis are not included.

Differences among reports may result from the demographics and epidemiologic features of populations from which case series are drawn, as well as differences specific to the reporting practice or institution. For example, the unusually high proportion of cases due to malignancy (52%) in a Scottish series [2] reflects the high incidence of lung cancer in that country. On the other hand, the very large percentage of postsurgical cases (75%) from a French tertiary referral center [3] is more likely a product of surgical specialization at the hospital and/or referral patterns, rather than any epidemiologic factor. Reports tally causes in relative terms, so such unusual distributions skew the relative frequency of other etiologies and leave an inaccurate impression of a rarity of other causes. For example, in the aforementioned French series, malignancy accounts for only 7% of cases of unilateral vocal fold paralysis. Conversely, in a series from a Veteran's Administration Medical Center, not included in the table because it makes no distinction between unilateral and bilateral cases, the high number of paralyses which result from medical causes (28%, principally from tuberculous lymphadenopathy) and malignancy (38%) [4] create the impression of a very low number of cases from surgical causes (10%). In the absence of absolute data regarding incidence, studies cannot be compared with one another except in the most general terms.

Despite such factors, it is possible to draw some generalizations regarding unilateral vocal fold paralysis. Vocal fold paralysis is the result of a peripheral neuropathy rather than a central nervous system process in the vast majority of cases. In most series, vocal fold paralysis tends to affect men more often than women, probably reflecting the underlying gender distribution of thoracic malignancy. In the single previous series in which most patients are women [5], the high proportion of benign thyroid disease and thyroid surgery likely accounts for the difference. Uniformly, the left vocal fold is affected more often than the right, in approximately a 60:40 ratio or greater, due to the greater length and more profound descent into the mediastinum of the left-sided nerve, and consequent greater vulnerability to disease and surgery. A comparison of right-sided (Table 3.3) and left-sided paralysis (Table 3.4) confirms that a left-sided paralysis is more likely to be related to malignancy than a right-sided one, although the difference is not nearly as clear as might be expected. The impression that the left fold is less likely to be paralyzed by surgery, on the other hand, is probably an artifact of the relatively high number of cases accounted for by malignancy. At any rate, the portion of right-sided paralysis due to malignancy is far from

Table 3.2. Relationship of left (RLN to ITA) Unilateral Vocal Fold Paralysis

Reference	Year	Number of cases	Male (%)	L/R (%)	Cause (%)						
					Malignancy	Trauma Surgical	Trauma Nonsurgical	Intubation	Neurologic[g]	Other medical	Idiopathic (incl. "viral")
[3]	2003	325	55	73/27	7	75	1	0	2	2	12
[2]	2002	77	66	83/17	52	22	0	5	0	9	12
[161]	2001	171	65	65/35	22	24	<1	13	4	8	28
[151]	2001	90	52	73/27	29	24	6	2	4	0	34[i]
[162]	1999	108	50	65/35	5	40	4	2	7	9[h]	33
[135]	1999	117[a]	56	69/31	31	32	0	2	5	15	15
[109]	1998	280	58	63/37	25	24	11	8	8	5	20
[145]	1998	98	67	70/30	32	30	7	4	8	3	16
[153]	1992	84	54	68/32	40	35	1	7	2	4	11
[160]	1983	519			18	22	2	10	1	4	42
[159]	1981	84			26	37	7	2	0	2	25
[134]	1981	80			53	11[e]	[e]	0	4	14	18 (14)
[155]	1979	210			22	37[e]	[e]	0	2	20	14
[136]	1974	127		57/43	24	16	10	3	8	11	27
[144]	1970	86	63	59/41	36	25	2	0	6	16	15
[126]	1963	97		59/41	28	34	0	0	8	11	19
[117]	1955	262	62	69/31	27	7	1	0	0	11	53[j]
[116]	1953	293[b]			39	21	2	0	[b]	9	29[k]
[152]	1943	210		70/30	31	15	2	0	2	23	26
[163]	1941	183	41		14	39	0	0	10	15	23
[150]	1933	173[c]	70		27	15[f]	1	0	4	36	17
[143]	1932	282[d]			31	11[f]	1	0	5	17	35

[a] Seventy-one patients with "abductor" paralysis, not otherwise defined, are excluded
[b] Excludes VFP of CNS etiology
[c] Two hundred twelve reported, but causes not given for 39
[d] Cases of known cause combined with those of unknown cause, reported separately in the original paper
[e] Distinction between surgical and nonsurgical trauma not made
[f] Does not distinguish between paralysis due to surgery and paralysis due to primary thyroid disease
[g] Includes CNS malignancy
[h] Six percent [7] due to glomus or vagal neuroma
[i] Includes 21% [19] attributed to "inflammation" not otherwise specified
[j] Includes 22% [58] originally reported due to "inflammatory" conditions, including upper respiratory infections
[k] Includes 17% [49] originally reported as due to "inflammatory" and "toxic" causes

Table 3.3. Left vocal fold paralysis

Reference	Year	Number of Cases	Male (%)	Cause (%)						
				Malignancy	Trauma		Intubation	Neurologic[g]	Other medical (incl. "viral")	Idiopathic
					Surgical	Nonsurgical				
[161]	2001	111		22	24	<1	13	4	8	28
[160]	1983	371		17	21	2	11	<1	5	42
[159]	1981	58		28	26	9	2	9	3	22
[126]	1963	57		30	25	0	0	12	19	14
[152]	1943	146		34	15	<1	0	2	27	21
[163]	1941	109	46	14	37	0	0	12	13	25
[150]	1933	128[a]	73	27	10[c]	1	0	5	39	18
[143]	1932	194[b]		28	9[c]	1	0	6	21	36

[a] One hundred sixty reported, but causes not given for 32
[b] Cases of known cause combined with those of unknown cause, reported separately in the original paper
[c] Does not distinguish between VFP due to surgery and VFP due to primary thyroid disease
[d] Includes CNS malignancy
[e] Includes "viral" and "inflammatory" not otherwise specified

Table 3.4 Right vocal fold paralysis

Reference	Year	Number of Cases	Male (%)	Cause (%) Malignancy	Trauma Surgical	Trauma Nonsurgical	Intubation	Neurologic[d,g]	Other medical (incl. "viral")	Idiopathic[e]
[161]	2001	60		17	35	2	7	8	0	32
[129]	2000	24	46	0	46	13	0	13	0	19
[160]	1983	148		11	26	2	8	3	2	41
[159]	1981	26		23	38	4	4		0	31
[128]	1963	40		25	48	0	0	3	0	25
[152]	1943	64		25	16	6	0	2	16	36
[163]	1941	74	34	14	42	0	0	7	5	10
[150]	1933	45[a]	62	27	19[c]	2	0	0	27	13
[143]	1932	88[b]		38	16[c]	1	0	5	8	34

[a] Fifty-two reported, but causes not given for 7
[b] Cases of known cause combined with those of unknown cause, reported separately in the original paper
[c] Does not distinguish between VFP due to surgery and VFP due to primary thyroid disease
[d] Includes CNS malignancy
[e] Includes "viral" and "inflammatory" not otherwise specified

negligible, and this should be kept in mind during diagnostic evaluation.

Iatrogenic sources of injury have multiplied over time, and thyroid surgery is no longer the sole procedure which places the recurrent nerve at risk (Table 3.5). It may be that thyroidectomy is safer now, but in all likelihood, most of the decrease in cases attributable to thyroid surgery is relative. The anterior approach to the cervical spine, carotid endarterectomy, and various cardiac and thoracic procedures have all become significant sources of laryngeal nerve injury. In addition, the potential for recurrent nerve damage from the cuffed endotracheal tube was recognized in the 1960s and early 1970s, and continues to account for cases of vocal fold immobility which are demonstrably neural in origin and not the result of cricoarytenoid joint disruption.

It seems that, in general, the evolution of computed tomography and magnetic resonance imaging has not had a marked impact on the incidence of idiopathic vocal fold paralysis. Benninger and colleagues [6] have suggested that normal radiography is nearly equivalent to computed tomography in the evaluation of the chest, and the historical trends appear to support this. However, as the penalty for an overlooked tumor is high, most physicians, including the present authors, continue to recommend computed tomographic imaging across the entire course of the affected nerve.

The most striking trend over time is the decreasing proportion of vocal fold paralysis due to nonmalignant medical conditions (Table 3.6). Historically, aortic aneurysm (largely due to syphilis), tuberculous lymphadenopathy, and several other infectious diseases occurred with greater frequency and accounted for a larger proportion of cases. Ortner's syndrome, or cardiovocal syndrome, is a rarity now, and cases are deemed worthy of publication, but it was a matter of course at the beginning of the twentieth century. Today, a noniatrogenic left vocal fold paralysis prompts a search for mediastinal tumor. However, in 1908, Bryson Delevan wrote, "In the minds of most practitioners, the discovery of fixation of the left side of the larynx is almost proof positive of the presence of an aortic aneurysm." [7, p 637]. In the absence of treatment of primary causes or survivable surgical options, aneurysms grew so large that they were occasionally responsible for *bilateral* paralysis [7, 8]. Vocal fold paralysis was also related to a series of infectious diseases that have become rare or nonexistent – diphtheria, puerperal fever, typhus, and particularly typhoid fever – as well as complications of untreated infectious diseases that are relatively uncommon since the advent of antibiotics, such as pleuritis, massive mediastinal lymphadenopathy, and pericardial effusion. Unchecked thyroid enlargement, usually due to benign disease, also used to account for a number of paralyzed vocal cords [7].

Although the surgeries and diseases which may cause vocal fold paralysis have changed, the broad categories – surgery/trauma, medical disease, and paralysis of unknown cause – have not, and provide a useful framework for a more specific review.

Surgery/Trauma

Surgery in the Neck

Thyroid Surgery

The close anatomical relationship of both the recurrent and superior laryngeal nerves with the blood vessels supplying the thyroid gland represents a well-recognized challenge to surgeons. Vocal fold paralysis does not result only from nerve section but also from nerve manipulation, sometimes minor; a paralyzed vocal fold has surprised many an experienced thyroid surgeon who is certain that nerve has been left intact.

In recent series, the number of patients experiencing temporary vocal fold dysfunction following thyroidectomy varies from 1.0 to 5.1%, and permanent paralysis from 0 to 5.8%, with most series reporting less than 3%, and in some cases less than 1% (Table 3.7). If this is judged as a percentage of nerves at risk rather than patients, a common means of tabulating this complication, the incidence may be up to 50% lower depending on the proportion of patients undergoing total thyroidectomy. Principal vari-

Table 3-5. Surgical causes of unilateral vocal fold paralysis. ACSS anterior cervical spine surgery

Reference	Year	Number of Cases	Surgical Cause (%)							
			Thyroid and parathyroid	ACSS	Carotid	Other cervical	Neurosurgery	Cardiac	Thoracic and mediastinal	Other
[3]	2003	243	44			6a	2	9	39	0
[2]	2002	17	24	6	18	0	0	12	41	0
[161]	2001	48	56							44[b]
[151]	2001	22	59							41[b]
[104]	1999	43	67	12	0	7	0	9	5	0
[135]	1999	37	22	19	27	0	11	0	16	0
[6]	1998	67	34							66[b]
[145]	1998	29	14			24[a]	31	0	31	0
[153]	1992	29	24							76[b]
[160]	1983	116	53	<1	0	3	0	16	27	0
[136]	1974	20	50							50[b]
[164]	1970	21	86	0	0	0	0	0	14	0
[126]	1963	33	91							9[b]
[117]	1955	18	94							6[b]
[116]	1953	61	97							3[b]
[152]	1943	32	88							13[b]
[163]	1941	71	99							1[b]
[150]	1933	26	100							
[143]	1932	26	100							

[a] Nonthyroid cervical cases not further described
[b] Nonthyroid cases not further described

Table 3.6. Nontraumatic causes of unilateral vocal fold paralysis (excluding surgery, trauma, and intubation)

Reference	Year	Number of Cases	Malignancy[b] (%)	Neurologic/CNS (%)	Pulmonary nonmalignant (%)	Cardiac and vascular (%)	Other medical (%)	Idiopathic (%)
[3]	2003	78	31	9		0	0	10	50
[2]	2002	56	72	0		0	0	13	16
[104]	1999	59	8	14		0	0	17	61
[135]	1999	78	46	8		0	13	10	23
[6]	1998	161	43	14		2	7	0	34
[160]	1983	325	29	2		5	2	<1	67
[136]	1974	89	35	11		0	9	7	38
[164]	1970	63	49	8		3	10	10	21
[128]	1963	64	42	13		9	6	<1	28
[117]	1955	241	29	0		5	0	7	46[e]
[116]	1953	225	50	c		d	d	12d	38e
[152]	1943	172	38	2		10	15	3	31
[163]	1941	112	22	16		8	7	9	38
[150]	1933	144[a]	32	5		17	26	a	20
[143]	1932	249	33	6		4	13	2	40

[a] Causes not given for 39 cases
[b] Includes both thoracic and extrathoracic malignancy
[c] Excludes VFP of CNS etiology
[d] Medical etiology not further specified
[e] Twenty-four percent originally reported as "inflammatory" and "toxic" causes

Table 3.7. Vocal fold paralysis after thyroid surgery: recent series

Reference	Year	Number of Cases	Temporary (%)	Permanent (%)	Total (%)
[10]	2005	521	5.1	0.9	6.0
[125]	2005	1020	1.4	0.4	1.8
[146]	2004	14,939	2.0	1.0	3.0
[12][a,b]	2004	301			8.6
[114][a,b]	2004	834	2.3	1.1	3.4
[130]	2003	2100			7.7
[15][b]	2003	1636	1.9	0.9	2.8
[124][a,b]	2003	1789	1.9	0.4	2.3
[165][a]	2002	102	1.0	0	1.0
[115]	2001	312		2.9	
[110]	1998	1192	2.9	0.5	3.4
[133]	1997	361		2.4	
[141]	1997	253	2.4	2.8	5.1
[149]	1995	186		0.9	
[132]	1994	797	3.1	0.5	3.6
[157]	1994	1026	2.5	2.4	5.9
[166][b,c]	1993	124		0.8	
[127]	1991	335			2.3
[139]	1985	514		5.8	

Incidences reported are based on number of patients/operations rather than nerves at risk
[a] Benign disease only
[b] Total thyroidectomy only
[c] Malignant disease only

ables which affect the comparison of reported studies include the original pathology and the extent of the surgery performed. Most studies agree that the risk of recurrent nerve complications is considerably increased in re-operative surgery, whether for benign or malignant disease [9–11]. Many authors also report a higher incidence of complications with malignant pathology [9–11], hyperthyroidism [12], or Graves disease [10]. It is also clear that identification of the nerve during thyroidectomy decreases the possibility of injury [9, 13–15], and routine nerve exposure is to be pursued in every case where this is possible without undue additional tissue dissection. Several intraoperative identification and monitoring techniques have been introduced as adjuncts to this task, but there has been no clear evidence that their routine use results in decrease of the incidence of recurrent nerve injury [16, 17]. Their principal utility may lie in cases of higher risk, although even in such instances misleading results may be obtained [18]. It appears that regardless of surgical circumstances, there is no substitute for a thorough familiarity with the anatomy and its variants, precise dissection, and prudence.

The vocal fold may be paralyzed before surgery by primary thyroid disease in as many as 1.2% of patients [19], a factor which argues in favor of routine preoperative evaluation of the larynx. The vocal fold is far more likely to be paralyzed when the underlying thyroid mass is malignant, but the majority of paralyzed vocal folds are caused by benign disease [19, 20]. In these instances, there is a potential for nerve recovery after decompression by thyroidectomy. The presence of vocal fold paralysis in a patient with thyroid carcinoma, even of the well-differentiated variety, is a marker of locally advanced disease and a poor prognostic indicator [21].

Anterior Approach to the Cervical Spine

Anterior exposure of the cervical spine requires separation of the laryngopharyngeal complex from the lateral tissues of the neck, including the carotid sheath. The recurrent nerve is thus necessarily stretched between its vagal origin and its end organ. Because the right-sided nerve is both shorter and has a more oblique trajectory, it is held to be more susceptible to such an injury than the left [22, 23]. The predominance of right-sided lesions (15 of 16) in the series of Netterville et al. seems to be in accord with this [24], but not all series feature such an asymmetrical distribution of cases. An alternate explanation attributes the vocal cord paralysis to endolaryngeal pressure on the terminal branches of the recurrent nerve from the endotracheal tube cuff, which is pressed against the side of the larynx and pulled against the underside of the vocal fold as the larynx is displaced laterally by the Cloward retractor [25]. A simple maneuver consisting of deflating the cuff and repositioning the tube following placement of the retractor was successful in decreasing the incidence of vocal fold paralysis from 6.4 to 1.7%, a difference which was statistically significant.

The incidence of vocal fold paralysis following an anterior approach to the cervical spine may be about 3%, decreasing to 0.3–2.7% over time (Table 3.8). It is interesting that a systematic laryngoscopic assessment of all patients 3–7 days following surgery revealed a surprisingly high incidence of vocal fold paralysis [26], the majority of which was asymptomatic. Approximately 70% of these cases resolved over 3 months. It is possible that many more cases of vocal fold paralysis occur than is generally accepted, and either are asymptomatic or resolve in the period of time during which dysphonia is dismissed as a routine aftereffect of intubation. This course would be expected in a mild traction or compression injury, and may be typical in many scenarios of iatrogenic vocal fold injury. Such findings also underline the effect of the time of evaluation on the incidence of vocal fold injury observed, and this poorly controlled variable should be kept in mind throughout this review.

Dysphagia is not infrequent following this operation, but it is not always due to vocal fold paralysis. Lateral displacement of the laryngopharyngeal complex from the anterior surface of the spine may disrupt the pharyngeal plexus.

Table 3.8. Vocal fold paralysis after anterior approach to the cervical spine

Reference	Year	Number of Cases	Temporary (%)	Permanent (%)
[26]	2005	120	20.8[a]	6.6[b]
[112]	2001	328		2.7
[25]	2000	900	3.0	0.3
[111]	1989	450		1.1

[a] 8.3% symptomatic, 12.5% asymptomatic
[b] At 3-month follow-up: 2.5% symptomatic; 4.2% asymptomatic

This denervation, followed by uneven or disorganized reinnervation in a muscular system that requires a high degree of coordination and sequential contraction for a normal swallow, probably accounts for many of these cases. Where there is also glottic insufficiency from an immobile vocal fold, there may be a greater potential for aspiration than one expects with recurrent nerve paralysis alone, a clinical feature that of which the physician should be aware.

Carotid Endarterectomy

Injury of the vagus or its branches during carotid endarterectomy may result from skeletonization and mobilization of the vessel, or retraction, electrocautery or inadvertent vagal compression by loops or clamps placed for vascular control. Necessary operative exposure frequently must extend close to the base of skull, and probably as a result, patients undergoing endarterectomy are at high risk for multiple cranial nerve deficits (Table 3.9). Various studies have reported injury of the hypoglossal, the glossopharyngeal, and the spinal accessory nerves, and Horner's syndrome, in addition to vagal nerve dysfunction. For similar reasons, a so-called "high vagal" injury, affecting the superior as well as the recurrent laryngeal nerve, probably occurs more often than in other surgeries in the neck. These factors, sometimes

Table 3.9. Vocal fold paralysis after carotid endarterectomy

Reference	Year	Number[a] of Cases	Vagal/recurrent (%)		Hypoglossal (%)	
			Temporary	Permanent	Temporary	Permanent
[118]	2004	1739	1.0		1.6	
[138]	2000	269	2.6		3.3	
[122]	1999	1415	2.5		3.7	
[121]	1999	76	4.0	4.0		
[108]	1999	200	4.0		5.5	
[148]	1997	183	7.7		4.4	
[119]	1997	50	6.0	2.0		
[123]	1995	656	1.2	0.2	10.7	0.2
[137]	1991	336	6.0		4.8	
[147]	1990	411	7.1	2.7		
[107]	1988	52	5.8		13.5	
[167]	1987	129	4.9		2.3	
[154]	1985	192	1.0		2.6	
[140]	1984	158	5.1		8.2	
[120]	1983	43	25		5	
[27][b]	1981	40	27	5.0	20	2.5
[128]	1980	240	5.8		5.4	

[a] Reported as number of operations/nerves at risk
[b] Initial evaluation at postoperative day 2

combined with additional deficits following stroke, another known complication, place the patient undergoing carotid endarterectomy at unusual risk for aspiration.

Vocal fold paralysis follows 1.0–7.7% of carotid endarterectomies. Once again, as in the case of cervical spine surgery, prompt systematic evaluation of the larynx 2 days following surgery has revealed a much higher incidence (27%) than in other reports [27]. This declines over the following months to a figure consistent with those reported elsewhere. Most cranial nerve injuries following carotid endarterectomy resolve or compensate; which is not entirely certain from available material.

A special concern in carotid surgery has to do with the frequent need for contralateral surgery. Should the first side be paralyzed, injury of the opposite side may result in an airway emergency, completely unexpected if the initial injury is undiagnosed. It is prudent to evaluate the larynx between operations. If the vocal fold is paralyzed, experience indicates that a delay of a few months is likely to restore mobility, and contralateral surgery will be safer.

Vagal Nerve Stimulator

Implantation of a vagal nerve stimulator for control of seizure disorders requires the placement of a coil-like electrode around the main trunk of the vagus in the neck, so it should be no surprise that vocal fold dysfunction is not rare in this population. Both the exact incidence and prognosis of vocal fold paralysis following placement of the vagal nerve stimulator remains to be established, but the most commonly reported side effect is hoarseness, occurring in as many as 35% of patients [28]. Shaffer et al. [29] found that 2 of 10 patients recruited from among those who had undergone the procedure had immobile vocal folds, and 6 of 10 had electromyographic changes suggestive of denervation and/or recovery. In the experience of the author, 6 of 8 patients with vocal fold immobility following stimulator placement recovered spontaneously within 4 months of surgery. It is noteworthy that not all dysphonia in vagal nerve stimulator patients is related to surgical injury, as the electrical activity of the stimulator itself causes vocal fold hypomobility and/or involuntary adduction during stimulation [29, 30]. As of this writing, the vagal nerve stimulator is undergoing federal review for treatment of drug-resistant depression. If approved, it could become a more significant source of vocal fold paralysis.

Other Neck Procedures

The recurrent nerve may be injured during cricopharyngeal myotomy near the cricothyroid joint as it enters the larynx. Newer endoscopic approaches to Zenker's diverticulum were initially thought to obviate this potential complication entirely, but this has not proved to be the case [31].

Surgery in the Chest

Lung Surgery

Vocal fold paralyses may follow left-sided pneumonectomy or lobectomy because of trauma to the nerve during perihilar dissection. The incidence of this complication varies from 6.7 to 31% in reported series [32, 33]. In many patients, the nerve must be intentionally sacrificed because of oncologic concerns. Glottic insufficiency adds to the compromised pulmonary function of these patients and creates a significant increase in postoperative morbidity. For this reason, some authors have recommended immediate medialization, under the same anesthetic, in patients in whom the injury is recognized intraoperatively [34, 35].

Mediastinal Procedures

Vocal fold paralysis occurs following instrumentation of the mediastinum in about 1% of cases [36–38].

Cardiac and Great Vessel Surgery

The incidence of vocal fold paralysis is 0.7–1.9% [39] during coronary artery bypass and valve repair or replacement. In addition to the possibility of direct injury during manipulations of the aortic stem, and traction injuries transmitted to the recurrent nerve via the great vessels, many of these appear to be related to ice slushing for cardiac protection. Abandonment of pericardial ice slushing reduced the incidence of vocal fold paralysis from 1.6 to 0.4% at one hospital [40]. Dimarakis and Protopapas [39] have also proposed that harvesting of the proximal internal mammary artery may place the recurrent nerve at risk, but as the vast majority of affected vocal folds are left-sided, trauma from other mediastinal manipulation cannot be excluded.

The left recurrent nerve may be injured in up to a third of patients undergoing repair of thoracic aortic aneurysm, with a low recovery rate compared with vocal fold paralysis following other surgeries [41, 42]. The incidence of left vocal fold paralysis in children undergoing ligation of a patent ductus arteriosus has been reported to be between 4.2 and 8.8% [43].

Esophageal Surgery

Esophagectomy is associated with a relatively high rate (15–45%) of vocal fold paralysis, of which an unusually high proportion (10–27%) is bilateral, a fact readily explained by anatomy [44–47]. Some of these cases may be present preoperatively as a result of the primary tumor, but this number has not been defined. As in lung surgery, a paralyzed vocal fold adds significantly to the normal post-operative morbidity of these patients, both in the short term and later, because it increases the severity of the dysphagia normally expected after esophagectomy [46].

Surgery at the Skull Base

As in carotid surgery, multiple cranial nerve deficits are not rare following skull base surgery and add to the challenges of rehabilitation, particularly in the elderly [48]. Netterville et al. reported vocal fold paralysis in all 40 of their cases of vagal paraganglioma, even with preservation of the vagus [49]. Jackson reported that 25% of paraganglioma patients developed vocal fold paralysis after surgery, in addition to the 30% who presented with the deficit [50]. As in thoracic surgery, early medialization has been advocated, but aspiration remains a problem in a significant number of patients [51].

Other Procedures and Interventions

Endotracheal Intubation

Vocal fold paralysis occasionally follows surgery that does not place the nerve at risk. Such cases have been occasionally attributed to cricoarytenoid dislocation, but damage to this well-supported joint has been shown by anatomical study to be extremely unlikely [52, 53], especially when no note was made of difficulty at intubation. Careful dissection has shown that the anterior branch of the recurrent laryngeal nerve is subject to compression between a "high-riding" endotracheal tube cuff and the thyroid cartilage, particularly if the cuff is overinflated [54, 55]. Brief reflection on the number of intubations in comparison with the frequency of this cause of paralysis suggests that it is an extremely rare occurrence. No study has been made of its natural history, but as a neurapraxic injury, spontaneous resolution is probably the rule. As noted previously, it is entirely possible that many short-lived paralyses go undiagnosed, attributed to routine voice change following intubation.

Venous Access and Other Instrumentation

Individual cases of vocal fold paralysis have been reported to result from central venous catheterization via the internal jugular or the subclavian vein [56, 57]. Such injuries of the recurrent nerve sometimes originate outside the medical setting among intravenous drug users [58, 59]. Vocal fold paralysis, distinct from cricoarytenoid dislocation, has been reported following nasogastric tube insertion [60, 61] and placement of an esophageal stethoscope [62]. It is attributed in these cases to local pressure palsies and local infection related to mucosal erosions.

Radiation

Radiation causes fibrosis in and around the nerve which may interfere with blood supply, compress the nerve, or otherwise compromise axonal flow. Cases of vocal fold paralysis have been documented following radiation treatment of nasopharyngeal carcinoma (along with other cranial neuropathies) [63–65] and mediastinal irradiation for the treatment of mediastinal tumors or breast cancer [66, 67]. Vocal fold paralysis has also been related to radioactive iodine treatment of thyroid malignancy [68–70]. A unique feature of vocal fold paralysis in this scenario is its latency: it may occur from 12 months to 34 years following radiation.

Drugs and Other Toxicities

Neurotoxic antimetabolites may cause peripheral neuropathy affecting the vocal folds. Vinca alkaloids (vincristine/vinblastine) and cisplatin are known to cause vocal fold paralysis, which is generally believed to be dose dependent and reversible upon withdrawal of the drug [71–75]. In the majority of such cases, the vocal fold paralysis is not isolated, and other neuropathies, including autonomic and sensory deficits, help signal systemic toxicity.

Organophosphates found in chemical warfare agents and commercially available pesticides inhibit acetylcholinesterase, causing massive parasympathetic discharge and muscle weakness in acute toxicity. Low or intermediate dose exposure may produce a more subtle muscle weakness and bilateral vocal fold paralysis which contributes to the distress caused by dysfunction of the muscles of respiration [76, 77, 131]. Like other chemical toxicities, this tends to be reversible, although intubation is occasionally necessary to secure the airway.

Medical Disease

Malignancy

Traumatic causes of vocal fold paralysis are generally apparent from the history and require little or no further diagnostic evaluation. Of the remainder of cases, 29–50% are caused by malignancy. Because of the obvious change in voice, vocal fold paralysis is often the presenting symptom for occult cancer. In modern series, mediastinal metastases from primary pulmonary tumors account for the large majority of such cases. Esophageal cancer is a less important cause. Older series featured a relatively large number of advanced thyroid carcinomas, and this has diminished markedly with the development of techniques for early diagnosis and safe surgical intervention. A small number of cases continue to be caused by lymphoma and unusual neoplasms, some of which affect the recurrent nerve or the vagus in the neck. Diagnostic imaging of patients with vocal fold paralysis is not complete without imaging of the base of skull through the level of the mediastinum and aortic arch.

Vocal fold paralysis due to malignancy has a very poor prognosis. Moreover, surgical management of the disease, when possible, usually requires nerve sacrifice. Under such circumstances, delay in the treatment of vocal fold paralysis is a disservice to the patient. Early restoration of adequate voice and swallowing in this context is an important quality-of-life issue, and usually does not interfere with oncologic treatment. The presence of foreign bodies, such as medialization implants in a radiated field or an area planned to be radiated, is potentially hazardous the heightened potential for extrusion, usually into the airway, has been noted [78].

Nonmalignant Disease

The recurrent nerve may be affected by mediastinal lymphadenopathy from nonmalignant disease, usually granulomatous processes such as tuberculosis and sarcoidosis. Effective treatment sometimes results in recovery [79, 80]. Dilatation of the aorta and the right subclavian artery can result in a stretch injury of either recurrent nerve [81, 82], and vocal fold paralysis may even evolve acutely during aortic dissection [83, 84]. Both tuberculosis and aortic aneurysm have been important and well-recognized sources of vocal fold paralysis in the past, but are now rare, their incidence decreased by advances in medicine and surgery. Other sources of nerve compression include benign thyroid disease in the neck, as noted above. Vocal fold paralysis has been documented in cases of pleural disease such as silicosis [85].

Stroke

Vocal fold paralysis may appear in the wake of a stroke, almost always in conjunction with other deficits [86]. Lateral medullary infarct (Wallenberg syndrome) is a well-known complex of neural injury featuring vocal fold paralysis, dysphagia, vertigo, ataxia, Horner's syndrome, and hemifacial sensory deficit and/or pain. The vocal fold paralysis may improve over weeks to months, although measures may need to be taken in the short term to prevent aspiration.

Other Neurologic Disease

The vocal fold paralysis in Arnold-Chiari malformation, resulting from vagal nerve root traction, is well known among otolaryngologists, and important to recognize promptly because it is reversible with timely hindbrain decompression. Even in patients without Arnold-Chiari malformation, vocal fold paralysis may present as a sign of ventriculoperitoneal shunt failure, along with ataxia and incontinence. Charcot-Marie-Tooth disease and its variants are a heterogeneous group of hereditary motor and sensory neuropathies. Laryngeal nerve involvement may be more widespread among the subtypes of the disease that have been previously suspected [87]. When present, neural compromise of the vocal fold appears to evolve slowly but relentlessly, and may demonstrate considerable asymmetry. Because of the gradual progression, patients generally compensate well until the paralysis is very dense. Vocal fold paralysis may evolve as a complex of bulbar deficits resulting in dysphagia, dysphonia, and dysarthria in post-polio syndrome, a degenerative neurologic condition seen many decades after the acute disease [88, 89].

Idiopathic Vocal Fold Paralysis

Vocal fold paralysis of unclear cause has been the subject of speculation and debate for a century and a half. The relationship between vocal fold paralysis and infectious disease became apparent to physicians early, and most explanations centered around mechanisms of nerve injury by infectious agents. Allowing for the discovery of viral pathogens, speculation continues to run in a similar channel today. Based on serologies, cases have been attributed to Lyme borreliosis [90], herpes zoster [91–94], herpes simplex [95, 96], Epstein-Barr virus [97], West Nile Virus [142], and cytomegalovirus in the immunocompromised patient [98]. Moreover, several authors have documented a transient increase in the number of cases of idiopathic vocal fold paralysis in the wake of the Hong Kong flu in the winter of 1969–1970 both in Europe [99–101] and Japan [102]. Even though a causal relationship remains to be established, these clinical relationships are convincing, but they still do not explain the majority of cases of idiopathic vocal fold paralysis in which serologies are normal and there is no antecedent history of viral disease.

With respect to recovery, most series suggest that 20–40% of patients with idiopathic vocal fold paralysis recover full mobility (Table 3.10), and an additional percentage regain acceptable voice. Occasionally, both figures are much higher [103–105]. No features of these latter reports suggest an explanation for the discrepancy. The delay in diagnosis, typically 4 weeks or more, probably dooms anti-inflammatory treatment, as used for Bell's palsy or sudden sensorineural hearing loss, to ineffectiveness.

Recovery generally takes place between 1 and 9 months after onset, with rare cases returning after 1 year. Postma and Shockley have pointed out even more short-lived paralyses, and it is likely that some cases resolve before the patient seeks medical attention [106].

Conclusion

The anatomical course of the recurrent laryngeal nerve determines the potential causes of

Table 3.10. Idiopathic vocal fold paralysis

Reference	Year	Number of Cases	Recovery of motion (%)	Recovery of voice without motion (%)
[3]	2003	40	35	
[2]	2002	9	44	
[161]	2001	50	14	72
[104]	1999	36	75	14
[6]	1998	50	24	
[145]	1998	16	19	6
[156]	1997	67	39	15
[158]	1989	28	22	25
[99][a]	1973	16	31	
[113]	1972	21	48	
[105]	1959	29	83	
[163]	1941	8	25	

[a] Combined unilateral and bilateral cases

vocal fold paralysis, which varies considerably from series to series based on local variations in disease frequency and particulars of practice. Disparate classification schemes and outcome standards make comparison among reports challenging. Nevertheless, broad conclusions are possible: vocal fold paralysis is a peripheral neuropathy which affects men more than women, and affects the left side more often than the right. The laryngeal nerves are vulnerable in a number of neck and chest procedures, as well as disease processes affecting those parts of the body. Each clinical scenario has its unique potential for morbidity, based on associated cranial nerve deficits and underlying medical conditions, and for recovery, based on the mechanism and severity of the initial injury. Despite a century and a half of clinical experience, significant questions remain about the pathophysiology underlying idiopathic paralysis and recovery rates.

References

1. Stewart JD (2000) Focal peripheral neuropathies, 3rd edn. Lippincott, Williams and Wilkins, Philadelphia
2. Loughran S, Alves C, MacGregor FB (2002) Current aetiology of unilateral vocal fold paralysis in a teching hospital in the West of Scotland. J Laryngol Otol 116:907–910
3. Laccourreye O, Papon JF, Kania R, Ménard M, Brasnu D, Hans S (2003) Paralysies laryngeés unilatérales: Données épidemiologiques et évolution thérapeutique. Presse Med 32:781–786
4. Titche LL (1976) Causes of recurrent laryngeal nerve paralysis. Arch Otolaryngol 102:259–261
5. Work WP (1941) Paralysis and paresis of the vocal cords: a statistical review. Arch Otolaryngol 34:267–280
6. Benninger MS, Gillen JB, Altman JS (1998) Changing etiology of vocal fold immobility. Laryngoscope 108:1346–1350
7. Delevan DB (1908) The etiology of paralysis of the recurrent laryngeal nerves of peripheral origin. Ann Otol Rhinol Laryngol 17:631–644
8. Casselberry WE (1908) Recurrent and abductor paralysis of the larynx: diagnosis and treatment. Ann Otol Rhinol Laryngol 17:607–630

9. Dralle H, Sekulla C, Haerting J, Timmermann W, Neumann HJ, Kruse E, Grond S, Muhlig HP, Richter C, Voss J, Thomusch O, Lippert H, Gastinger I, Brauckhoff M, Gimm O (2004) Risk factors of paralysis and functional outcome after recurrent laryngeal nerve monitoring in thyroid surgery. Surgery 136:1310–1322
10. Chiang FY, Wang LF, Huang YF, Lee KW, Kuo WR (2005) Recurrent laryngeal nerve palsy after thyroidectomy with routine identification of the recurrent laryngeal nerve. Surgery 137:342–347
11. Testini M, Nacchiero M, Portincasa P, Miniello S, Piccinni G, Venere B di, Campanile L, Lissidini G, Bonomo GM (2004) Risk factors of morbidity in thyroid surgery: analysis of the last 5 years of experience in a general surgery unit. Int Surg 89:125–130
12. Zambudio AR, Rodriguez J, Riquelme J, Soria T, Canteras M, Parrilla P (2004) Prospective study of postoperative complications after total thyroidectomy for multinodular goiters by surgeons with experience in endocrine surgery. Ann Surg 240:18–25
13. Sturniolo G, D'Alia C, Tonante A, Gagliano E, Taranto F, Lo Schiavo MG (1999) The recurrent laryngeal nerve related to thyroid surgery. Am J Surg 177:485–488
14. Thomusch O, Machens A, Sekulla C, Ukkat J, Lippert H, Gastinger I, Dralle H (2000) Multivariate analysis of risk factors for postoperative complications in benign goiter surgery: prospective multicenter study in Germany. World J Surg 24:1335–1341
15. Tartaglia F, Sgueglia M, Muhaya A, Cresti R, Mulas MM, Turriziani V, Campana FP (2003) Complications in total thyroidectomy: our experience and a number of considerations. Chir Ital 55:499–510
16. Robertson ML, Steward DL, Gluckman JL, Welge J (2004) Continuous laryngeal nerve integrity monitoring during thyroidectomy: Does it reduce risk of injury? Otolaryngol Head Neck Surg 131:596–600
17. Beldi G, Kinsbergen T, Schlumpf R (2004) Evaluation of intraoperative recurrent nerve monitoring in thyroid surgery. World J Surg 28:589–591
18. Hermann M, Hellebart C, Freissmuth M (2004) Neuromonitoring in thyroid surgery: prospective evaluation of intraoperative electrophysiological responses for the prediction of recurrent laryngeal nerve injury. Ann Surg 240:9–17
19. Rowe-Jones JM, Rosswick RP, Leighton SE (1993) Benign thyroid disease and vocal cord palsy. Ann R Coll Surg 75:241–244
20. McCall AR, Ott R, Jarosz H, Lawrence AM, Paloyan E (1987) Improvement of vocal cord paresis after thyroidectomy. Am Surg 53:377–379
21. Chan WF, Lo CY, Lam KY, Wan KY (2004) Recurrent laryngeal nerve palsy in well-differentiated thyroid carcinoma: clinicopathologic features and outcome study. World J Surg 28:1093–1098
22. Ebraheim NA, Lu J, Skie M, Heck BE, Yeasting RA (1997) Vulnerability of the recurrent laryngeal nerve in the anterior approach to the lower cervical spine. Spine 22:2664–2667
23. Weisberg NK, Spengler DM, Netterville JL (1997) Stretch-induced nerve injury as a cause of paralysis secondary to the anterior cervical approach. Otolaryngol Head Neck Surg 116:317–326
24. Netterville JL, Koriwchak MJ, Winkle M, Courey MS, Ossoff RH (1996) Vocal fold paralysis following the anterior approach to the cervical spine. Ann Otol Rhinol Laryngol 105:85–91
25. Apfelbaum RI, Kriskovich MD, Haller JR (2000) On the incidence, cause, and prevention of recurrent laryngeal nerve palsies during anterior cervical spine surgery. Spine 15:2906–2012
26. Jung A, Schramm J, Lehnerdt K, Herberhold C (2005) Recurrent laryngeal nerve palsy during anterior cervical spine surgery: a prospective study. J Neurosurg Spine 2:123–127
27. Liapis CD, Satiani B, Florance CL, Evans WE (1981) Motor speech malfunction following carotid endarterectomy. Surgery 89:56–59
28. Ramsay RE, Uthman BM, Augustinsson LE, Upton AR, Naritoku D, Willis J, Treig T, Barolat G, Wernicke JF (1994) Vagus nerve stimulation for treatment of partial seizures, vol 2. Safety, side effects, and tolerability. First International Vagus Nerve Stimulation Study Group. Epilepsia 35:627–636
29. Shaffer MJ, Jackson CE, Szabo CA, Simpson CB (2005) Vagal nerve stimulation: clinical and electrophysiological effects on vocal fold function. Ann Otol Rhinol Laryngol 114:7–14
30. Zalvan C, Sulica L, Wolf S, Cohen J, Gonzalez-Yanes O, Blitzer A (2003) Laryngopharyngeal dysfunction from the implant vagal nerve stimulator. Laryngoscope 113:221–225
31. Chang CY, Payyapilli RJ, Scher RL (2003) Endoscopic staple diverticulostomy for Zenker's diverticulum: review of the literature and experience in 159 consecutive cases. Laryngoscope 113:957–965
32. Sugarbaker DJ, Jaklitsch MT, Bueno R, Richards W, Lukanich J, Mentzer SJ, Colson Y, Linden P, Chang M, Capalbo L, Oldread E, Neragi-Miandoab S, Swanson SJ, Zellos LS (2004) Prevention, early detection, and management of complications after 328 consecutive extrapleural pneumonectomies. J Thorac Cardiovasc Surg 128:138–146
33. Filaire M, Mom T, Laurent S, Harouna Y, Naamee A, Vallet L, Normand B, Escande G (2001) Vocal cord dysfunction after left lung resection for cancer. Eur J Cardiothorac Surg 20:705–711

34. Mom T, Filaire M, Advenier D, Guichard C, Naamee A, Escande G, Llompart X, Vallet L, Gabrillargues J, Courtalhiac C, Claise B, Gilain L (2001) Concomitant type I thyroplasty and thoracic operations for lung cancer: preventing respiratory complications associated with vagus or recurrent laryngeal nerve injury. J Thorac Cardiovasc Surg 121:642–648
35. Bhattacharyya N, Batirel H, Swanson SJ (2003) Improved outcomes with early vocal fold medialization for vocal fold paralysis after thoracic surgery. Auris Nasus Larynx 30:71–75
36. Puhakka HJ (1989) Complications of mediastinoscopy. J Laryngol Otol 103:312–315
37. Martin de Nicolas Serrahima JL, Garcia Barajas S, Marron Fernandez C, Diaz-Hellin Gude V, Larru Cabrero E, Oteo Lozano M, Perez Anton JA, Toledo Gonzalez J (1999) Technical complications in the surgical inspection of the mediastinum in the staging of cancer of the lung. Arch Bronchoneumol 35:390–394
38. Stenborg R (1973) Casas of recurrent nerve paralysis in Gothenburg from 1968 to 1971. Acta Otolaryngol 75:364–365
39. Dimarakis I, Protopapas AD (2004) Vocal cord palsy as a complication of adult cardiac surgery: surgical correlations and analysis. Eur J Cardiothoracic Surg 26:773–775
40. Ishimoto S, Kondo K, Ito K, Oshima K (2003) Hoarseness after cardiac surgery: possible contribution of low temperature to the recurrent nerve paralysis. Laryngoscope 113:1088–1089
41. Ishimoto S, Ito K, Toyama M, Kawase I, Kondo K, Oshima K, Niimi S (2002) Vocal cord paralysis after surgery for thoracic aortic aneurysm. Chest 121:1911–1915
42. Teixedo MT, Leonetti JP (1990) Recurrent laryngeal nerve paralysis associated with thoracic aortic aneurysm. Otolaryngol Head Neck Surg 102:140–144
43. Zbar RI, Chen AH, Berendt DM, Bell EF, Smith RJ (1996) Incidence of vocal fold paralysis in infants undergoing ligation of patent ductus arteriosus. Ann Thoracic Surg 61:814–816
44. Nishimaki T, Suzuki T, Kanda T, Obinata I, Komukai S, Hatakeyama K (1999) Extended radical esophagectomy for superficially invasive carcinoma of the esophagus. Surgery 125:142–147
45. Gockel I, Kneist W, Keilmann A, Junginger T (2005) Recurrent laryngeal nerve paralysis (RLNP) following esophagectomy for carcinoma. Eur J Surg Oncol 31:277–281
46. Baba M, Natsugoe S, Shimada M, Nakano S, Noguchi Y, Kawachi K, Kusano C, Aikou T (1999) Does hoarseness of voice from recurrent nerve paralysis after esophagectomy for carcinoma influence patient quality of life? J Am Coll Surg 188:231–236
47. Hulscher JB, van Sandick JW, Devriese PP, van Lanschot JJ, Obertop H (1999) Vocal cord paralysis after subtotal oesophagectomy. Br J Surg 86:1583–1587
48. Netterville JL, Civantos FJ (1993) Rehabiliation of cranial nerve deficits after neurotologic skull base surgery. Laryngoscope 113 (Suppl 60):45–54
49. Netterville JL, Jackson CG, Miller FR, Wanamaker JR, Glasscock ME (1998) Vagal paraganglioma: a review of 46 patients treated during a 20-year period. Arch Otolaryngol Head Neck Surg 124:1133–1140
50. Jackson CG (2001) Glomus tympanicum and glomus jugulare tumors. Otolaryngol Clin N Am 34:941–970
51. Bielamowicz S, Gupta A, Sekhar LN (2000) Early arytenoid adduction for vagal paralysis after skull base surgery. Laryngoscope 110:346–351
52. Paulsen FP, Rudert HH, Tillman BN (1999) New insights into the pathomechanism of postintubation arytenoid subluxation. Anesthesiology 91:659–666
53. Paulsen FP, Jungman K, Tillmann BN (2000) The cricoarytenoid joint capsule and its relevance to endotyracheal intubation. Anesth Analg 90:180–185
54. Cavo JW (1985) True vocal cord paralysis following intubation. Laryngoscope 95:1352–1359
55. Brandwein M, Abramson AL, Shikowitz MJ (1986) Bilateral vocal cord paralysis following intubation. Arch Otolaryngol Head Neck Surg 112:877–882
56. Salman M, Potter M, Ethel M, Myint F (2004) Recurrent laryngeal nerve injury: a complication of central venous catheterization – a case report. Angiology 55:345–346
57. Martin-Hirsch DP, Newbegin CJ (1995) Right vocal fold paralysis as a result of central venous catheterization. J Laryngol Otol 109:1107–1108
58. Hillstrom RP, Cohn AM, McCarroll KA (1990) Vocal cord paralysis resulting from neck injections in the intravenous drug use population. Laryngoscope 100:503–506
59. Raz S, Ramanathan V (1984) Injection injuries of the recurrent laryngeal nerve. Laryngoscope 94:197–200
60. Sofferman RA, Haisch CE, Kirchner JA, Hardin NJ (1990) The nasogastric tube syndrome. Laryngoscope 100:962–968
61. Ibuki T, Ando N, Tanaka Y (1994) Vocal cord paralysis associated with difficult gastric tube insertion. Can J Anaesth 41:431–434
62. Friedman M, Toriumi DM (1989) Esophageal stethoscope. Another possible cause of vocal cord paralysis. Arch Otolaryngol Head Neck Surg 115:95–98
63. Chaudhry MR, Akhtar S (1995) Bilateral vocal cord paralysis following radiation therapy for na-

sopharyngeal carcinoma. ORL J Otorhinolaryngol Relat Spec 57:48–49
64. Takimoto T, Saito Y, Suzuki M, Nishimura T (1991) Radiation-induced cranial nerve palsy: hypoglossal and vocal cord palsies. J Laryngol Otol 105:44–45
65. Lin YS, Jen YM, Lin JC (2002) Radiation-related cranial nerve palsy in patients with nasopharyngeal carcinoma. Cancer 95:404–409
66. Johansson S, Svensson H, Denekamp J (2000) Timescale of evolution of late radiation injury after postoperative radiotherapy of breast cancer patients. Int J Radiat Oncol Biol Phys 48:745–750
67. Johansson S, Lofroth DO, Denekamp J (2001) Left sided vocal cord paralysis: a newly recognized late complication of mediastinal irradiation. Radiother Oncol 58:287–294
68. Craswell PW (1978) Vocal cord paresis following radioactive iodine therapy. J Nucl Med 19:975–976
69. Snyder S (1978) Vocal cord paralysis after radioiodine therapy. J Nucl Med 19:975–976
70. Robson AM (1981) Vocal cord paralysis after treatment of thyrotoxicosis with radioiodine. Br J Radiol 54:632
71. Anghelescu DL, De Armendi AJ, Thompson JW, Sillos EM, Pui CH, Sandlund JT (2002) Vincristine-induced vocal cord paralysis in an infant. Paediatr Anaesth 12:168–170
72. Taha H, Irfan S, Krishnamurthy M (1999) Cisplatin induced reversible bilateral vocal cord paralysis: an undescribed complication of cisplatin. Head Neck 21:78–79
73. Ryan SP, DelPrete SA, Weinstein PW, Erichson RB, Bar MH, Lo KM, Cohen NS, Tepler I (1999) Low-dose vincristine-associated bilateral vocal cord paralysis. Conn Med 63:583–584
74. Burns BV, Shotton JC (1998) Vocal fold palsy following vinca alkaloid treatment. J Laryngol Otol 112:485–487
75. Delaney P (1982) Vincristine-induced laryngeal nerve paralysis. Neurology 32:1285–1288
76. da Silva HJ, Sanmuganathan PS, Senanayake N (1994) Isolated bilateral recurrent laryngeal nerve paralysis: a delayed complication of organophosphorus poisoning. Hum Exp Toxicol 13:171–173
77. Thompson JW, Stocks RM (1997) Brief bilateral vocal cord paralysis after insecticide poisoning. A new variant of toxicity syndrome. Arch Otolaryngol Head Neck Surg 123:93–96
78. Netterville JL, Stone RE, Luken ES, Civantos FJ, Ossoff RH (1993) Silastic medialization and arytenoid adduction: the Vanderbilt experience. A review of 116 phonosurgical procedures. Ann Otol Rhinol Laryngol 102:413–424
79. Meral M, Akgun M, Kaynar H, Mirici A, Gorguner M, Saglam L, Erdogan F (2004) Mediastinal lymphadenopathy due to mycobacterial infection. Jpn J Infect Dis 57:124–126
80. Rafay MA (2000) Tuberculous lymphadenopathy of superior mediastinum causing vocal cord paralysis. Ann Thorac Surg 70:2142–2143
81. Ishii H, Muto J, Kamei T, Harada O, Yasuoka Y (1971) Inflammatory paralysis of the larynx. Jpn J Otol Tokyo 74:1562–1571
82. Thirlwall AS (1997) Ortner's syndrome: a centenary review of unilateral recurrent laryngeal nerve palsy secondary to cardiothoracic disease. J Laryngol Otol 111:869–871
83. Charbel S, Sargi Z, Rassi B (2004) Cardiovocal syndrome: a rare case of painless aortic dissection presenting as isolated dysphonia. Otolaryngol Head Neck Surg 131:332–333
84. Woodson GE, Kendrick B (1989) Laryngeal paralysis as the presenting sign of aortic trauma. Arch Otolaryngol Head Neck Surg 115:1100–1102
85. Lardinois D, Gugger M, Balmer MC, Ris HB (1999) Left recurrent laryngeal nerve palsy associated with silicosis. Eur Respir J 14:720–722
86. Venketasubramanian N, Seshadri R, Chee N (1999) Vocal cord paresis in acute ischemic stroke. Cerebrovasc Dis 9:157–162
87. Sulica L, Blitzer A, Lovelace RE, Kaufmann P. Vocal fold paresis of Charcot-Marie-Tooth disease. Ann Otol Rhinol Laryngol. 2001 Nov;110(11):1072–6
88. Driscoll BP, Gracco C, Coelho C, Goldstein J, Oshima K, Tierney E, Sasaki CT (1995) Laryngeal function in postpolio patients. Laryngoscope 105:35–41
89. Cannon S, Ritter FN (1987) Vocal cord paralysis in postpoliomyelitis syndrome. Laryngoscope 97:981–983
90. Schroeter V, Belz GG, Blenk H (1988) Paralysis of recurrent laryngeal nerve in Lyme disease. Lancet 2:1245
91. Wu CL, Linne OC, Chiang CW (2004) Herpes zoster laryngis with prelaryngeal skin erythema. Ann Otol Rhinol Laryngol 113:113–114
92. Nishizaki K, Onoda K, Akagi H, Yuen K, Ogawa T, Masuda Y (1997) Laryngeal zoster with unilateral laryngeal paralysis. ORL J Otorhinolaryngol Relat Spec 59:235–237
93. Randel RC, Kearns DB, Nespeca MP, Scher CA, Sawyer MH (1996) Vocal cord paralysis as a presentation of intrauterine infection with Varicella zoster virus. Pediatrics 97:127–128
94. Rothschild MA, Drake W III, Scherl M (1994) Cephalic zoster with laryngeal paralysis. Ear Nose Throat J 73:850–852
95. Bachor E, Bonkowsky V, Hacki T (1996) Herpes simplex virus type I reactivation as a cause of a unilateral temporary paralysis of the vagus nerve. Eur Arch Otorhinolaryngol 253:297–300

96. Pou A, Carrau RL (1995) Bilateral abductor vocal cord paralysis in association with herpes simplex infection: a case report. Am J Otolaryngol 16:216–219
97. Parano E, Pavone L, Musumeci S, Giambusso F, Trifiletti RR (1996) Acute palsy of the recurrent laryngeal nerve complicating Epstein-Barr virus infection. Neuropediatrics 27:164–166
98. Small PM, McPhaul LW, Sooy CD, Wofsy CB, Jacobson MA (1989) Cytomegalovirus infection of the laryngeal nerve presenting as hoarseness in patients with acquired immunodeficiency syndrome. Am J Med 86:108–110
99. Fex S, Elmqvist D (1973) Endemic recurrent laryngeal nerve paresis. Acta Otolaryngol 75:368–369
100. Hefter E, Bildstein P (1970) Endemieartiges Auftreten von Rekurrensparesen im Winter 1969/70. Z Laryngol Rhinol Otol 49:787
101. Wirth G, Leypoldt R (1970) Gehäuftes Auftreten von Stimmbandlähmung während der Grippeepidemie im Winter 1969/70. Z Laryngol Rhinol Otol 49:777
102. Ishii K, Adachi H, Tsubaki K, Ohta Y, Yamamoto M, Ino T (2004) Evaluation of recurrent nerve paralysis due to thoracic aortic aneurysm and aneurysm repair. Laryngoscope 114:2176–2181
103. León X, Venegas MP, Orús C, Quer M, Maranillo E, Sañudo JR (2001) Inmovilidad glótica: Estudio retrospectivo de 229 casos. Acta Otorrinolaringol Esp 52:486–492
104. Havas T, Lowinger D, Priestly J (1999) Unilateral vocal fold paralysis: causes, options and outcomes. Aust N Z J Surg 69:509–513
105. Williams RG (1959) Idiopathic recurrent laryngeal nerve paralysis. J Laryngol Otol 73:161–166
106. Postma GN, Shockley WW (1998) Transient vocal fold immobility. Ann Otol Rhinol Laryngol 107:236–240
107. Aldoori MI, Baird RN (1988) Local neurological complication during carotid endarterectomy. J Cardiovasc Surg (Torino) 29(4):432–436
108. Ballotta E, Da Giau G, Renon L, Narne S, Saladini M, Abbruzzese E, Meneghetti G (1999) Cranial and cervical nerve injuries after carotid endarterectomy: a prospective study. Surgery 125:85–91
109. Benninger MS, Crumley RL, Ford CN et al. (1994) Evaluation and treatment of the unilateral paralyzed vocal fold. Otolaryngol Head Neck Surg 111:497–508
110. Bergamaschi R, Becouarn G, Ronceray J, Arnaud JP (1998) Morbidity of thyroid surgery. Am J Surg 176:71–75
111. Bertalanffy H, Eggert HR (1989) Complications of anterior cervical discectomy without fusion in 450 consecutive patients. Acta Neurochir (Wien) 99:41–50
112. Beutler WJ, Sweeney CA, Connolly PJ (2001) Recurrent laryngeal nerve injury with anterior cervical spine surgery risk with laterality of surgical approach. Spine 26:1337–1342
113. Blau JN, Kapadia R (1972) Idiopathic palsy of the recurrent laryngeal nerve: a transient cranial mononeuropathy. Br Med J 4:259–261
114. Bron LP, O'Brien CJ (2004) Total thyroidectomy for clinically benign disease of the thyroid gland. Br J Surg 91:569–574
115. Chow TL, Chu W, Lim BH, Kwok SP (2001) Outcomes and complications of thyroid surgery: retrospective study. Hong Kong Med J 7:261–265
116. Clerf LH (1953) Unilateral vocal cord paralysis. J Am Med Assoc 151:900–903
117. Cunning DS (1955) Unilateral vocal cord paralysis. Ann Otol Rhinol Laryngol 64:487–494
118. Cunningham EJ, Bond R, Mayberg MR, Warlow CP, Rothwell PM (2004) Risk of persistent cranial nerve injury after carotid endarterectomy. J Neurosurg 101:445–448
119. Curran AJ, Smyth D, Sheehan SJ, Joyce W, Hayes DB, Walsh MA (1997) Recurrent laryngeal nerve dysfunction following carotid endarterectomy. J R Coll Surg Edinb 42:168–170
120. Dehn TC, Taylor GW (1983) Cranial and cervical nerve damage associated with carotid endarterectomy. Br J Surg 70:365–368
121. Espinoza FI, MacGregor FB, Doughty JC, Cooke LD (1999) Vocal fold paralysis following carotid endarterectomy. J Laryngol Otol 113:439–441
122. Ferguson GG, Eliasziw M, Barr HW, Clagett GP, Barnes RW, Wallace MC, Taylor DW, Haynes RB, Finan JW, Hachinski VC, Barnett HJ (1999) The North American Symptomatic Carotid Endarterectomy Trial: surgical results in 1415 patients. Stroke 30:1751–1758
123. Forssell C, Kitzing P, Bergqvist D (1995) Cranial nerve injuries after carotid artery surgery. A prospective study of 663 operations. Eur J Vasc Endovasc Surg 10:445–449
124. Friguglietti CU, Lin CS, Kulcsar MA (2003) Total thyroidectomy for benign thyroid disease. Laryngoscope 113:1820–1826
125. Goncalves Filho J, Kowalski LP (2005) Surgical complications after thyroid surgery performed in a cancer hospital. Otolaryngol Head Neck Surg 132:490–494
126. Hagan PJ (1963) Vocal cord paralysis. Ann Otol Rhinol Laryngol 72:206–222
127. Herranz-Gonzalez J, Gavilan J, Matinez-Vidal J, Gavilan C (1991) Complications following thyroid surgery. Arch Otolaryngol Head Neck Surg 117:516–518
128. Hertzer NR, Feldman BJ, Beven EG, Tucker HM (1980) A prospective study of the incidence of in-

128. jury to the cranial nerves during carotid endarterectomy. Surg Gynecol Obstet 151:781–784
129. Hughes CA, Troost S, Miller S, Troost T (2000) Unilatearl true vocal fold paralysis: cause of right-sided lesions. Otolaryngol Head Neck Surg 122:678–680
130. Ignjatovic M, Cuk V, Ozegovic A, Cerovic S, Kostic Z, Romic P (2003) Early complications in surgical treatment of thyroid diseases: analysis of 2100 patients. Acta Chir Iugosl 50:155–175
131. Indudharan R, Win MN, Noor AR (1998) Laryngeal paralysis in organophosphorous poisoning. J Laryngol Otol 112:81–82
132. Jatzko GR, Lisborg PH, Muller MG, Wette VM (1994) Recurrent nerve palsy after thyroid operations: principal nerve identification and a literature review. Surgery 115:139–144
133. Kasemsuwan L, Nubthuenetr S (1997) Recurrent laryngeal nerve paralysis: a complication of thyroidectomy. J Otolaryngol 26:365–367
134. Kearsley JH (1981) Vocal cord paralysis: an aetiologic review of 100 cases over 20 years. Aust N Z J Med 11:663–666
135. Kelchner LN, Stemple JC, Gerdeman B, LeBorgne W, Adam S (1999) Etiology, pathophysiology, treatment choices and voice results for unilateral adductor vocal fold paralysis: a 3-year retrospective. J Voice 13:592–601
136. Maisel RH, Ogura JH (1974) Evaluation and treatment of vocal cord paralysis. Laryngoscope 84:302–316
137. Maniglia AJ, Han DP (1991) Cranial nerve injuries following carotid endarterectomy: an analysis of 336 procedures. Head Neck 13:121–124
138. Maroulis J, Karkanevatos A, Papakostas K, Gilling-Smith GL, McCormick MS, Harris PL (2000) Cranial nerve dysfunction following carotid endarterectomy. Int Angiol 19:237–241
139. Martensson H, Terins J (1985) Recurrent laryngeal nerve palsy in thyroid gland surgery related to operations and nerves at risk. Arch Surg 120:475–477
140. Massey EW, Heyman A, Utley C, Haynes C, Fuchs J (1984) Cranial nerve paralysis following carotid endarterectomy. Stroke 15:157–159
141. Moulton-Barrett R, Crumley R, Jalilie S, Segina D, Allison G, Marshak D, Chan E (1997) Complications of thyroid surgery. Int Surg 82:63–66
142. Myssiorek D (2004) Recurrent laryngeal nerve paralysis: anatomy and etiology. Otolaryngol Clin N Am 37:25–44
143. New GB, Childrey JH (1932) Paralysis of the vocal cords: a study of two hundred and seventeen medical cases. Arch Otolaryngol 16:143–159
144. Parnell FW, Brandenburg JH (1970) Vocal cord paralysis: a review of 100 cases. Laryngoscope 80:1036–1045
145. Ramadan HH, Wax MK, Avery S (1998) Outcome and changing cause of unilateral vocal cord paralysis. Otolaryngol Head Neck Surg 118:199–202
146. Rosato L, Avenia N, Bernante P, Palma M de, Gulino G, Nasi PG, Pelizzo MR, Pezzullo L (2004) Complications of thyroid surgery: analysis of a multicentric study on 14,934 patients operated on in Italy over 5 years. World J Surg 28:271–276
147. Sannella NA, Tober RL, Cipro RP, Pedicino JF, Donovan E, Gabriel N (1990) Vocal cord paralysis following carotid endarterectomy: the paradox of return of function. Ann Vasc Surg 4:42–45
148. Schauber MD, Fontenelle LJ, Solomon JW, Hanson TL (1997) Cranial/cervical nerve dysfunction after carotid endarterectomy. J Vasc Surg 25:481–487
149. Shindo ML, Sinha UK, Rice DH (1995) Safety of thyroidectomy in residency: a review of 186 consecutive cases. Laryngoscope 105:1173–1175
150. Smith AB, Lambert VF, Wallace HL (1933) Paralysis of the recurrent laryngeal nerve: a survey of 235 cases. Edinburgh Med J 40:344–354
151. Srirompotong S, Sae-Seow P, Srirompotong S (2001) The cause and evaluation of unilateral vocal fold paralysis. J Med Assoc Thai 84:855–858
152. Suehs OW (1943) Paralysis of the larynx: a study of 270 cases. Texas State J Med 38:665–671
153. Terris DJ, Arnstein DP, Nguyen HH (1992) Contemporary evaluation of unilateral vocal cord paralysis. Otolaryngol Head Neck Surg 107:84–90
154. Theodotou B, Mahaley MS Jr (1985) Injury of the peripheral cranial nerves during carotid endarterectomy. Stroke 16:894–895
155. Tucker HM (1980) Vocal cord paralysis – 1979: etiology and management. Laryngoscope 585–590
156. Verhulst J, Lecoq M, Marraco M, Maurice C (1997) Paralysie recurrentielle idiopahtique: analyse retrospective de 67 cas. Rev Laryngol Otol Rhinol 118:263–265
157. Wagner HE, Seiler C (1994) Recurrent laryngeal nerve palsy after thyroid gland surgery. Br J Surg 81:226–228
158. Willatt DJ, Stell PM (1989) The prognosis and management of idiopathic vocal cord paralysis. Clin Otolaryngol 14:247–250
159. Woodson GE, Miller RH (1981) The timing of surgical intervention in vocal cord paralysis. Otolaryngol Head Neck Surg 89:264–267
160. Yamada M, Hirano M, Ohkubo H (1983) Recurrent laryngeal nerve paralysis. A 10-year review of 564 patients. Auris Nasus Larynx 10:S1–S15
161. León X, Venegas MP, Orús C, Quer M, Maranillo E, Sañudo JR (2001) Inmovilidad glótica: studio

retrospective de 229 casos. Acta Otorrinolarimgol Esp 52:486–492
162. Havas T, Lowinger D, Priestly J (1999) Unilateral vocal cord paralysis: causes, options and outcomes. Aust N Z J Surg 69:509–513
163. Work WP (1941) Paralysis and paresis of the vocal cords: a statistical review. Arch Otolaryngol 34:267–280
164. Parnell FW, Brandenburg JH (1970) Vocal cord paralysis: a review of 100 cases. Laryngoscope 80:1036–1045
165. Dener C (2002) Complication rates after operations for benign thyroid disease. Acta Otolaryngol. 122:679–683
166. Ley PB, Roberts JW, Symmonds RE Jr, Hendricks JC, Snyder SK, Frazee RC, Smith RW, McKenney JF, Brindley GV Jr (1993) Safety and efficacy of total thyroidectomy for differentiated thyroid carcinoma: a 20-year review. Am Surg 59:110–114
167. Knight FW, Yeager RM, Morris DM (1987) Cranial nerve injuries during carotid endarterectomy. Am J Surg 154:529–532

Chapter 4

Evaluation of Vocal Fold Paralysis

C. Blake Simpson, Esther J. Cheung

History

Vocal Quality and Swallowing

The evaluation of unilateral vocal fold paralysis (UVFP) involves a thorough history and physical exam. The symptoms of UVFP are well known to all otolaryngologists. These symptoms are related to glottic insufficiency resulting from some degree of lateral displacement of the paralyzed vocal fold. The primary symptom of UVFP is dysphonia, or hoarseness. This symptom is what typically leads the patient to seek medical care. The voice can vary from simple vocal fatigue in mild or well-compensated cases, to almost complete aphonia in severe cases. Much of the quality of the voice is determined by the muscular tone of the affected vocal fold and each patient's unique glottal compensatory strategy to phonate. An atrophic and poorly compensated vocal fold paralysis typically presents with a breathy, weak voice due to air escape. The voice may also have a "wet" or "gurgly" quality to it if secretions are retained in the pyriform sinus, as is typical in high vagal injuries. With time, most patients will eventually progress to a stronger voice using various compensatory strategies. In males particularly, supraglottic hyperfunction is common. These patients constrict the supraglottic tract either laterally, apposing the false folds, or in an anterior-posterior dimension, apposing the epiglottis to the arytenoids or the epiglottis to the contralateral false fold. This hyperfunctional muscular contraction leads to a characteristic rough, pitch-locked, low-frequency voice. This voice can sound quite similar to a patient with primary muscular tension dysphonia, and the diagnosis of vocal fold paralysis may not be suspected [1]. Unloading of the voice, as described later in this chapter, is used to help analyze these patients. In contrast, other patients, often females, may develop an unnaturally high-pitched voice that is breathy in quality. This has been referred to as a "paralytic falsetto," and is characterized by a mean increase in fundamental frequency of 85 Hz above "natural" pitch. This condition is thought to be caused by compensatory contraction of the ipsilateral cricothyroid (CT) muscle which remains innervated in isolated RLN paralysis [2]. Swallowing difficulties are often encountered, specifically aspiration of liquids, along with a weak and ineffective cough. Some dysphagia for solids may also be present, especially in brainstem or high vagal injuries, due to the concomitant denervation of the pharyngeal constrictors. Risk of aspiration is heightened in these instances as well, due to the loss of ipsilateral laryngeal sensation from SLN involvement.

Vocal Inventory

It is important to obtain an inventory of the patient's voice responsibilities, both work related and social. If patients are a vocal professionals, they rely on a serviceable voice for their livelihood. These patients should be questioned regarding their upcoming work schedule to help determine the urgency of early surgical intervention. Most professional voice users opt for temporizing vocal augmentation (collagen, Gelfoam, etc.) so that they can return to work as soon as possible.

Airway

A patient with UVFP may occasionally complain of being "short of breath"; however, careful history will show that the patient is not experiencing airway obstruction, as seen with bilateral vocal fold paralysis. These patients are actually reporting a breathlessness that occurs principally during conversation and is due to air leakage because of inefficient laryngeal closure. The same mechanism impairs the capacity to project the voice. Many patients increase respiratory effort and laryngeal muscle activity in an attempt to force glottal closure, raise subglottic pressure, and achieve a louder voice. These compensatory behaviors are mostly ineffective, leading to fatigue. In addition, exertional activity that requires lifting, pushing, and pulling may be difficult for patients with UVFP, because glottic closure is essential to an effective Valsalva mechanism.

Medical History: Establishing an Etiology

When UVFP is found on physical exam, it is imperative to take a complete history which considers all etiologic possibilities [3]. Specifically, one must inquire whether the patient's hoarseness followed a surgical procedure or trauma. Table 4.1 lists the cervical and thoracic surgeries that may lead to VFP and the proposed mechanism of injury. If the onset of hoarseness immediately follows any of these procedures, it is reasonable to assume an iatrogenic cause as the etiology. Endotracheal intubation has been implicated as a cause in VFP [4], but the mechanism is not well understood. Intubation trauma can also lead to CA joint effusion, and in rare cases, may cause CA joint subluxation/dislocation. Indications in the history which may suggest joint dislocation are: difficult and/or traumatic intubation and prolonged sore throat or odynophagia greater than 48 h after intubation [5]. External trauma can lead to vocal fold immobility, either by arytenoid dislocation or injury to the vagus.

A history of stroke should be solicited, as should concomitant neurologic signs, including weakness in the extremities, ataxia, dysarthria, velopharyngeal insufficiency (VPI), or dysphagia. A remote history of polio should raise the possibility of a post-polio syndrome, in which patients may develop laryngeal weakness and/or paresis 20–30 years after the onset of polio [6]. Exposure to any neurotoxic medications, such as vincristine, vinblastine, and occasionally cisplatin, should be noted [7]. Information about onset of hoarseness after an upper or lower respiratory tract infection may be elicited, and helps support a diagnosis of viral neuropathy in cases of "unexplained" VFP [8].

Table 4.1. Surgical/iatrogenic causes of vocal fold paralysis

Surgery/procedure	Mechanism of nerve injury/relevant anatomy
Anterior cervical fusion	Retraction; stretch injury of RLN (right more common) [20]
Esophagectomy	RLN injury in tracheoesophageal groove
Carotid endarterectomy	Vagal injury during dissection
Mediastinoscopy	RLN injury, usually left
Coronary artery bypass grafting	Retraction/direct injury to vagus/RLN during internal mammary artery harvest for grafting [21]
	Hypothermic nerve injury from ice cardioplegia [22]
Pulmonary resection	Usually left upper lobe/RLN injury
Endotracheal intubation	Possible pressure neuropraxia from compression of anterior rami of RLN due to a high-riding endotracheal cuff in the subglottis [23]

Physical Examination

General

Examination of the neck for adenopathy and thyroid masses should be performed. Vagal or recurrent nerve compression and infiltration by a neck or thyroid neoplasm can lead to VFP in advanced cases. Palatal movement when phonating /a/ should be noted. Palatal paralysis in combination with ipsilateral VFP may indicate a "high" vagal lesion. In the case of palatal paralysis, the palate retracts toward the uninvolved "good" side (e.g., in a left vagal paralysis, the palate retracts to the right). A complete cranial nerve exam should evaluate for other involved nerves, especially CN XI and XII, due to the close proximity these have to CN X at the skull base. Involvement of these adjacent cranial nerves warrants a thorough radiographic evaluation of the base of the skull.

Laryngeal

The appropriate evaluation for VFP starts with the recognition of unilateral vocal fold immobility on fiberoptic laryngoscopy. Indirect (mirror) laryngoscopy and rigid 70 or 90 degree laryngoscopy are helpful but do not replace fiberoptic laryngoscopy. Fiberoptic laryngoscopy is the only method to view vocal fold mobility in its natural state. Tongue protrusion, and the dynamic changes produced by grasping it with a gauze during indirect and rigid office laryngoscopy, changes the biomechanics of the larynx and may affect laryngeal exam findings, particularly with respect to glottic closure, which is a critical parameter in therapeutic decision-making. It is important to obtain an unencumbered, extended viewing period of the vocal folds during a variety of tasks. The best way to obtain this is fiberoptic laryngoscopy [9].

When evaluating for suspected UVF paralysis/paresis, a useful task is the "ee-sniff" maneuver, in which the patient alternates between phonating an "e" vowel and sniffing vigorously. This causes the vocal folds to alternately adduct and abduct maximally and is an excellent way to judge the degree of paresis/paralysis [9]. Any abduction of the affected vocal fold indicates incomplete paralysis (paresis), which generally has a better prognosis than total paralysis. It is important not to falsely attribute a small amount of adduction of the affected vocal fold as representing evidence of partial innervation. The RLN sectioning leads to paralysis of the ipsilateral thyroarytenoid, posterior cricoarytenoid, and lateral cricoarytenoid, but not the interarytenoid. The interarytenoid is a midline muscle, and has dual innervation from both RLNs; therefore, some residual adduction may be present in complete unilateral VFP, due to innervation from the contralateral RLN.

A completely immobile vocal fold can rest in a variety of positions, traditionally designated lateral (cadaveric), median, paramedian, and intermediate; these do not correspond to any particular neurologic lesion, but are clinical conventions used to describe the approximate position of an immobile vocal fold. In reality, the fold may lie in any position along its sweep of motion. For most of the twentieth century, it was thought that the position of the paralyzed vocal fold had some topognostic significance (e.g., that lateral vocal fold position indicated complete CN X paralysis due to combined RLN and SLN involvement). This theory was later disproved by both Woodson [10] and Koufman et al. [11]. The position of the vocal fold after nerve injury seems to be due entirely to the degree of reinnervation and synkinesis present, and nothing else.

Some authors focus on the position of the arytenoid when evaluating vocal fold immobility. In most cases it is much more fruitful to focus on the vocal fold movement itself, rather than the arytenoid, in determining vocal fold immobility. But sometimes an overhanging arytenoid obscures the observation of the underlying vocal fold and makes it impossible to ignore its position in cases of VF immobility. This overhanging, anteriorly displaced arytenoid is sometimes taken to indicate an arytenoid dislocation; however, EMG data from patients with an immobile vocal fold accompanied by an "overhanging arytenoid" typically shows complete denervation or poor reinnervation of the TA muscle [12]; therefore, in non-traumatic cases, anterior displacement or an overhanging, sagging arytenoid should not raise suspicion for arytenoid dislocation.

The actual incidence of arytenoid subluxation and dislocation is a source of much debate. Many investigators believe it is an exceedingly rare clinical entity, and almost exclusively due to external trauma associated with motor vehicle crashes and penetrating injuries. Some laryngologists feel that intubation-related cricoarytenoid dislocation is virtually non-existent, owing to the extremely strong supporting cricoarytenoid ligaments (J.L. Netterville, personal communication); however, a handful of small case reports have demonstrated endotracheal intubation-associated arytenoid dislocations. A study by Sataloff et al. [13] has described 26 CA dislocations and subluxations over a 9-year period, but only 6 cases related to intubation were EMG confirmed.

Clues that may raise the suspicion of an arytenoid dislocation when evaluating unilateral vocal fold mobility include the following:
1. Arytenoid edema.
2. Difference in vocal fold level. (Generally, an anterior arytenoid dislocation would result in a lower vertical position of the vocal process on the affected side.) Note that vocal fold height differences are also commonly seen with VFP.
3. Absence of a "jostle sign." ("Jostle sign" is a brief lateral movement of the arytenoid on the immobile side during glottic closure due to contact from the mobile arytenoid), although this is also likely to be absent in a paralyzed vocal fold with good preserved or reinnervated muscle tone.)

Because none of the above scenarios are pathognomonic for arytenoid dislocation, a high degree of suspicion is needed.

In some patients with UVFP, compensatory supraglottic contraction (i.e., "dysphonia plica ventricularis") obscure vocal fold movement. In these cases the author advocates that the patient phonate with an easy onset such as a "sigh," or be instructed to "hum through the nose." This technique, described by Koufman as "unloading," is useful for removing any unwanted compensatory supraglottic hyperfunction that obscures vocal fold visualization [9]. This technique is invaluable in many cases of compensated, longstanding VFP and glottic incompetence that have been misdiagnosed as "muscle tension dysphonia" or "dysphonia plica ventricularis."

Videostroboscopy is a helpful part of the work-up of vocal fold movement abnormalities. Videostroboscopy may show incomplete closure or a large glottal gap in uncompensated VFP and, in these cases, no useful information can be gleaned from the stroboscopic exam because periodic vibration of the vocal folds cannot be initiated. In many cases, however, the paralyzed vocal fold shows increased amplitude of vibration due to the atrophic, "floppy" nature of the denervated vocalis muscle [14]. In cases of mild or moderate vocal fold paresis, the increased amplitude seen on stroboscopy may be the only sign of vocal fold weakness. Other potentially useful information obtained via stroboscopy concerns vocal fold height differences and the status of vocal process contact during phonation. These parameters help determine the need for arytenoid adduction, which changes vocal fold height and adjusts vocal process position, when evaluating patients for laryngoplastic phonosurgery.

A simple test to evaluate the degree of vocal disability and glottic insufficiency is measuring the patient's maximal phonation time (MPT). This is done by simply instructing the patient to take a deep breath and phonate an "ee" vowel for as long as possible. Normal MPT for a healthy adult is approximately 25 s. In cases of VFP, the MPT is reduced to 10 s or less. Shorter MPT values indicate more severe glottic incompetence, worse voice, and increased vocal fatigue. The MPT values of 5 or less indicate severe, uncompensated VFP that may need arytenoid adduction in addition to medialization laryngoplasty [15]. Poor pulmonary reserve from asthma or chronic obstructive pulmonary disease may reduce MPT significantly, so results need to be taken in context of the patient's pulmonary status. The MPT should be expected to improve (i.e., increase) after successful medialization surgery for VFP.

Lastly, it is noted that "unilateral vocal fold immobility" is a physical finding, and not a diagnosis. One must determine the cause. In the vast majority of cases of unilateral vocal fold immobility, laryngeal paralysis is the cause. In a small number of cases, the etiology may be cricoarytenoid joint arthritis (Rheumatoid arthritis, gout), cricoarytenoid joint effusion/subluxation/dislocation (external trauma/traumatic endotracheal intubation), or neoplastic infiltration ("occult" squamous cell carcinoma in the ventricle/paraglottic space). In general, the history will suggest whether CA joint derangements are the culprit, and careful fiberoptic laryngoscopy combined with CT scan will reveal neoplastic infiltration as the cause of vocal fold immobility. In cases where one cannot confidently exclude the CA joint involvement or neoplasm in cases of unilateral vocal fold immobility, an electromyographic examination or laryngoscopy with palpation for passive mobility of the vocal folds is warranted.

Work-up

Serology

There is little yield from screening laboratory tests such as chemistry panel, complete blood count, urinalysis, VDRL/FTA-ABS, thyroid function tests, autoimmune panels, or erythrocyte sedimentation rate. In a study by Terris et al. [16], serologic studies had 0% yield in determining the etiology in 84 patients with UVFP. If elements of the history and physical exam point towards a systemic process as the cause of UVFP, then certain lab tests may be needed; however, a general "shotgun" approach to the work-up of uncomplicated UVFP is unnecessary and wasteful.

Imaging Studies

As screening tools, barium swallow and thyroid scans have virtually no yield in determining the etiology of VFP and are not advocated in the diagnostic work-up [16]. In contrast, a modified barium swallow to evaluate swallowing and aspiration risk is frequently helpful in managing patients with dysphagia and VFP.

In cases where a clear-cut temporal relation exists between surgical iatrogenic trauma and VFP, no radiologic work-up is necessary. In cases where no cause can be found for the VFP, adequate imaging studies are essential. There is some disagreement as to what constitutes an "adequate" radiologic assessment for unexplained VFP. Most investigators agree that a CT (with contrast) or MRI encompassing the base of skull through the upper chest is adequate [14]. The radiologist should be informed that the entire course of the vagus down to the take-off point of the RLN needs to be included in the study. Benninger and colleagues have argued that computed tomography (CT) or magnetic resonance imaging (MRI) of the neck combined with chest radiography constitutes an adequate workup [14]. They noted that 100% of pulmonary or mediastinal malignancies associated with VFP were detected on routine chest radiography, and that imaging of the chest by CT was unnecessary. Other authors disagree with this approach. Glazer et al. demonstrated that of 18 metastatic mediastinal masses seen on CT, only five were visualized on routine CXR [17]. Koufman et al. advocates the addition of MRI of the brainstem in cases of obvious "high vagal" lesion (palatal paralysis + VFP), because this is a difficult area to image and small lesions may be missed [18].

In cases of suspected aspiration or significant dysphagia due to VFP, a modified barium swallow should be obtained. Evaluation of all stages of swallow by a qualified speech pathologist will provide valuable information regarding any associated laryngopharyngeal sensory deficits or pharyngeal weakness, as well as assessing the patient's risk of aspiration. Swallowing guidelines and immediate swallow therapy can also be instituted. As an alternative, a fiberoptic endoscopic evaluation of swallowing (FEES) can be performed which is useful (especially in concert with fiberoptic endoscopic evaluation of swallowing with sensory testing) in assessing aspiration risk [19].

Perhaps one of the more controversial aspects of VFP evaluation is the role of laryngeal electromyography (LEMG). Some authors advocate LEMG for all cases of VFP and others find it of little or no utility. The present au-

Fig. 4.1. Evaluation of unilateral vocal fold paralysis (UVFP)

* Anterior cervical fusion, esophagectomy, thyroidectomy, carotid endarterectomy, mediastinoscopy, CABG, aortic surgery, pulmonary resection, endotracheal intubation

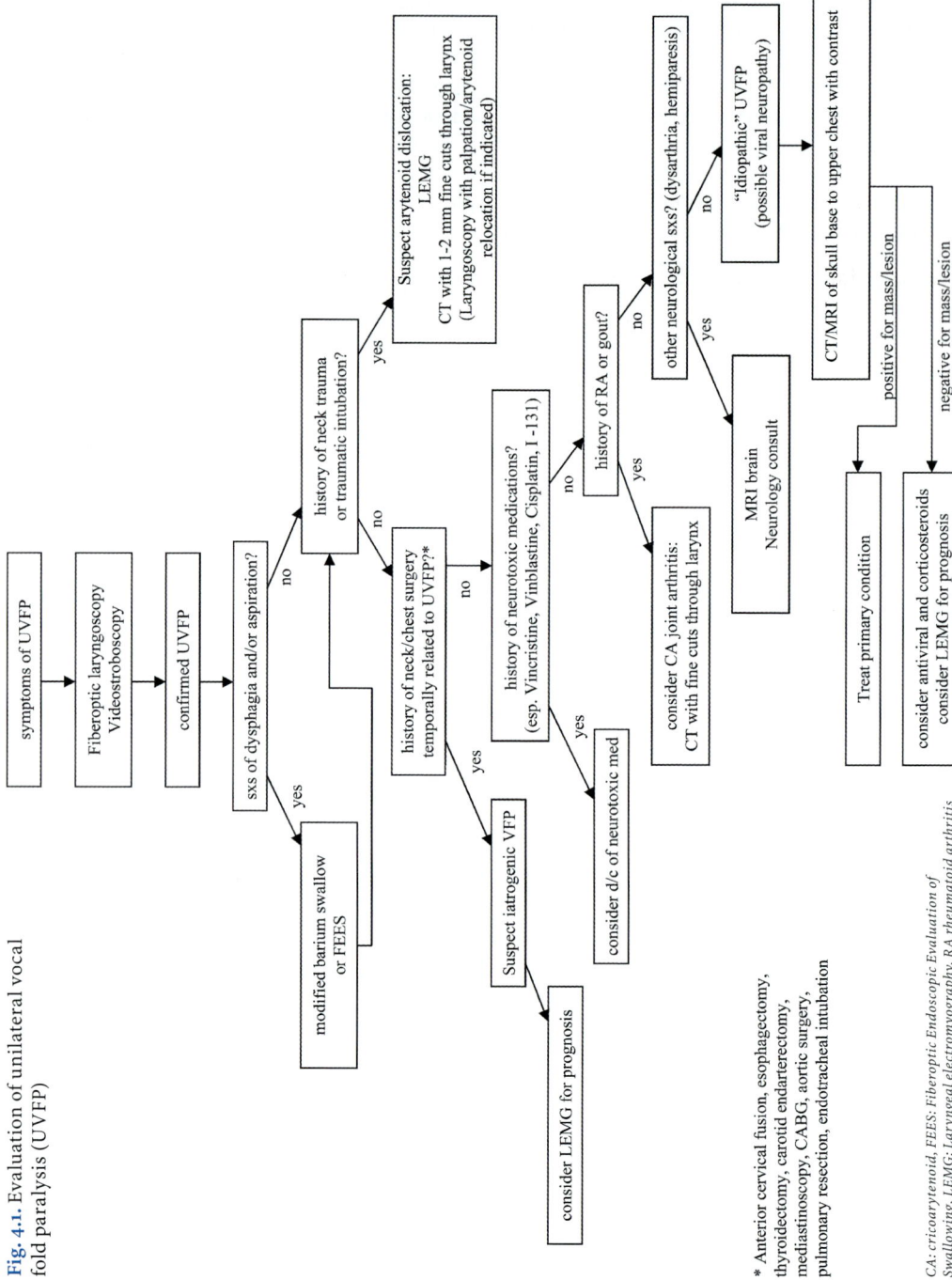

CA: cricoarytenoid, FEES: Fiberoptic Endoscopic Evaluation of Swallowing, LEMG: Laryngeal electromyography, RA rheumatoid arthritis

thors believe that it may help give prognostic information regarding the chance of recovery in some instances of VFP, and can be useful in cases of suspected arytenoid dislocation. The topic of LEMG is covered in another chapter in this book.

Conclusion

The evaluation for unilateral vocal fold immobility is relatively straight-forward (Fig. 4.1), and a thorough history often reveals the etiology of the condition. Quite commonly there is a temporal relation between the patient's onset of hoarseness and an surgical injury, and in these cases no further diagnostic studies are needed. In the case of unexplained UVFP, however, radiographic evaluation with CT or MRI of the neck and upper chest is essential to rule out an occult malignancy, especially bronchogenic carcinoma. Routine serologic tests are unnecessary and add no significant diagnostic information. In those patients with dysphagia and suspected aspiration, evaluation with either a modified barium swallow or a FEES is also important. Laryngeal EMG can be a useful guide in determining the prognosis for recovery in cases of UVFP, and evaluation for suspected arytenoid dislocation. Although arytenoid dislocation/subluxation is a potential cause of unilateral vocal fold immobility, it is a distinctly uncommon phenomenon, and is mostly limited to external laryngeal trauma.

References

1. Koufman JA, Postma GN, Cummins MM, Blalock PD (2000) Vocal fold paresis. Otolaryngol Head Neck Surg 122:537–541
2. Lundy DS, Casiano RR (1995) Compensatory falsetto: effects on vocal quality. J Voice 9:439–442
3. Simpson CB, Fleming DJ (2000) Medical and vocal history in the evaluation of dysphonia. Otolaryngol Clin North Am 33:719–729
4. Ellis PD, Pallister W (1975) Recurrent laryngeal nerve palsy and endotracheal intubation. J Laryngol Otol 89:823–826
5. Quick CA, Merwin GE (1978) Arytenoid dislocation. Arch Otolaryngol Head Neck Surgery 104:267–270
6. Robinson LR, Hillel AD, Waugh PF (1998) New laryngeal muscled weakness in post-polio syndrome. Laryngoscope 108:732–734
7. Annino DJ, MacArthur CJ, Friedman EM (1992) Vincristine-induced recurrent laryngeal nerve paralysis. Laryngoscope 102:1260–1262
8. Flowers RH, Kernodle DS (1990) Vagal mononeuritis caused by herpes simplex virus: association with unilateral vocal cord paralysis. Am J Med 88:686–688
9. Koufman JA (1995) Evaluation of laryngeal biomechanics by fiberoptic laryngoscopy. In: Rubin JS, Sataloff RT, Korovin GS, Gould WJ (eds) Diagnosis and treatment of voice disorders. Igaku-Shoin, New York, pp 122–134
10. Woodson GE (1993) Configuration of the glottis in laryngeal paralysis. I: Clinical study. Laryngoscope 103:1227–1234
11. Koufman JA, Walker FO, Joharji GM (1995) The cricothyroid muscle does not influence vocal fold position in laryngeal paralysis. Laryngoscope 105:369–372
12. Blitzer A, Jahn AF, Keider A (1996) Semon's law revisited: an electromyographic analysis of laryngeal synkinesis. Ann Otol Rhinol Laryngol 105:764–769
13. Sataloff RT, Bough ID, Spiegel JR (1994) Arytenoid dislocation: diagnosis and treatment. Laryngoscope 104:1353–1361
14. Benninger MS, Crumley RL, Ford CN et al. (1994) Evaluation and treatment of the unilateral paralyzed vocal fold. Otolaryngol Head Neck Surg 111:497–508
15. Woo P (2000) Arytenoid adduction and medialization laryngoplasty. Otolaryngol Clin North Am 33:817–839
16. Terris DJ, Arnstein DP, Nguyen HH (1992) Contemporary evaluation of unilateral vocal cord paralysis. Otolaryngol Head Neck Surg 107:84–90
17. Glazer HS, Aronberg DJ, Lee JKT, Sagel SS (1983) Extralaryngeal causes of vocal cord paralysis: CT evaluation. AJR 141:527–531
18. Koufman JA, Postma GN, Whang CS et al. (2001) Diagnostic laryngeal electromyography: the Wake Forest experience 1995–1999. Otolaryngol Head Neck Surg 124:603–606
19. Aviv JE (2000) Prospective, randomized outcome study of endoscopy versus modified barium swallow in patients with dysphagia. Laryngoscope 110:563–574
20. Weisberg NK, Spengler DM, Netterville JL (1997) Stetch-induced nerve injury as a cause of paralysis secondary to the anterior cervical approach. Otol Laryngol Head Neck Surg 116:317–326

21. Phillips TG, Green GE (1987) Left recurrent laryngeal nerve injury following internal mammary artery bypass. Ann Thorac Surg 43:440
22. Shin-ichi I, Kenji K, Ken I et al. (2003) Hoarseness after cardiac surgery: possible contribution of low temperature to the recurrent nerve paralysis. Laryngoscope 113:1088–1089
23. Cavo JW (1985) True vocal cord paralysis following intubation. Laryngoscope 95:1352–1359

Chapter 5

Diagnostic Electromyography for Unilateral Vocal Fold Dysmotility

Allen Hillel, Lawrence Robinson

Introduction

Electromyography (EMG) is a diagnostic technique that is about 100 years old. Even before electromyography became an accepted clinical tool, Weddell [1], in 1944, published the first report of laryngeal EMG when he tried to investigate the activity of the laryngeal muscles in four patients who had suffered injuries to the larynx. It was 1 year later when the first EMG machine designed specifically for clinical use was made by Golseth [2, 3]. During the next 30 years, EMG gradually became accepted as the clinical standard for investigating the status of a nerve after an injury. By the mid 1980s, EMG had become a mature field and a routine part of any diagnostic and prognostic evaluation of the neuromuscular system.

In the mid-1950s Faaborg-Andersen and Buchthal [4] published a detailed treatise in which they described the activity in many of the laryngeal muscles during both phonatory and nonphonatory tasks. In the following years, as the field of diagnostic EMG progressed, the newer findings of motor unit morphology was applied to EMG studies in the larynx [5, 6]. Many authors in recent years have worked to further define the expected findings of EMG studies in a great number of clinical conditions [7–21]. Laryngeal EMG has become a routine test in many clinical laryngology laboratories and has been used not only to diagnose peripheral nerve injuries, but also to diagnose systemic nervous system disorders such as myasthenia gravis, Charcot-Marie Tooth, and laryngeal dystonia [10, 22–26].

The use of EMG guidance for injections of botulinum toxin to the larynx has made laryngeal electromyography for localization a routine technique for many laryngologists [27–29]; however, broad acceptance and adoption of laryngeal EMG as the standard of care to evaluate the injured larynx has only recently begun to occur. This chapter presents the technique and clinical value of laryngeal EMG, with the hope that its clinical use will become more widespread.

Definition of Immobility

Visual examination of the larynx provides much information regarding the etiology of an abnormal voice. The increasingly common use of videostroboscopy offers the opportunity to visualize the physical factors causing the abnormal voice in the vast majority of cases. The ability to review recorded examinations without the added burden of simultaneously manipulating the laryngoscope allows the examiner to examine the results in detail. The mobility of each vocal fold can be better assessed and distinguished from incidental movement caused by respiration and interarytenoid muscle activity; however, the etiology of a vocal fold dysmotility cannot be determined by visual examination. While visual exams can determine immobility and dysmotility, they cannot determine if the underlying cause is paralysis or paresis. Paralysis and paresis are neurologic entities which can only be definitively diagnosed by neurophysiologic testing.

Definition of Electromyography

Electromyography is the study of the electrical activity in muscles. Based on the findings, an examiner is able to deduce a number of features relating to the condition of muscle and efferent motor nerve. Although much information can be gathered objectively from EMG testing, electromyography has the greatest power when it is interpreted in conjunction with the clinical findings. This interpretation of objective EMG findings in the context of the clinical findings is often referred to as "The Art of Electromyography".

In the following sections of this chapter, the different varieties of electromyographic tests are presented as well as recommendations for specific tests that can provide the most information for a specific clinical presentation.

Techniques of Electromyography

The field of electromyography employs numerous testing algorithms that are directed to various clinical situations [30]. Laryngeal electromyography generally uses three testing techniques:
1. Diagnostic needle testing
2. Fine-wire electromyography
3. Repetitive stimulation

Simple recruitment looks for electrical activity from motor units as the muscle is voluntarily recruited. Recruitment as an isolated test is primarily used to localize needle placement for chemodenervation with botulinum toxin. More information is obtained from this test when it is part of a full diagnostic EMG. Diagnostic needle testing closely examines the type of electrical activity present in the muscles of the larynx both at rest and during voluntary recruitment. The specific waveforms are diagnostic of the condition of the efferent motor nerve. In some cases the waveforms can demonstrate ongoing or recent denervation or, in other cases, predict the onset of recovery. For vocal fold dysmotility disorders, this technique provides the most information.

Fine-wire electromyography employs multiple fixed fine-wire electrodes and is valuable in particular for examining the presence and timing of activity in many muscles simultaneously. This technique is used for examination of patients with suspected synkinesis and patients with laryngeal dystonia.

Repetitive stimulation records the compound action potential of a muscle as the nerve is stimulated. This technique supersedes voluntary control as all muscle fibers contract synchronously due to the electrical stimulation of the nerve by the examiner. The compound action potential is a relatively stable response in the presence of a fixed hooked-wire electrode. This technique is particularly useful in suspected cases of myasthenia gravis.

For the purposes of evaluating unilateral dysmotility, diagnostic needle EMG provides the best information. The remainder of this chapter focuses on diagnostic needle EMG.

EMG Waveforms: How They Are Derived, and What They Mean

The interpretation of diagnostic morphology is based on the waveform of a normal motor unit action potential (MUAP; Fig. 5.1). This normal waveform represents the electrical activity of the muscle fibers controlled by one nerve fiber and has a characteristic appearance and sound. Other types of waveforms are seen during injury. They can be characterized into three categories: (a) injury; (b) recovery; and (c) evidence of old injury.

Nerve injury leaves muscle fibers without innervation. Soon after denervation, as acetylcholine hypersensitivity develops in the muscle fibers, they start to discharge spontaneously, especially after the physical stimulation of the needle as it is inserted into the muscle. They generate two primary waveforms: positive sharp waves and fibrillations (Fig. 5.2). The presence of these waveforms indicates that an injury has occurred to the nerve, that the muscle fibers have not yet been "contacted" by a nerve sprout, and that the muscle fiber has not yet become fibrosed or died due to chronic lack of innervation. Positive sharp waves and fibrillations are signs of either recent or ongoing denervation.

When muscle fibers are "contacted" by a nerve sprout, they then contract voluntarily under control of that nerve; however, the new nerve sprouts have slower conduction than mature nerves, and the newly enervated muscle

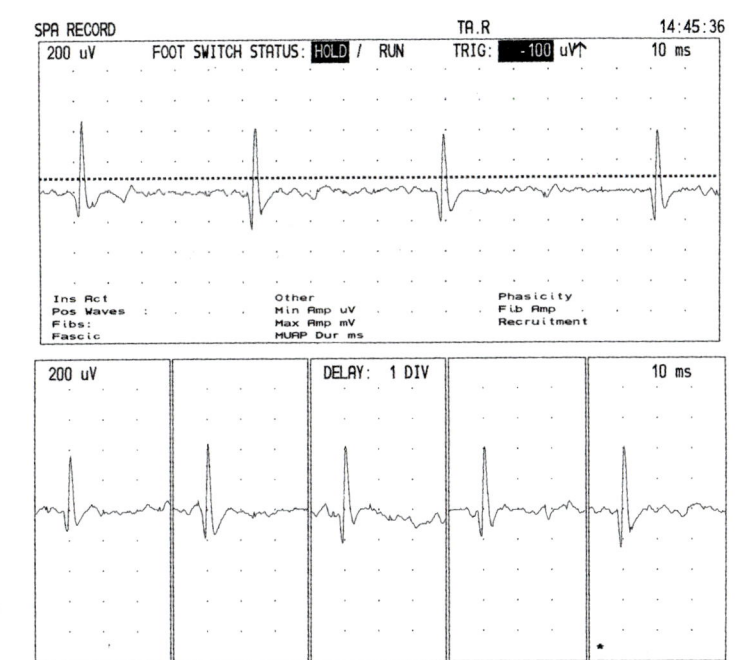

Diagnostic Electromyography for Unilateral Vocal — Chapter 5

Fig. 5.1. A normal motor unit from the TA muscle. Note that the amplitude is about 700 mV (200 mV/division) and the duration is about 7 ms (10 ms/division).

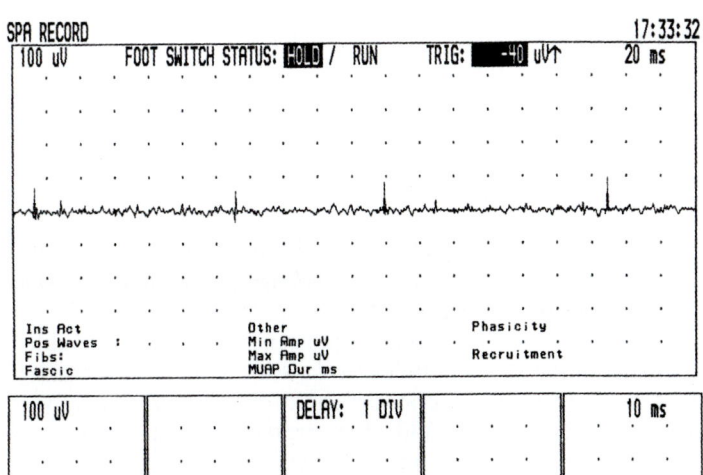

Fig. 5.2. Fibrillations potentials. Note that the duration of this waveform is about 1 ms.

fibers will be slightly delayed in activating. The combination of the early firing by the muscle fibers innervated by the mature part of the nerve fiber and the later firing by the newly innervated muscle fibers creates a complex, longer-duration waveform that is called a polyphasic potential (Fig. 5.3). Polyphasic potentials are a sign that reinnervation is occurring and may be a good prognostic sign for recovery.

When the new nerve sprouts to the previously denervated muscle fibers mature, they begin to conduct at a normal speed. The delay seen with polyphasic potentials resolves since all the muscle fibers will receive the signal to contract at the same time. The motor unit will no longer be as spread out over time; however, this "mature" polyphasic potential reflects the discharge of more muscle fibers than a normal motor unit, and although it has the normal triphasic appearance, it is much larger in amplitude. These large-amplitude motor units (Fig. 5.4) are a sign that a peripheral nerve injury occurred some time ago, but that reinnervation has occurred and is now stable. Large-amplitude motor units are a sign of an old, but stable, peripheral nerve injury.

Additional features of diagnostic LEMG are the number of motor units and the rate of firing. In a normal muscle with a normal nerve, voluntary recruitment is accompanied by many motor units firing in a dense pattern (Fig. 5.5). If there are few motor units firing, each faster than normal, it is a sign that the central nervous system is driving a reduced number of available motor units at a fast pace in order to generate muscle performance. Few motor units firing fast is a sign of a peripheral nerve injury (Fig. 5.6). In contrast, if there are many motor units firing slowly, that is a sign that the central nervous system might be impaired (Fig. 5.7).

The above explanation of diagnostic waveforms is simplified but does offer a basic understanding of the techniques of EMG interpretation. It is beyond expectation that a laryngologist will be able to provide consistent, reliable, accurate interpretations of EMG tracings. An experienced electromyographer should be able to recognize these patterns as well as other patterns such as myokymia and complex repetitive discharges. The combination of a laryngologist who understands the anatomy and clinical presentation with an electromyographer who understands neurophysiology and can interpret the EMG waveforms is the ideal team for LEMG.

How LEMG Defines Dysmotility and Refines the Diagnosis

When presented with abnormal vocal fold movement, EMG can provide important information to help with management decisions. Generally, LEMG is performed when an intervention is considered, or, less commonly, when information is needed to reassure a patient. Since an LEMG can only detect recovery that has occurred at the time of the test, it cannot rule out later recovery. Regenerating peripheral nerves are considered to grow about 1 mm/day, so theoretically, the recurrent nerve could take up to a year before demonstrating electrical reinnervation patterns; therefore, the results of early LEMGs usually do not affect management unless the laryngologist is considering early intervention. If early intervention is considered, an LEMG can provide some guiding results. If there is no recruitment, then it is reasonable to undertake a corrective procedure with the understanding that recovery, although considerably less likely, might still occur within the year. Medialization with an injectable or with an external approach can be chosen depending on the clinical situation and the laryngologist's preference. If polyphasic potentials are present, a delay in intervention or a choice of an absorbable injectable substance might be preferable.

Another case for early LEMG is the concern for a cricoarytenoid dislocation. A paralyzed vocal fold often presents with an appearance of an arytenoid that is tipped forward over the glottis. Before attempting to "reduce" the dislocation surgically, an LEMG is important to rule out paralysis. If paralysis is present, the surgical procedure can be avoided.

At about 1 year after onset, LEMG can definitively characterize the underlying pathophysiology behind an immobility or dysmotility. Although changes can occur theoretically up to 2 years post-injury, the 1-year findings can be

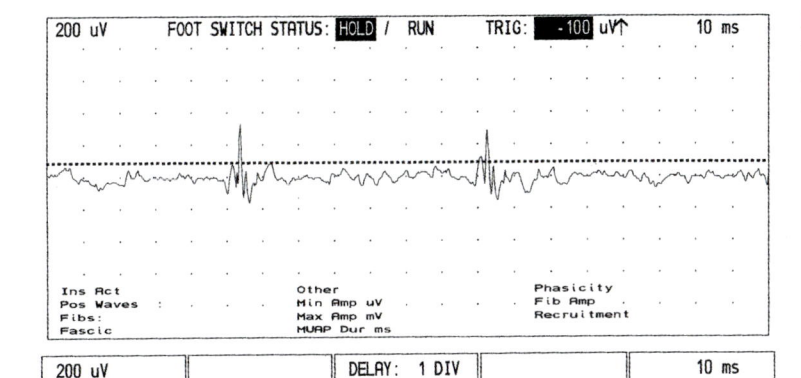

Fig. 5.3. Polyphasic potentials. Note that there are at least five "turns" in the tracing, and that the duration is prolonged at about 12 ms.

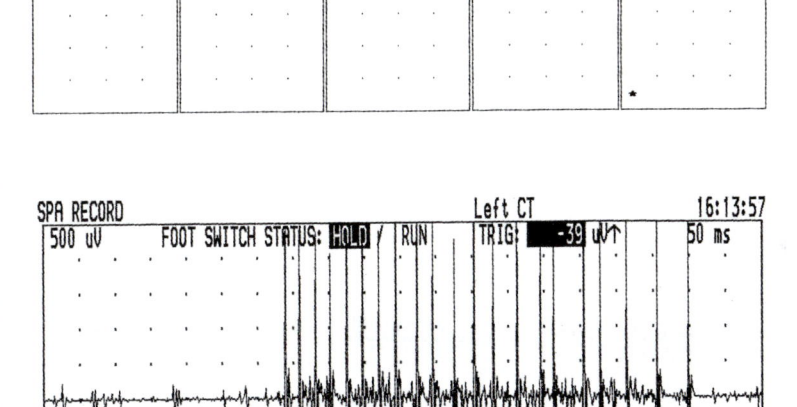

Fig. 5.4. Large-amplitude motor unit depicting an old but stable peripheral nerve injury. The amplitude is about 4 mV (200 mV/division) with under 2 mV being the normal range. Note that the waveform is triphasic and that the duration of the waveform is about 7 ms.

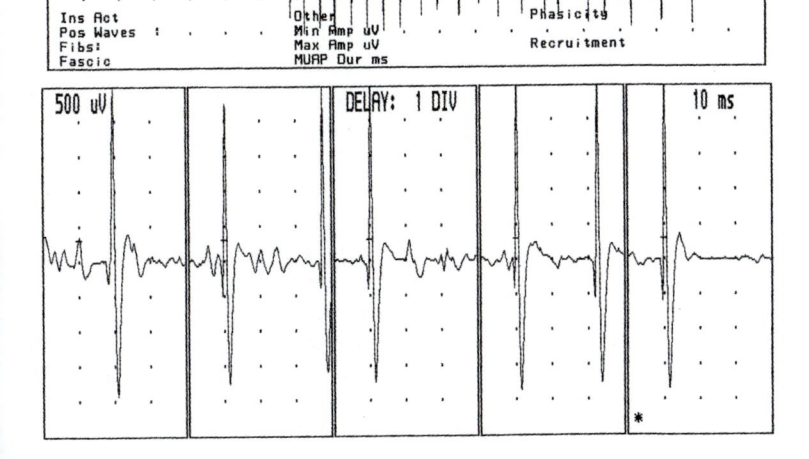

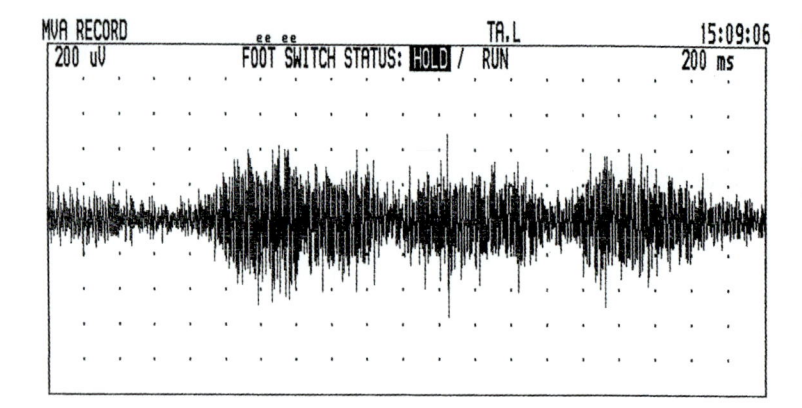

Fig. 5.5. Normal recruitment pattern during the phonation task of "eee,eee,eee" (/i,i,i/). Note the dense recruitment representing the firing of many motor units.

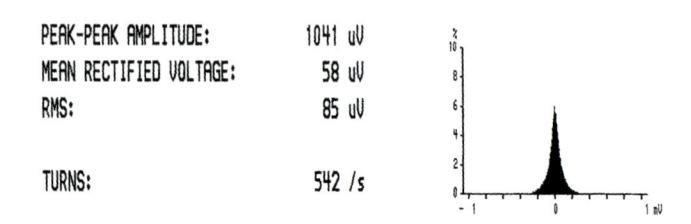

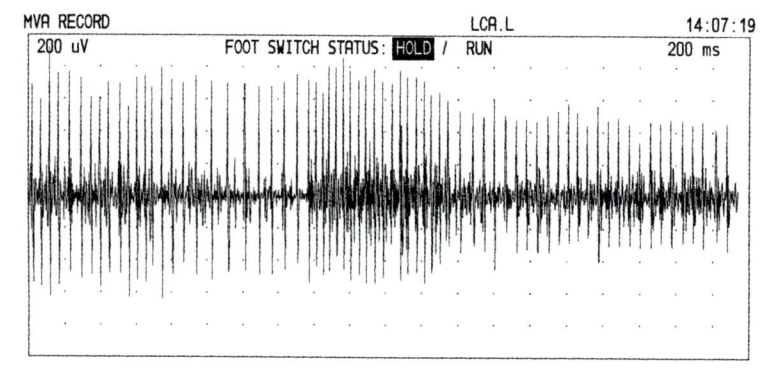

Fig. 5.6. Few motor units firing fast indicating evidence of a peripheral nerve injury. Note that the recruitment pattern is less dense than in Fig. 5.5. Also note that in contrast to Fig. 5.5, individual motor units can be seen and are repetitive at a rate indicating fast firing. This condition is known as "few motor units firing fast."

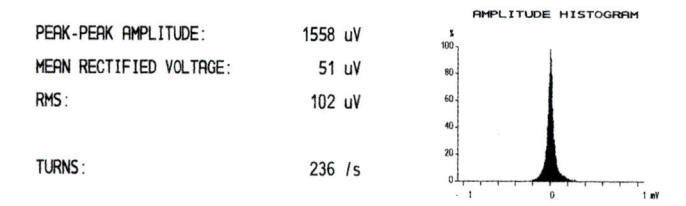

considered «final» for most clinical purposes when dealing with peripheral nerve injuries [30]. Central nervous system injuries classically have a longer recovery time.

The findings at 1 year can be broadly grouped into four categories:

1. Dense peripheral nerve injury with no recruitment

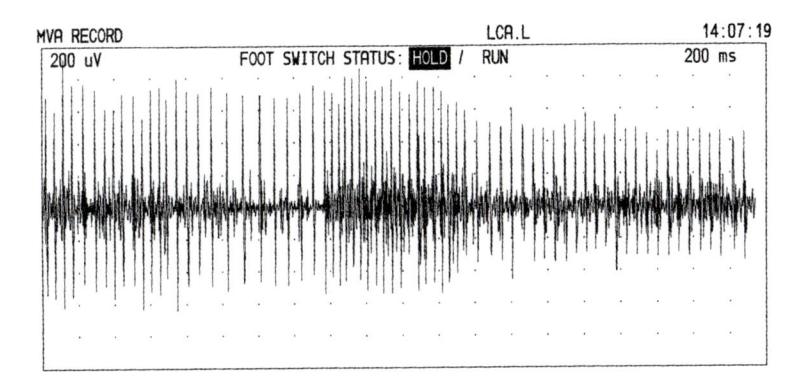

MVA RECORD   LCA.L   14:07:19
200 uV   FOOT SWITCH STATUS: HOLD / RUN   200 ms

Fig. 5.7. Many motor units firing slowly indicating concern for a central deficit. Note that the recruitment pattern is not as full as in Fig. 5.5, and that the motor units do not seem to be rapidly repetitive as in Fig. 5.5. This condition is characterized as "many motor units firing slowly."

PEAK-PEAK AMPLITUDE:	1558 uV
MEAN RECTIFIED VOLTAGE:	51 uV
RMS:	102 uV
TURNS:	236 /s

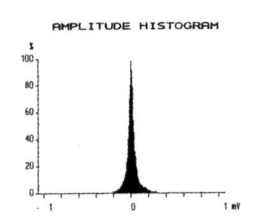

AMPLITUDE HISTOGRAM

2. A severe peripheral nerve injury with a few motor units, usually firing fast
3. A moderate peripheral nerve injury with many motor units but decreased recruitment
4. Normal recruitment.

These four groups can further be characterized by the types of motor units present and the timing of their activity associated with phonation. If polyphasic potentials are present, it is important to consider that ongoing recovery is occurring and that a delay in definitive treatment might be indicated. If large-amplitude motor units are present, the examiner can have some confidence that the recovery has matured and is stable. When examining the timing of responses, synkinesis can be diagnosed if the PCA is active with simple phonation, or the TA/LCA is more active with a sniff than during voice tasks [8].

How LEMG Can Guide Treatment

Unilateral vocal fold immobility is frequently managed without LEMG. Therapeutic choices among voice therapy, vocal fold medialization, arytenoid repositioning procedures, injection medialization, and reinnervation are based on the visual exam and physician preference; however, decisions are made and outcomes are assessed without a clear understanding of the underlying injury.

The LEMG provides information about the pathophysiology of vocal fold immobility and dysmotility. With this information, the physician can make therapeutic choices based on an understanding of the etiology of the disorder [17, 21, 31]. In the previous section, an example of suspected arytenoid dislocation was discussed. Rather than proceed to a general anesthetic and attempted operative intervention, the physician can observe the patient if an LEMG demonstrates paralysis. In the case of immobility due to cricoarytenoid joint fixation, a normal LEMG would deter one from performing a reinnervation procedure that would likely worsen the voice. In the case of dense paralysis, the physician might be directed toward a reinnervation.

A lack of understanding of the pathophysiology of vocal fold movement has led to the reporting of widely varying reports of success with the same procedures. For example, in the case of studies of the duration of collagen or fat as an injectable agent for medialization, reports vary from a few months to years [32–37]; however, the endpoint in determining the outcome of injectables in many studies is voice quality. It is very likely the differences in outcomes between studies are due to the random percentage of patients who happen to have spontaneous recovery of nerve function after their injections. Patients who have good voice due to neural recovery, even synkinetic recovery, could be erroneously judged as having had a permanent response to an injection even if the substance had been completely resorbed.

Surgeons who do not use LEMG can also suffer from the lack of understanding in the underlying pathophysiology as they try to evaluate unsatisfactory results of procedures. It might be that a medialization failed to provide an excellent voice because the surgeon was not aware of a contralateral paresis. The surgeon might be guided by his visual exam to do a revision medialization with a similar poor result, rather than perform a medialization on the contralateral paretic side.

The LEMG allows the treating physician to discover the mechanism of disease before treatment, even if it sometimes does not affect treatment choice. The validity of outcome measures is lost without accurate treatment indications. The advancement of laryngology depends upon the refinement of our empirical treatment and study to include an objective evaluation of the neurophysiology of immobility and dysmotility. It is recommended that all laryngologists work to develop a good program of LEMG so that clinical decisions and treatment outcomes can be evaluated with an understanding of the underlying mechanism of disease.

Philosophy of LEMG

Laryngeal electromyography offers the best diagnostic examination to evaluate the pathophysiology of vocal fold dysmotility. With experience, an otolaryngologist can gather information that can affect treatment planning and operative decisions. The findings of LEMG can also help the practitioner evaluate the outcomes of therapies with an understanding of the specific disease process. This understanding can lead to a tremendous improvement in both diagnostic and therapeutic skills of the individual practitioner, and overall, can significantly advance the field of laryngology as studies of therapeutic outcomes are related to specific diagnoses.

Case Examples

Case 1

A 37-year-old man presented with an 18-month history of weak voice. There was not particular event at the onset of his voice difficulties. He had undergone numerous examinations with the findings of a normal laryngeal exam. Videostroboscopy in our clinic demonstrated normal mobility; however, in one short sequence, there was a suggestion of increased amplitude of the mucosal wave on the left side. Laryngeal EMG was performed and demonstrated the presence of "few motor units firing fast" (Fig. 5.8). No fibrillations or positive sharp waves were found that would indicate ongoing denervation and no polyphasic potentials were found that would indicate ongoing reinnervation. Based on these findings and a normal CT scan, the patient agreed to a vocal fold medialization with resolution of his voice fatigue.

Case 2

A 33-year-old man presented to clinic with a 2-week history of voice loss without an antecedent event. Examination showed a hoarse, breathy voice with a strobe exam demonstrating left true vocal fold atrophy with bowing and incomplete glottic closure. The LEMG at 1 month after the onset of symptoms showed findings of many motor units firing slowly in the left TA muscle. Examination of the left CT muscle also demonstrated normal motor units with a decreased rate of firing (Figs. 5.9, 5.10). These findings were judged to be consistent with an upper motor neuron lesion. Both an MRI and neurological examinations were normal. Based on the results of the LEMG, the patient received speech therapy as his only intervention. The patient returned at 4 months with a significant improvement in his voice. The LEMG demonstrated a rate near normal with good recruitment (Fig. 5.11).

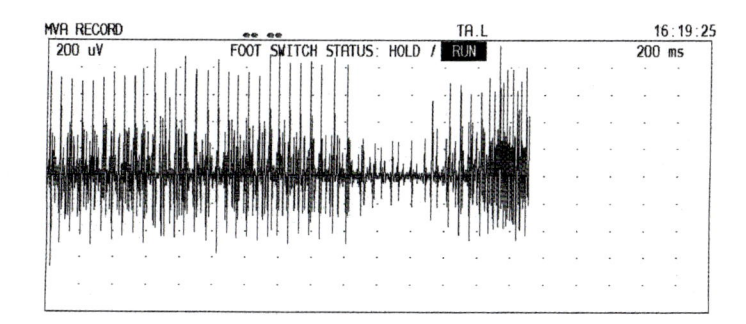

Fig. 5.8. Few motor units firing fast indicating a peripheral recurrent nerve injury.

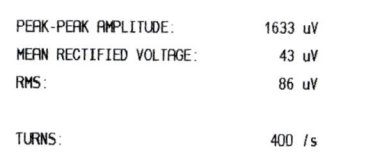

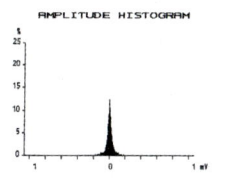

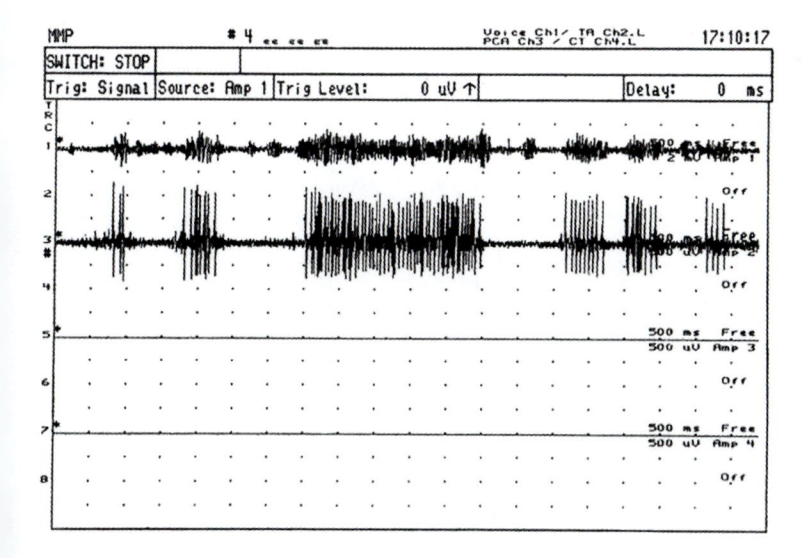

Fig. 5.9. This EMG is 1 month after the onset of the patient's hoarseness. The upper channel in this tracing is a signal from a microphone recording the patient's voice. The second channel shows normal motor units firing slowly in the left TA muscle, indicative of a central nervous system injury.

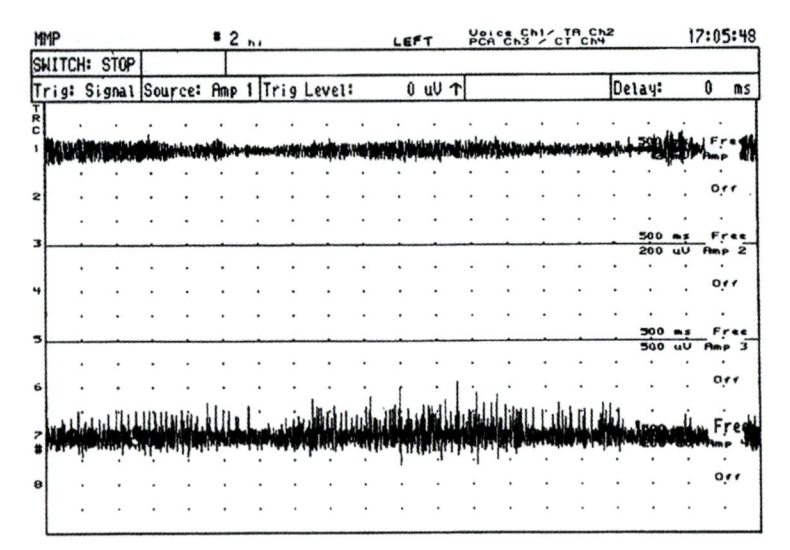

Fig. 5.10. This EMG is 1 month after the onset of the patient's hoarseness. The upper channel in this tracing is a signal from a microphone recording the patient's voice. The lower channel shows normal motor units firing slowly in the left CT muscle, indicative of a central nervous system injury.

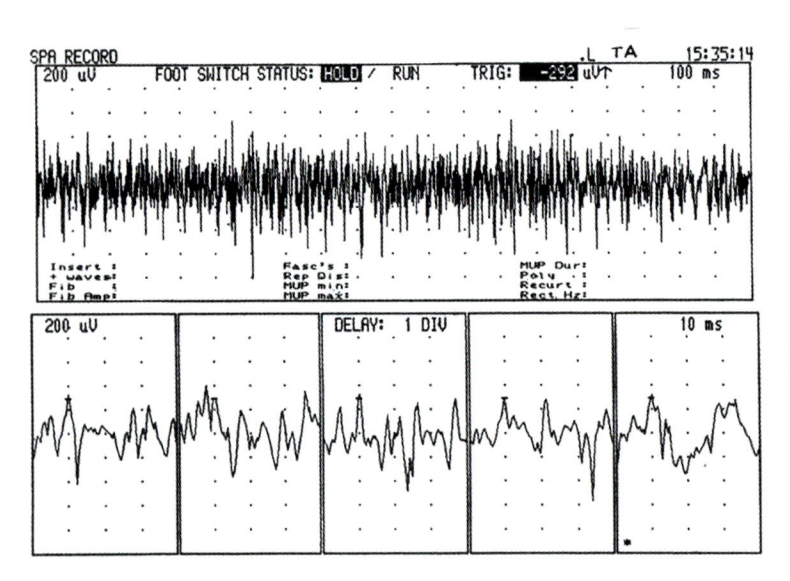

Fig. 5.11. This EMG of the left TA is 4 months after the onset of the patient's hoarseness. At this time the patient reported significant improvement of his voice and was again able to sing. The EMG tracing demonstrates improved recruitment with an increased rate of firing when compared with the tracing at 1 month (see Fig. 5.9).

References

1. Weddell G, Feinstein B, Paattle R (1944) The electrical activity of voluntary muscle in man under normal and pathological conditions. Brain 67:178–242
2. Golseth JG (1950) Diagnostic contributions of the electromyogram. Calif Med 73:355–357
3. Golseth JG (1957) Electromyographic examination in the office. Calif Med 87:298–300
4. Faaborg-Andersen K, Buchthal F (1956) Action potentials from internal laryngeal muscles during phonation. Nature 177:340–341
5. Buchthal F (1959) Electromyography of intrinsic laryngeal muscles. Q J Exp Physiol 44:137–148
6. Hiroto I, Hirano M, Tomita H (1968) Electromyographic investigation of human vocal cord paralysis. Ann Otol 77:296–304
7. Maronian N et al. (2003) Electromyographic findings in recurrent laryngeal nerve reinnervation. Ann Otol Rhinol Laryngol 112:314–323

8. Maronian NC et al. (2004) A new electromyographic definition of laryngeal synkinesis. Ann Otol Rhinol Laryngol 113:877–886
9. Maronian NC et al. (2004) Tremor laryngeal dystonia: treatment of the lateral cricoarytenoid muscle. Ann Otol Rhinol Laryngol 113:349–355
10. Hillel AD (2001) The study of laryngeal muscle activity in normal human subjects and in patients with laryngeal dystonia using multiple fine-wire electromyography. Laryngoscope 111(Suppl 97):1–47
11. Hillel AD et al. (1999) Evaluation and management of bilateral vocal cord immobility. Otolaryngol Head Neck Surg 121:760–765
12. Hillel AD, Robinson LR, Waugh P (1997) Laryngeal electromyography for the diagnosis and management of swallowing disorders. Otolaryngol Head Neck Surg 116:344–348
13. Dray TG, Robinson LR, Hillel AD (1999) Idiopathic bilateral vocal fold weakness. Laryngoscope 109:995–1002
14. Benninger MS et al. (1994) Evaluation and treatment of the unilateral paralyzed vocal fold. Otolaryngol Head Neck Surg 111:497–508
15. Heman-Ackah YD, Batory M (2003) Determining the etiology of mild vocal fold hypomobility. J Voice 17:579–588
16. Koufman JA et al. (2001) Diagnostic laryngeal electromyography: the Wake Forest experience 1995–1999. Otolaryngol Head Neck Surg 124:603–606
17. Koufman JA et al. (2000) Vocal fold paresis. Otolaryngol Head Neck Surg 122:537–541
18. Mostafa BE et al. (2004) The role of laryngeal electromyography in vocal fold immobility. ORL J Otorhinolaryngol Relat Spec 66:5–10
19. Sulica L, Blitzer A (2004) Electromyography and the immobile vocal fold. Otolaryngol Clin North Am 37:59–74
20. Sulica L (2003) Vocal fold paralysis and electromyography. Arch Phys Med Rehabil 84:1906; author reply 1906
21. Jacobs IN, Finkel RS (2002) Laryngeal electromyography in the management of vocal cord mobility problems in children. Laryngoscope 112:1243–1248
22. Dray TG, Robinson LR, Hillel AD (1999) Laryngeal electromyographic findings in Charcot-Marie-Tooth disease type II. Arch Neurol 56:863–865
23. Hillel AD et al. (2004) Treatment of the interarytenoid muscle with botulinum toxin for laryngeal dystonia. Ann Otol Rhinol Laryngol 113:341–348
24. Klotz DA et al. (2004) Findings of multiple muscle involvement in a study of 214 patients with laryngeal dystonia using fine-wire electromyography. Ann Otol Rhinol Laryngol 113:602–612
25. Sulica L et al. (2001) Vocal fold paresis of Charcot-Marie-Tooth disease. Ann Otol Rhinol Laryngol 110:1072–1076
26. Mao VH et al. (2001) Laryngeal myasthenia gravis: report of 40 cases. J Voice 15:122–130
27. Blitzer A et al. (1986) Botulinum toxin (BOTOX) for the treatment of «spastic dysphonia» as part of a trial of toxin injections for the treatment of other cranial dystonias. Laryngoscope 96:1300–1301
28. Blitzer A et al. (1988) Localized injections of botulinum toxin for the treatment of focal laryngeal dystonia (spastic dysphonia). Laryngoscope 98:193–197
29. Gibbs SR, Blitzer A (2000) Botulinum toxin for the treatment of spasmodic dysphonia. Otolaryngol Clin North Am 33:879–894
30. Dumitru D, Zworts MJ, Amato AA (2001) Electrodiagnostic medicine, 2nd edn. Elsevier, Amsterdam
31. Woo P (1998) Laryngeal electromyography is a cost-effective clinically useful tool in the evaluation of vocal fold function. Arch Otolaryngol Head Neck Surg 124:472–475
32. Remacle M et al. (1987) Correction of a glottis gap by injection of collagen. Apropos of 25 cases. Ann Otolaryngol Chir Cervicofac 104:37–43
33. Hill AN et al. (2003) Treatment of hypophonia with collagen vocal cord augmentation in patients with parkinsonism. Mov Disord 18:1190–1192
34. Umeno H et al. (2005) Analysis of voice function following autologous fat injection for vocal fold paralysis. Otolaryngol Head Neck Surg 132:103–107
35. Shindo ML, Zaretsky LS, Rice DH (1996) Autologous fat injection for unilateral vocal fold paralysis. Ann Otol Rhinol Laryngol 105:602–606
36. McCulloch TM et al. (2001) Long-term follow-up of fat injection laryngoplasty for unilateral vocal cord paralysis. Laryngoscope 112:1235–1238
37. Havas TE, Priestley KJ (2003) Autologous fat injection laryngoplasty for unilateral vocal fold paralysis. Aust N Z J Surg 73:938–943

Part II

Treatment

Chapter 6
Decision Points in the Management of Vocal Fold Paralysis *77*
Lucian Sulica, Andrew Blitzer

Chapter 7
Voice Therapy for Unilateral Vocal Fold Paralysis *87*
Celia F. Stewart, Elizabeth Allen

Chapter 8
Injection Augmentation *97*
Karen A. Cooper, Charles N. Ford

Chapter 8.1
Autologous Fat for Vocal Fold Injection *105*
Clark A. Rosen

Chapter 8.2
Collagen in Vocal Fold Injection *111*
Mark S. Courey

Chapter 8.3
Treatment of Glottal Insufficiency Using Micronized Human Acellular Dermis (Cymetra) *117*
Albert L. Merati

Chapter 8.4
Vocal Fold Augmentation with Calcium Hydroxylapatite *123*
Peter C. Belafsky, Gregory N. Postma

Chapter 8.5
Treatment of Glottal Insufficiency Using Hyaluronan *127*
Stellan Hertegård, Åke Dahlqvist, Lars Hallén, Claude Laurent

Chapter 9
Principles of Medialization Laryngoplasty *135*
C. Blake Simpson, Lucian Sulica

Chapter 9.1
Silastic Medialization Laryngoplasty *145*
C. Blake Simpson

Chapter 9.2
Medialization Thyroplasty Using the Montgomery Thyroplasty System *153*
Mark A. Varvares, Rebecca M. Brandsted

Chapter 9.3
Medialization Thyroplasty Using the VoCoM Vocal Cord Medialization System *159*
Tanya K. Meyer, Andrew Blitzer

Chapter 9.4
Titanium Medialization Implant *165*
Berit Schneider

Chapter 9.5
Medialization Laryngoplasty with Gore-Tex (Expanded Polytetrafluoroethylene) *169*
Timothy M. McCulloch, Henry T. Hoffman

Chapter 10
Arytenoid Repositioning Surgery *177*
Gayle E. Woodson

Chapter 6

Decision Points in the Management of Vocal Fold Paralysis

Lucian Sulica, Andrew Blitzer

Introduction

Decisions regarding therapeutic intervention in cases of vocal fold paralysis are guided by concerns regarding morbidity, principally from dysphagia and aspiration, and expectations and assumptions about the eventual outcome for the patient if left untreated. In turn, expectations concerning prognosis are influenced by the apparent cause of the paralysis and the time that has elapsed since onset. Electrophysiologic testing, in the form of laryngeal electromyography, has also been used to predict outcome, but a surprising amount of uncertainty regarding its utility still persists.

The ideal management strategy for unilateral vocal fold paralysis would offer timely treatment to patients whose disability is permanent, while sparing those who are likely to recover spontaneously from an unneeded surgery. As a secondary goal, it would offer effective temporary relief from dysphonia and swallowing difficulties to this second group of patients while they await improvement. Existing strategies emphasize expectant management, preferring to err on the side of delay in the treatment of patients with permanent deficits. These approaches, which have been legitimized by time, tend to assign less importance to the costs and limitations of an extended period of dysphonia, although these may be considerable. An expectant approach is appropriate if rehabilitation techniques are unsatisfactory, unpredictable, or risky, and if very little is known about prognosis.

However, advances in the understanding of laryngeal neurophysiology and the accumulation of clinical information have both yielded some insight, albeit incomplete, into mechanisms of recovery from vocal fold paralysis. Laryngeal electromyography has matured to become a practical clinical tool which yields valuable prognostic information in many cases. Interventions for vocal fold paralysis are generally safe, most techniques not even requiring a general anesthetic. They may be tailored to each case of vocal fold paralysis to achieve significant improvement in voice and other symptoms in the majority of patients. Many are reversible or revisable without undue difficulty, and dangerous complications are uncommon. In this new context, a critical examination of the factors which inform the decision to treat unilateral vocal fold paralysis may make it possible to modify the traditional approach to better serve the needs of the patient and come closer to the ideal.

Dysphagia and Aspiration

Most clinicians agree that clinically significant dysphagia in patients with vocal fold paralysis overrides concerns about unnecessary intervention and mandates early intervention. Such symptoms are usually evident and readily diagnosable from elements of the history such as coughing with eating or drinking, weight loss and episodes of pneumonia, and examination findings such as marked glottic insufficiency and observed pooling and aspiration of secretions. The modified barium swallow and endoscopic evaluation of swallowing exist to supplement the clinical assessment of such patients and to help guide treatment.

Aspiration has been identified in 18–38% of patients with unilateral vocal fold paralysis from all causes [1–3], although troublesome aspiration is probably more likely in certain clinical situations. These include combined recurrent and superior laryngeal nerve injury [4], either by discrete distal injury of both nerves or as part of a so-called "high vagal" injury, as well as situations in which vocal fold paralysis exists alongside other cranial nerve injuries, particularly the hypoglossal. Such a scenario is especially likely after skull base surgery but may also follow carotid endarterectomy and other surgeries in the neck requiring cephalad dissection, as well as stroke and other central nervous system injury or insult. In addition, surgeries that affect pulmonary reserve, as do most thoracic procedures, appear to carry a higher risk of aspiration with vocal fold paralysis. Age may also be an independent risk factor [5].

Algorithms featuring prompt medialization have been proposed after skull base surgery [6, 7] and thoracic surgery [8–10]. Laryngoplasty and injection appear to be equally effective in improving swallowing dysfunction [2]. It is worth noting that a significant proportion of patients remain troubled by aspiration even after a medialization procedure [6, 11], probably a reflection of the multifactorial nature of the problem. Again, it is likely that laryngeal anesthesia from a superior laryngeal nerve injury is probably an important reason for continued dysphagia. Woodson [12] has suggested that the addition of arytenoid adduction and cricopharyngeal myotomy may be of benefit in these persistent cases.

Prognosis

Perhaps the most significant impediment to efficient management of vocal fold paralysis has been a lack of clear information regarding prognosis. There is no equivalent of Pietersen's landmark studies [13, 14] of facial palsy to clarify the natural history of the paralyzed vocal fold. Clearly, the potential for spontaneous improvement varies from clinical scenario to clinical scenario, but even reports addressing vocal fold paralysis from the same cause can be difficult to reconcile with one another because of important differences in data collection and reporting. These differences consist principally of:

1. heterogeneity in clinical series resulting from differences in the time elapsed from the onset of the paralysis to examination.
2. variable definitions of recovery.
3. an oversimplified, "all-or-none" concept of paralysis and paralytic dysphonia presented in many reports.

The first difficulty arises from the clinical nature of vocal fold paralysis. A comparison with facial palsy, another peripheral cranial mononeuropathy which may result from surgery, medical disease, or unknown etiology, is instructive. Facial hemiplegia is immediately evident and alarming, and affected patients typically rush to seek medical attention. Vocal fold paralysis, however, is not always so obvious, symptoms being proportional to the degree of glottic insufficiency; an immobile vocal fold resting close to the midline may not generate significant dysphonia. Even when patients are severely dysphonic, they are capable of dismissing symptoms as "laryngitis" for weeks, if not months, before seeing a physician.

The time which has elapsed from onset to examination has an impact on observations. Prompt examination is likely to reveal a higher rate of paralysis than an examination performed weeks or months later, as well as a higher rate of recovery. Conversely, delayed examination yields a lower rate of paralysis, as some cases will have already improved, and a lower rate of recovery, as only the more profound neuropathies will have persisted to be identified. This is borne out in studies regarding vocal fold paralysis following carotid endarterectomy presented in Chap.3 (see Table 9): systematic immediate examination revealed a rate of paralysis of 27%, far higher than the more typically reported rate of 1–6%. This same effect is probably also present to some extent after nonsurgical vocal fold paralysis, as short-lived vocal fold paralysis has been identified in several clinical contexts [15]. To date, only reports in which all patients undergo laryngeal examination after a surgery which puts the vocal fold at risk have succeeded in controlling this variable. Many other studies do not even report information regarding the relation of the time of examination to the onset of the complaint.

Another important point of confusion stems from the fact that, in some cases, acceptable voice returns in the absence of vocal fold motion. Studies suggest that this is due to maintenance or restoration of vocal fold muscular tone and bulk, and thus adequate glottic closure in adduction, by reinnervation which is not sufficient or specific enough to restore motion [16, 17]. Vocal fold motion and voice function are, therefore, not entirely synonymous. Reports usually assess recovery in terms of either motion or voice quality, but only rarely both. Most articles in the otolaryngology literature consider "recovery" to mean a return of vocal fold motion, and make only passing mention of voice quality. These articles probably understate the rate of clinical recovery, although the information regarding physiologic reinnervation is accurate. Others, usually in the general surgery or medicine literature, declare outcome favorable if voice has returned, but do not systematically assess vocal fold motion in these cases. It is possible to argue convincingly that this second group of studies, which effectively categorize nonmobile but well-apposed vocal folds as favorable outcomes, provide more clinically useful information, since, as of this writing, surgical interventions can offer no better result.

Finally, vocal fold motion and voice function are often treated strictly as all-or-none phenomena: either the vocal fold is paralyzed or it is not, and either the voice has returned to normal or it has not. However, it is probably correct to view neural compromise of glottic function as a continuum of disability. It is clear that both partial paralysis (paresis) and incomplete recovery of complete paralysis are possible, as is a wide variability in the extent of phonatory dysfunction. While the potential for partial recovery is generally acknowledged, it is rarely incorporated into tabulations and discussions of nontreated outcomes of cases of vocal fold paralysis. This cannot be attributed to a lack of means of measuring voice quality. Reports of voice improvement following surgical treatment are detailed, typically featuring a number of qualitative and quantitative means of voice assessment. In comparison, data regarding voice in cases of vocal fold paralysis allowed to evolve naturally are crude. Considerable detail, and possibly some insight into mechanisms of recovery, are lost as a result. At the very least, this compromises our ability to compare spontaneous evolution with the effects of treatment.

Given these limitations, it should come as no surprise that information about the natural history of vocal fold paralysis is approximate. Prognosis for both vocal fold motion and voice following paralysis due to mediastinal nerve compression by malignancy is so poor that it is taken as a matter of course that these patients do not recover. The same is generally true of nerve section. Lest the latter observation seem too self-evident, it is useful to recall that experience with recurrent nerve section for spasmodic dysphonia has shown that the vocal fold has a robust tendency for reinnervation, even when a sizable length of nerve is removed. A surprising number of these cases show evidence of reinnervation (without return of vocal fold motion), and in fact, this may account for treatment failure in the majority of cases [18, 19]. However, the general clinical impression of poor prognosis remains valid.

Prognosis following various types of surgical injury is highly variable and no doubt affected by differences in the definition of recovery, as described above. A review of recent series of vocal fold paralysis following thyroidectomy show that 46–100% of paralyses identified after surgery recover, although most reports fall into the range of 65–85% (see Chap. 3, Table 7). In vocal fold paralysis after cervical spine surgery via an anterior approach, 18–90% recovered [20–23], the rate exceeding 60% in most reports. Injury during carotid endarterectomy improves in 0–86% (see Chap. 3, Table 9), and early reports indicate that recovery occurs in most cases which follow implantation of the vagal nerve stimulator. A similar pattern appears to follow vocal fold paralysis ascribed to intubation [24, 25], as might be expected in a case of neurapraxic injury. The rate of recovery following intrathoracic surgery is not well documented but may well be lower, in part because of the need to sacrifice the nerve during pneumonectomy for oncologic reasons. Recovery following skull base surgery is generally deemed to be poor [26].

The natural evolution of idiopathic vocal fold paralysis has been of considerable interest, and outcomes are generally reported more scrupulously and in somewhat more detail than for other clinical scenarios. In most series, 20–40% of patients regain vocal fold mobility and an additional number recover voice without motion, so that 25–50% of patients (see Chap. 3, Table 10) experience substantial improvement evident 1–9 months following the onset of the problem, although recovery has been reported as late as 18 months [27]. Selected studies report higher rates of recovery, either of voice [28] or vocal fold motion [29], but no factor to account for the discrepancy is obvious.

Thus, apart from vocal fold paralysis from malignancy and nerve section, prognosis for vocal fold paralysis remains variable and difficult to extrapolate except in the broadest way from the clinical scenario in which it occurs. It is this uncertainty that probably accounts for the persistence of the traditional delay of 6–12 months prior to intervention. A review of the literature reveals that the evidence supporting these intervals is limited and subject to all of the ambiguities reviewed above. Most otolaryngologists who have treated patients with vocal fold paralysis can recall cases that have not conformed to these expectations.

Laryngeal Electromyography

In the absence of conclusive information about prognosis and time required for recovery, clinical neurophysiologic testing may be especially useful. Laryngeal electromyography measures electrical activity in muscle by means of needle electrodes. Technical aspects and findings are described in Chap. 5. Laryngeal electromyography is able to identify normal innervation, absence of innervation, reinnervation, and even synkinetic reinnervation by virtue of characteristic electrical signals. Criteria for assignment of prognosis in vocal fold paralysis can vary, but generally, preservation of normal motor unit waveforms, activation of motor units during appropriate voluntary tasks, and preservation of a brisk degree of recruitment have been considered indicative of good prognosis. The presence of spontaneous activity and the absence of normal motor unit waveforms and recruitment are signs of poor prognosis. Time is also a highly relevant factor. The earlier favorable signs are identified, the more likely it is that spontaneous recovery will take place, although extremely early electromyographic assessment may exaggerate the degree of injury [30, 31]. Beyond 6 months, electromyography seems to be of limited use, as the potential for recovery is uniformly poor [32–34].

Laryngeal electromyography has been criticized as being "subjective." While this is true of certain aspects, particularly judgments regarding the integrity or impairment of recruitment with voluntary activity, most electromyographic findings – such as fibrillations, positive sharp waves, and polyphasic motor unit potentials – are clear, both in appearance and significance. Electromyography might be more properly described as qualitative rather than subjective: electromyographic findings require interpretation by a knowledgeable physician. In this regard it does not differ from laryngoscopy and stroboscopy, for example, except inasmuch as training and familiarity allows otolaryngologists to use these studies routinely and comfortably in daily practice. Strictly speaking, in fact, electromyography exceeds both of these in its ability to definitively – and objectively – diagnose vocal fold paralysis, as opposed to immobility.

The practical clinical difficulty has been that laryngeal electromyography appears to be unreliable in predicting recovery. That is, the appearance of unambiguous signs of reinnervation does not always lead to return of function. In fact, both animal and human studies have shown that a paralyzed vocal fold is only sometimes a denervated fold [16, 36, 37]. In many – perhaps most – cases, vocal fold muscles are reinnervated, but that reinnervation is often dysfunctional. This includes not only misdirected adductor and abductor innervation but also changes in neural organization peripherally and centrally (see Chap. 2). The complex, highly specialized nature of the laryngeal neuromotor system probably leaves many ways in which reinnervation may miscarry. Laryngeal electromyography is not able to reveal all of these subtleties, so that electromyographic evidence of nerve regrowth is not synonymous with vocal fold motion. Probably for this reason, laryngeal electromyography continues to occupy an indeterminate position in the evaluation of vocal fold paralysis in the minds of some practitioners.

The power of electromyography in revealing the failure of reinnervation is often overlooked in the eagerness to predict recovery. In this context, there are no physiologic ambiguities, and electromyographic findings reflect glottic function more reliably. Over time, the resting potential of a muscle cell that receives no neural input falls to near the depolarization threshold. From time to time, it crosses this threshold, and the single cell fires, depolarizes, and then repeats this cycle. On electromyography, this manifests as fibrillation potentials or positive sharp waves which occur spontaneously. These characteristic electrical features of denervation leave little to be misinterpreted and strongly suggest that (a) the initial injury is profound, and (b) there is little reinnervation of any sort. The more time that elapses from injury, the more definitive the finding becomes. Although potentially misleading very early in the course of the paralysis [30], spontaneous activity, with absent or scant voluntary motor unit activation, appears to be a highly accurate predictor of nonrecovery significantly earlier than 6 months [35, 38, 39, 40, 41]. A review of comparable studies of electromyographic assessment of vocal fold paralysis of less than 6 months duration (Table 6.1) reveals that accurate prediction of recovery does not exceed 80%, and has been reported to be as low as 13% when strict criteria for recovery of full range of motion are used. However, when determination of poor prognosis rests on the presence of spontaneous activity and absence (or scant presence) of motor units, laryngeal electromyography is an accurate predictor of the failure of recovery (75–100%).

This is clinically useful information that can be used to identify patients for early definitive intervention, eliminating a several-month wait for a vocally disabled person, or eliminating the need for a temporary intervention when a definitive one is likely to be ultimately necessary. At our centers, failure of reinnervation as demonstrated by electromyography has been a reliable finding as early as 3 months. Appropriately designed studies are needed to refine this observation further and determine more precisely how early such findings may be deemed to be significant.

Adjusting the Treatment Algorithm

The means of treating unilateral vocal fold paralysis are usually divided into temporary and definitive techniques. Temporary medialization is nearly synonymous with injection augmentation, as injectable substances do not persist reliably in the vocal fold. Polytetrafluoroethylene polymer (Teflon, Polytef), which has fallen into disfavor because of adverse tissue response, and calcium hydroxylapatite

Table 6.1. Laryngeal electromyography and unilateral vocal fold paralysis of <6 months duration

Reference	Year	Number of Cases	Accurate prediction	Accurate predition of recovery (%) of no/limited
[41]	2003	31[a]	80	80
[39]	2001	111	13	94
[30]	1993	18	70	75
[34]	1991	29[a]	63	80
[40]	1985	18	80	100

[a] Paralysis of less than 6 months duration

UVFP: Unilateral Vocal Fold Paralysis
EMG: Electromyography

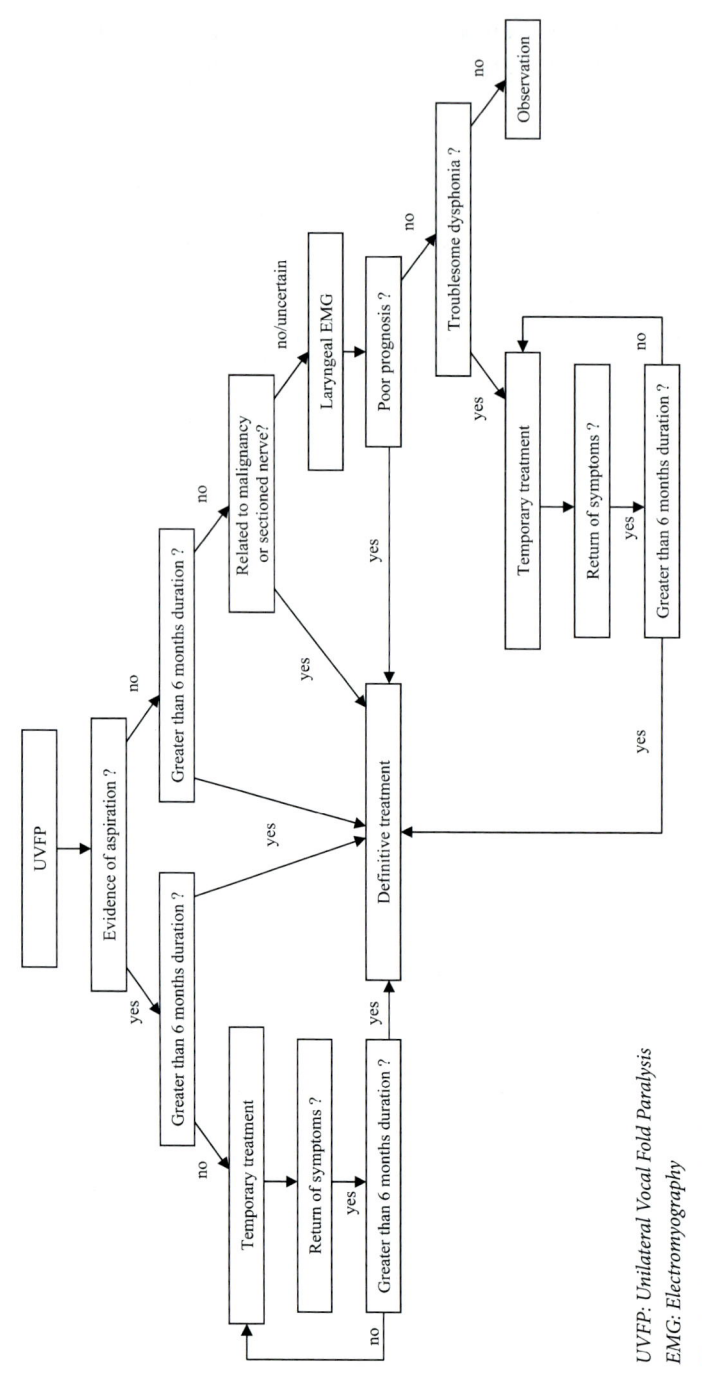

Fig. 6.1. Treatment of unilateral vocal fold paralysis

(Radiesse), which is undergoing evaluation for durability at the time of this writing, are the only exceptions to this. Definitive medialization therefore comprises medialization laryngoplasty and arytenoid repositioning procedures. Although absent from the algorithm presented here (Fig. 6.1), voice and swallowing therapy may prove useful in addition to these surgical measures in the symptomatic patient.

Because of potentially life-threatening consequences, the presence or absence of aspiration remains the most important consideration in patients with vocal fold paralysis. Selection of treatment depends on the duration of paralysis. In practice, patients with dysphagia present shortly after the onset of paralysis, making injection augmentation of a temporary substance a particularly suitable means of addressing their problems. Injection has been criticized as ineffective for closing posterior glottic gaps due to arytenoid malposition. If such an insufficiency appears to be a significant problem, framework surgery may be considered regardless of the time elapsed since the onset of paralysis.

In patients without significant dysphagia, and with unilateral vocal fold paralysis of long duration, framework surgery may be performed without further work-up. Although our algorithm specifies 6 months, the time interval after which medialization laryngoplasty becomes appropriate is not precisely established. Some surgeons prefer to wait as long as 12 months, both because of the potential for recovery, and because atrophy or reinnervation may shift the position of the vocal fold, even when mobility does not return. Since laryngoplasty provides a stable degree of medial vocal fold displacement, it is advantageous that the neuromuscular status of the vocal fold stabilize prior to the surgery. There is no information regarding the amount of time this takes, but obviously, the more time that is allowed to pass since onset, the likelier it is that there will be little further change.

Patients with vocal fold paralysis due to tumor compression or invasion, or nerve section, may also be treated early because of the dismal prospect for recovery of vocal fold motion. Atrophy may be more likely in these patients, a factor which may need to be taken into account, particularly if a medialization laryngoplasty is being performed soon after onset.

Laryngeal electromyography is useful to evaluate patients who present within a few months of the onset of their dysphonia, and in iatrogenic cases of vocal fold paralysis when status of the nerve is unknown or presumed to be intact. In most practices, the majority of patients fall into this category. Patients with poor prognosis should be considered for early definitive treatment. On the other hand, patients with good or indeterminate prognosis may be observed, or, if dysphonia is bothersome, may undergo injection augmentation. If dysphonia returns after the injectate resorbs, medialization laryngoplasty provides a long-term remedy.

Conclusion

An assessment of certain simple aspects of each case of vocal fold paralysis, combined with a choice of surgical techniques, allows the development of a rational treatment strategy that approaches the ideal proposed in the introduction. There is no doubt that it could be further refined by additional information regarding the natural history of vocal fold paralysis, which, in many respects, remains poorly defined despite more than a century of clinical study. More sophisticated electrodiagnostic techniques, combined with a better understanding of laryngeal neurophysiology, is needed to understand the phenomenon of inappropriate reinnervation in the larynx and its clinical implications.

References

1. Tabaee A, Murry T, Zschommler A, Desloge RB (2005) Flexible endoscopic evaluation of swallowing with sensory testing in patients with unilateral vocal fold immobility: incidence and pathophysiology of aspiration. Laryngoscope 115:565–569
2. Bhattacharyya N, Kotz T, Shapiro J (2002) Dysphagia and aspiration with unilateral vocal cord immobility: incidence, characterization, and response to surgical treatment. Ann Otol Rhinol Laryngol 111:672–679

3. Heitmiller RF, Tseng E, Jones B (2000) Prevalence of aspiration and laryngeal penetration in patients with unilateral vocal fold motion impairment. Dysphagia 15:184–187
4. Flint PW, Purcell LL, Cummings CW (1997) Pathophysiology and indications for medialization thyroplasty in patients with dysphagia and aspiration. Otolaryngol Head Neck Surg 116:349–354
5. Baron EM, Soliman AMS, Gaughan JP, Simpson L, Young WF (2003) Dysphagia, hoarseness and unilateral true vocal fold motion impairment following anterior cervical diskectomy and fusion. Ann Otol Rhinol Laryngol 112:921–926
6. Bielamowicz S, Gupta A, Sekhar LN (2000) Early arytenoid adduction for vagal paralysis after skull base surgery. Laryngoscope 110:346–351
7. Netterville JL, Civantos FJ (1993) Rehabiliation of cranial nerve deficits after neurotologic skull base surgery. Laryngoscope 113 (Suppl 60):45–54
8. Bhattacharyya N, Batirel H, Swanson SJ (2003) Improved outcomes with early vocal fold medialization for vocal fold paralysis after thoracic surgery. Auris Nasus Larynx 30:71–75
9. Mom T, Filaire M, Advenier D, Guichard C, Naamee A, Escande G, Llompart X, Vallet L, Gabrillargues J, Courtalhiac C, Claise B, Gilain L (2001) Concomitant type I thyroplasty and thoracic operations for lung cancer: preventing respiratory complications associated with vagus or recurrent laryngeal nerve injury. J Thorac Cardiovasc Surg 121:642–648
10. Abraham MT, Bains MS, Downey RJ, Korst RJ, Kraus DH (2002) Type I thyroplasty for acute unilateral vocal fold paralysis following intrathoracic surgery. Ann Otol Rhinol Laryngol 111:667–671
11. Nayak VK, Bhattacharyya N, Kotz T, Shapiro J (2002) Patterns of swallowing failure following medialization in unilateral vocal fold immobility. Laryngoscope 112:1840–1844
12. Woodson G (1997) Cricopharyngeal myotomy and arytenoid adduction in the management of combined laryngeal and pharyngeal paralysis. Otolaryngol Head Neck Surg 116:339–343
13. Pietersen E (1982) The natural history of Bell's palsy. Am J Otol 4:107–111
14. Pietersen E (2002) Bell's palsy: The spontaneous course of 2500 peripheral facial nerve palsies of different etiologies. Acta Otolaryngol (Suppl) 549:4–30
15. Postma GN, Shockley WW (1998) Transient vocal fold immobility. Ann Otol Rhinol Laryngol 107:236–240
16. Blitzer A, Jahn AF, Keidar A (1996) Semon's law revisited: an electromyographic analysis of laryngeal synkinesis. Ann Otol Rhinol Laryngol 105:764–769
17. Crumley RL (2000) Laryngeal synkinesis revisited. Ann Otol Rhinol Laryngol 109:365–371
18. Netterville JL, Stone RE, Rainey C et al. (1991) Recurrent nerve avulsion for treatment of spastic dysphonia. Ann Otol Rhinol Laryngol 100:10–14
19. Aronson AE, Santo LW de (1983) Adductor spastic dysphonia: Three years after recurrent laryngeal nerve section. Laryngoscope 93:1–8
20. Apfelbaum RI, Kriskovich MD, Haller JR (2000) On the incidence, cause, and prevention of recurrent laryngeal nerve palsies during anterior cervical spine surgery. Spine 25:2906–2912
21. Morpeth JF, Williams MF (2000) Vocal fold paralysis after anterior cervical diskectomy and fusion. Laryngoscope 110:43–46
22. Netterville JL, Koriwchak MJ, Winkle M, Courey MS, Ossoff RH (1996) Vocal fold paralysis following the anterior approach to the cervical spine. Ann Otol Rhinol Laryngol 105:85–91
23. Jung A, Schramm J, Lehnerdt K, Herberhold C (2005) Recurrent laryngeal nerve palsy during anterior cervical spine surgery: a prospective study. J Neurosurg Spine 2:123–127
24. Woodson GE, Miller RH (1981) The timing of surgical intervention in vocal cord paralysis. Otolaryngol Head Neck Surg 89:264–267
25. Hahn FW, Martin JT, Lilliei JC (1970) Vocal cord paralysis with endotracheal intubation. Arch Otolaryngol 92:226–229
26. Netterville JL, Jackson CG, Miller FR, Wanamaker JR, Glasscock ME (1998) Vagal paraganglioma: a review of 46 patients treated during a 20-year period. Arch Otolaryngol Head Neck Surg 124:1133–1140
27. Tsunoda K, Kikkiwa YS, Kumada M, Higo R, Tayama N (2003) Hoarseness caused by unilateral vocal fold paralysis: How long should one delay phonosurgery? Acta Otolaryngol 123:555–556
28. León X, Venegas MP, Orús C, Quer M, Maranillo E, Sañudo JR (2001) Inmovilidad glótica: Estudio retrospectivo de 229 casos. Acta Otorrinolaringol Esp 52:486–492
29. Havas T, Lowinger D, Priestly J (1999) Unilateral vocal fold paralysis: causes, options and outcomes. Aust N Z J Surg 69:509–513
30. Gupta SR, Bastian RW (1993) Use of laryngeal electromyography in prediction of recovery after vocal cord paralysis. Muscle Nerve 16:977–976
31. Munin MC, Murry T, Rosen CA (2000) Laryngeal electromyography: diagnostic and prognostic applications. Otolaryngol Clin N Am 33:759–770
33. Hiroto I, Hirano M, Tomita H (1968) Electromyographic investigation of human vocal cord paralysis. Ann Otol Rhinol Laryngol 77:296–304
34. Hirano M, Nozoe I, Shin T, Maeyama T (1991) Electromyography for laryngeal paralysis. In: Hirano

M, Kirchner JA, Bless DM (eds) Neurolaryngology: recent advances. Singular, San Diego, pp 232–248
35. Min YB, Finnnegan EM, Hoffman HT, Luschei ES, McCulloch TM (1994) A preliminary study of the prognositic role of electromyography in laryngeal paralysis. Otolaryngol Head Neck Surg 111:770–775
36. Crumley RL, McCabe BF (1982) Regeneration of the recurrent laryngeal nerve. Otolaryngol Head Neck Surg 90:442–447
37. Zealear DL, Hamdan AL, Rainey CL (1994) The effects of denervation on posterior cricoarytenoid muscle physiology and histochemistry. Ann Otol Rhinol Laryngol 103:780–788
38. Mostafa BE, Gadallah NA, Nassar NM, Al-Ibiary HM, Fahmy HA, Fouda NM (2004) The role of laryngeal electromyography in vocal fold immobility. Otorhinol Laryngol 66:5–10
39. Sittel C, Stennert E, Thumfart WF, Dapunt U, Eckel HE (2001) Prognostic value of laryngeal electromyography in vocal fold paralysis. Arch Otolaryngol Head Neck Surg 127:155–160
40. Parnes SM, Satya-Murti S (1985) Predicitive value of laryngeal electromyography in patients with vocal cord paralysis of neurogenic origin. Laryngoscope 95:1323–1326
41. Munin MC, Rosan CA, Zullo T (2003) Utility of laryngeal electromyography in predicting recovery after vocal fold paralysis. Arch Phys Med Rehabil 84:1150–1153

Chapter 7

Voice Therapy for Unilateral Vocal Fold Paralysis

Celia F. Stewart, Elizabeth Allen

Introduction

Behavioral voice therapy can be helpful in rehabilitating the weak breathy voice quality often associated with vocal fold paralysis. Voice therapy has been found to be effective both as a stand-alone treatment and in conjunction with medical treatments. The remediation presented in this chapter will be based on the physiology of voice production and the associated rehabilitation procedures.

Assessment

Assessment of voice and swallowing is performed to identify the history of the disorder, the clinical symptoms of the paralysis, and the severity of these symptoms in order to develop a rehabilitation plan and estimate the prognosis. Evaluation focuses on determining the specific consequences of vocal fold paralysis on the patient's respiration, phonation, resonance, articulation, and swallowing, and the effect of the disorder on the patient's life. During assessment, the effectiveness of a range of potential compensatory strategies is evaluated [24]. Information can be obtained from a variety of sources: videostroboscopic visualization of the vocal folds; case history; perceptual assessment; self-ratings; and acoustic and aerodynamic evaluation [20, 47]. A multidimensional voice evaluation gives the most complete analysis of the disorder and best insight into therapy outcomes [20, 62, 66]. A detailed interview gathers facts about the nature and onset of the symptoms, typical pattern of voice use, swallowing symptoms, detection of vocal irritations such as throat clearing, pertinent medical information, and identification of factors that may interfere with rehabilitation [44].

Perceptual Assessment

The pitch, loudness, and quality of the voice are evaluated perceptually by having a patient read a passage, produce conversational speech, or describe a picture or event. Voice tasks such as pitch and loudness range, glissando, s/z ratio, and maximum phonation time are used to assess vocal range and control. Perceptual ratings are very complex and the accuracy of the ratings is related to the level of experience and sophistication of the listener [6, 37].

The voice samples are recorded and pitch, intensity, and quality are rated on scales such as the GRBAS [25], the Buffalo voice profile scale [74], and clinician-devised scales. The perceptual symptoms most frequently associated with paralyzed vocal folds are breathiness [4, 13], reduced loudness [63], roughness, diplophonia [18, 61], and weak cough [61]. The most common physiologic results of unilateral vocal fold paralysis are inadequate glottal closure and asymmetrical vibration [47]. Breathiness, reduced loudness, and weak cough have been associated with leakage of air through the glottis during the closed phase of vibration and roughness has been associated with asymmetrical vibration of the vocal folds (Fig. 7.1; Table 7.1) [4, 47].

Self-Ratings

We assess the severity of the disorder by identifying not only the voice symptoms but also the limitations the voice disorder imposes on com-

Table 7.1. Speech breakdowns [4]

Speech symptoms	Common speech symptoms
Respiration	Short breath groups
	Decreased loudness of speech
	Reduced precision of articulation
	Diminished intelligibility
Phonation	Altered pitch
	Decreased loudness of speech
	Abnormal quality
	Phonation breaks
	Diminished intelligibility
Resonation/articulation	Changes in nasality
	Reduced precision of articulation
	Altered rhythm of speech
	Diminished intelligibility

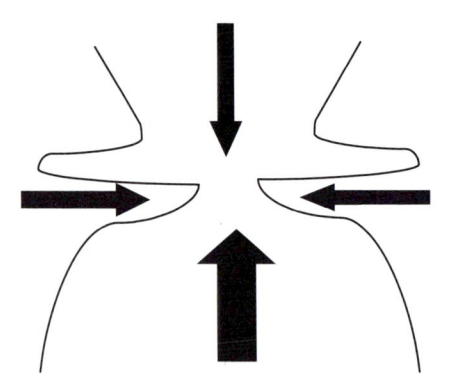

Fig 7.1. Back pressure during articulation of consonants. During production of consonants pressure is generated supraglottally by the closure of the vocal tract. This pressure increases the subglottal pressure that is necessary to generate vibration of the vocal folds. Consequently, the subglottal pressure must exceed the pressure from the medial compression of the vocal folds and the supraglottal pressure so that vibration will occur

munication. Voice disorders have long been associated with changes in self-image and with economic and social handicaps [73]. Patients report alterations in response to stress and frustration, withdrawal from social situations, depression, and changes at work [3, 53, 64]. Several new self-assessment tools have been developed to quantify the effect of dysphonia on quality of life: the Voice Handicap Index (VHI) [32], the Voice Outcome Survey [22], the Voice related Quality-of-Life Instrument [29], the Outcome Scale [17], and the Three-Item Outcome Scale [66]. The VHI has been the most widely investigated and has been shown to be effective for quantifying patient's perception of disability related to voice disorder [7, 9, 32, 53] and for identifying changes related to therapy [45].

Objective Measurements

Acoustic, aerodynamic, and physiologic assessments, such as jitter, shimmer, noise-to-harmonic ratio, pitch range, loudness range, vital capacity, maximum phonation time, average intensity of conversation, s/z ratio, quasi-open quotient, cepstrum analysis, and glottal air flow, have been used to measure the severity of disorders and treatment outcomes [12, 14, 24, 27, 39, 54]. In addition, acoustic analysis can be useful in quantifying the effects of treatments [11, 23, 27]. Unfortunately, some disordered voices cannot be analyzed acoustically because of their erratic vibration patterns. Acoustic and aerodynamic measures are most effective and give a more complete picture of voice production when used in conjunction with perceptual measures [15].

Compensations

The severity of the voice disorder can be exacerbated by the patient's response to the voice symptoms. These responses include changes in posture and muscle tone. A patient may use compensatory maneuvers to help the voice but inadvertently place strain on the voice production system [9]. Compensatory maneuvers that lead to vocal fatigue include increasing supraglottal constriction and increasing expiratory drive [8]. These activities can result in short-term improvement in voice production but can also lead to vocal fatigue, strident voice, and worsening of the voice symptoms. In addition, these hyperfunctional compensations can be the source of increased effort when speaking [8, 26, 35, 61]. Patients' self-assessment of their vocal performance is often related to their perception of the effort required to make functional voice. When effort increases, satisfaction can decrease (Table 7.2).

Guidelines for Planning Voice Therapy

Deciding whether to use medical, surgical, and behavioral therapies individually or jointly is determined by the patient's vocal performance and history. Perceptual and acoustic ratings are only moderately correlated with vocal fold vibration and consequently no single component of a voice evaluation is adequate to predict the overall response to rehabilitation [24, 66]. In addition, all relevant factors, such as reflux, allergies, and depression, should be addressed.

Guidelines for when to offer voice therapy have been offered based on laryngeal behavior, etiology, objective ratings, and the patient's gender [24]. A period of voice therapy should be considered for those patients with unilateral vocal fold paralysis, strong cough, and adequate airway protection [41]. In addition, female patients may have a better response to both behavioral and surgical intervention than males [24].

Patients with milder symptoms and adequate airway protection may be better candidates for voice therapy. Where the nerve has been preserved, voice therapy is recommended prior to restorative surgery [24, 61]. The possible benefit from voice therapy can be determined after one or two sessions of voice therapy. Several studies have suggested that 4–6 weeks is the minimum time required for patients to achieve sustained benefit from voice therapy [55, 59, 68]. The clinical standard has been to wait 6 months before surgical intervention to allow for reinnervation. It is beneficial to have a voice reassessment at the end of the 6-month period to determine if voice function has improved sufficiently so that the patient can benefit from voice therapy.

Voice therapy has also been found to be effective when implemented prior to medical intervention to augment the effectiveness of the surgical treatment [24, 61]. A patient who has relied on counterproductive compensatory vocal behaviors may not have optimal results following surgery because these compensations may not spontaneously resolve [24]. Behavioral therapy can decrease these hyperfunctional

Table 7.2. Counterproductive compensation and associated symptoms

Types of counterproductive behavior	Some symptoms of counterproductive compensation
Nonlinguistic effortful movements	Nonproductive throat clearing and coughing
Increased effort during speech	Strident, strained, rough voice quality with abrupt onset of voicing; vocal fatigue
Extraneous muscle activity in the head, neck, and shoulders	Supraglottal constriction, frown lines, cording of neck muscles, and elevated shoulders

compensations and reduce extraneous muscle activity so that the surgeon will get the best results [31]. Behavioral voice therapy is most effective when it is administered both shortly before and immediately after restorative surgery [24, 31].

Patterns of Vocal Symptoms

Two dominant patterns of voice symptoms have emerged: hypofunctional and hyperfunctional [24]. The hypofunctional pattern includes the symptoms that are directly related to the paralysis [4, 13]. The hyperfunctional pattern emerges as a counterproductive response to the underlying disorder and is associated with voice strain and fatigue [24, 31, 50]. Accurate identification of these two patterns allows appropriate treatment. The hyperfunctional compensations include supraglottic activity that is used to compensate for lack of glottic closure and may be associated with effortful voicing, fatigue, and laryngeal pain. Usually, these compensations are not eliminated by surgical intervention and the overall response to surgery may be enhanced by speech therapy [10, 24, 31, 51].

Rehabilitation Hypotheses

Behavioral rehabilitation hypotheses are developed based on the pattern of perceptual symptoms, objective voice measures, the vocal needs of the patient, the skill with which the patient generalizes the new voice production, the factors that interfere with improved production of voice, and the patient's compliance with vocal practice [47]. During therapy, rehabilitation hypotheses are revised in response to the patient's performance in therapy. For those patients with breathy, diplophonic voice, weak glottal coup, and shortness of breath during speech, the symptoms result from excessive air leakage between the vocal folds [48]. One way to help the patient compensate for these symptoms is to minimize the leak and maximize vocal production. On the other hand, symptoms of breathiness, stridency, high-pitched voice, reduced loudness, cording of the neck muscles, and stiffness in the neck and shoulder area lead to the hypothesis that the symptoms result from a combination of excessive air leakage through the glottis and hyperfunctional compensation for this symptom. This hypothesis can be tested by reducing or eliminating the compensations and then working to improve the voice by minimizing the leakage of air [24].

Therapy Procedures

Voice therapy tasks can be divided into indirect procedures, direct procedures [62], and electronic enhancements. Indirect procedures consist of ongoing collection of history information, counseling, education, vocal hygiene, and maximizing posture [43, 62]. Direct approaches include normalization of expiratory drive, decreasing transglottal pressure, enhancing projection, and optimizing medial compression of the vocal folds [24, 31, 62]. Electronic enhancements consist of using instruments, such as portable amplification devices and telephone amplifiers, to project the voice. Sellars et al. [62] found that two-thirds of voice therapy treatment time was used in indirect therapy including descriptions of voice production, counseling, and eliminating postural tension.

Indirect Rehabilitation

Indirect therapy is based on the case history information and patient observations. It includes collecting information about the history of the disorder, compensations, and stance and developing strategies to compensate for factors that can worsen the symptoms including reflux, depression, and allergies. Counseling and education encompasses describing normal physiology and the impact of vocal paralysis on voicing, relating the effect of vocal fold paralysis to airway protection, and exposing the compensations the patient is using to improve his voice.

Indirect therapy also addresses the problems that result when an individual attempts to compensate for a paralyzed vocal fold by performing effortful closure of the glottis before and during speech. Common hyperfunctional compensations include nonproductive throat clearing and coughing [43, 62]. These compensations develop because they can lead to momentary improvement in voice. The patient may have identified these behaviors accidentally when temporary relief occurred after throat clearing, lifting a heavy box, or stiffening his head and neck area. It may be difficult to stop the maladaptive behavior because it allows for improved voice in some situations; however, the use of the compensation can lead to a worsening of the voice disorder. The brisk closure caused by throat clearing and coughing can irritate the vocal folds and cause vocal fatigue. If a patient has been using nonproductive throat clearing and coughing for a number of years, stopping the behavior can be difficult [63].

Another compensatory behavior is changing stance and using extraneous muscle activity in the head, neck, and shoulder areas [43, 62]. Subtle postural changes can have a negative impact on voice production and are addressed in therapy [43, 62]. Postural muscle tension includes clenching the jaw, tightening the lips, furrowing the forehead, tilting the head, or stiffening the neck and shoulders. Subtle postural changes can result from ineffective compensation in reaction to forcing the voice or from unrelated injury. Postural changes are identified by observing a patient's stance and are reduced by making the patient aware of the location and having the patient consciously relax the muscle contraction. Decreasing the muscle tension in the head, neck, and chest areas can enhance control of expiratory drive and foster comfortable breathing during speech [16, 43, 63, 67].

Direct Rehabilitation

Direct therapy activities improve closure of the glottis [62]. One method focuses on increasing adduction of the vocal folds by pushing [13, 75] and was first introduced by Froeschels in 1955 [21]. Pushing exercises should be avoided because they may exacerbate hyperfunction and may cause collisional trauma which may result in vocal fatigue, air loss, neck discomfort, and strident voice quality [24, 43]. Other exercises are probably as effective and have less potential for harm [24, 60].

Inconsistent results have been reported about the effect of head position on voice production [42, 47, 72]. McFarlane reported that rapid and sometimes dramatic change could be precipitated by having a patient rotate his head toward the paralyzed vocal fold [42]. Watterson et al. [72] found an inconsistent and minor positive effect on glottal closure. In contrast, Paseman et al. [47] found no change in airflow, open quotient, or maximum flow declination rate with head rotation. The differences in response to the procedure may reflect the measurements that were used to identify the change. McFarlane et al. [42] measured vocal intensity associated with increased vocal effort, whereas Paseman measured aerodynamic changes [47].

Other direct therapies include procedures to maximize optimal phonation through modifying expiratory drive, medial compression of the vocal folds, and back pressure [62]. One way to decrease expiratory drive is to have the patient speak using a quiet confidential voice [43]. This therapy is based on the phenomena that the voice is clearer and carries better when it is softer and breathy such as the voice used in quiet confidential communication [43, 58]. When a patient speaks in a quiet confidential voice, the air pressure and air flow are decreased to match the resistance of the vocal folds. By controlling the pressure and flow of air, individuals can control the loudness of their voice, the breath groups used in speaking, and the pressure to articulate consonants [28, 46, 52, 71]. When the subglottal pressure is matched to the tension of the vocal folds, a more balanced relationship is established and vocal fold vibration improves. If the air flow is too weak, the vocal folds will not vibrate, and if the expiratory drive is too strong, the vocal fold is displaced laterally and the voice is compromised. In addition, a softer breathy voice is preferable because it „carries much better than does a louder, strained, and effortful voice" [43].

Manipulating the sounds in a syllable can alter the amount of glottal closure of the vocal folds. When syllables contain voiceless sounds, the vocal folds are partially abducted and medial compression is decreased. Conversely, when syllables contain voiced consonants and vowels, the medial compression is increased. Improved voicing has been associated with light glottal closure in larynxes with partial laryngeal paralysis [72]. Firm glottal closure is more likely to occur at conversational loudness and pitch than at elevated pitch or loudness [72]. This effect has been attributed to the greater mass per unit length and greater compliance of the vocal fold at lower pitches and loudness levels. Watterson et al. [72] speculated that this increased mass and compliance enhances medial approximation during the closed phase. They further theorized that decreased mass and compliance during high pitch and loudness could hamper glottal closure. Watterson et al. [72] also found that paralyzed folds usually have greater amplitude of vibration than healthy ones, probably due to decreased tension. Appropriate glottal closure can be facilitated by having a patient sustain vowels and produce glissandos in a quiet voice [43, 68].

Another way to modify the strength of glottal closure is by adjusting the pressure above the glottis. Back pressure is generated and manipulated by changing resonation, articulation of consonants. As air pressure builds behind a point of constriction or closure, pressure in the oral and pharyngeal cavities increases and equalizes the aerodynamic and myoelastic forces [18, 43]. Supraglottal pressure is directly related to the sounds that are being produced and require specific control of breathing [5, 40]. When there is increased pressure above the glottis and the pressure below the glottis remains unchanged, the pressure differential across the glottis decreases. In English, the greatest amount of oral and pharyngeal pressure is generated by producing stops and nasal sounds. Conversely, vowels generate the least back pressure. Furthermore, voiced stops are created with larger volumes of supraglottal air than voiceless stops [36, 38, 49]. Since consonants such as /b/ generate large amounts of back pressure, whereas vowels produce little back pressure, the pressure across the glottis can be controlled by manipulating the sounds in speech. Therapy tokens, such as /umhum/ and /mi, mi/ [19, 43], increase the back pressure and facilitate gentle vibration by decreasing the pressure change across the glottis [70].

Transfer of Skills

For the voice to be effective and efficient, a speaker must consistently and reliably modify his production to meet his vocal needs. For some speakers the performance demands are limited to conversational speech. The vocal demands for professional voice users include singing and dramatic speaking in a variety of contexts. The rehabilitation process must include consideration of the demands that the patient places on his voice and help the patient meet these demands. Transfer of the skills is easiest if the transfer begins early in the rehabilitation process.

Vocal Practice

When we provide behavioral voice therapy to a patient with a paralyzed vocal fold, only a small part of the practice occurs during the session. In order for therapy to be effective, a patient must practice frequently so that stamina is increased and so that the new manner of voice production becomes habitual; therefore, therapy sessions focus on identifying and perfecting voice production. Voice practice outside of the therapy session focuses on habituating the new vocal production in a variety of settings. The patient's compliance with the homework and therapy varies based on many factors including effectiveness of the therapy, patient's interest, adverse effects, ease of use, and health [1, 57].

Communicating in Noisy Environments

We live in a noisy world and need to be heard in many situations. Some of the most difficult situations are environments where multiple people are talking simultaneously such as classrooms or cafeterias. Unfortunately, one of the symptoms of vocal fold paralysis is decreased loudness of speech. Communication in noise can be enhanced in several ways: changing the situation; using amplification; and projecting the voice [43]. One of the best ways to change the environment is to improve the acoustics. If that is not possible, the individual can move closer to the listener when speaking and talk in smaller groups.

Unfortunately, it is not always possible to adjust the environment. Amplification by electronic devices is one solution to this difficult problem [33, 34, 43, 56, 57]. Both portable amplification devices and phone amplification are available. When decreased loudness is the only symptom, amplification is effective for enhancing the voice and improving overall voice clarity [38, 56, 57]. Jonsdottir et al. [34] and Roy et al. [56] speculated that using amplification helped patients to produce the strongest voice with the least effort. Improvements in technology, through the use of hands-free cell phones and wireless microphones, have made amplification devices smaller, more available, and socially acceptable.

A third way to enhance voice production in noise is using increased resonance to project the voice [62, 69]. Even though the voice is weakened, therapy can focus on maximizing the projection so that the voice will be as effective as possible. Voice resonance is enhanced when the phonation threshold pressure is reduced and appropriate breath support is provided [69]. Projection should be done without respiratory, glottal, or extraneous effort [69]. Voice projection for patients with paralyzed vocal folds relies on coordinating gentle production of voice by speaking in a quieter breathy voice, decreasing the air flow and the subglottal air pressure, and decreased medial compression of the vocal folds with focusing the voice in front of the lips. By placing the confidential voice in front of the lips, the voice will be stronger, carry farther, and be effortless.

Results

Prognosis for benefit from therapy can be estimated by testing a patient's response to therapy procedures. Patients usually have a good response to therapy if they have improved voice or a reduction in physiologic effort after one or two sessions of therapy. Coordination of the systems of respiration, phonation, and resonation, articulation allows the voice to be produced with less effort and as efficiently and effectively as possible [30]. When the speech actions are not coordinated, effort increases and breakdown occurs. Patients' self-assessment of satisfaction with vocal performance is often inversely related to the amount of effort that is required to produce voice. Good results to voice therapy were reported in patients who had unilateral recurrent laryngeal nerve paralysis following thoracic surgery and in patients with superior laryngeal nerve paresis [2, 61].

Conclusion

Treating patients with paralyzed vocal folds can be very gratifying. Almost all patients who have some residual movement and adequate airway protection improve in response to treatment. Therapy procedures focus on maximizing the efficiency of voice production by ensuring that all appropriate medical treatments have been explored, minimizing compensations that are counterproductive, educating the patient about the voice disorder, balancing the pressures in the vocal tract, and transferring the enhanced voice production to a variety of vocal situations [62]. Using a combination of techniques for assessment and treatment allows for identification of factors that cause and perpetuate the voice disorder and enables the clinician to adjust the therapy as needed [72]. Remediation focuses on maximizing the efficiency with which the patient uses the voice so that optimal voice production can occur with the least effort.

References

1. Ackerstaff AH, Hilgers FJ, Balm AJ, Tan IB (1998) Long-term compliance of laryngectomized patients with a specialized pulmonary rehabilita-

tion device: Provox Stomafilter. Laryngoscope 108:257–260
2. Anderson T, Sataloff RT (2002) The power of voice therapy. Ear Nose Throat J 81:433–434
3. Aronson AE (1969) Speech pathology and symptom therapy in the interdisciplinary treatment of psychogenic aphonia. J Speech Hear Disord 34:321–341
4. Aronson AE (1990) Clinical voice disorders, 3rd edn. Thieme, New York
5. Bailey EF, Hoit JD (2002) Speaking and breathing in high respiratory drive. J Speech Lang Hear Res 45:89–99
6. Bassich CJ, Ludlow CL (1986) The use of perceptual methods by new clinicians for assessing voice quality. J Speech Hear Disord 51:125–133
7. Behrman A, Sulica L, He T (2004) Factors predicting patient perception of dysphonia caused by benign vocal fold lesions. Laryngoscope 114:1693–1700
8. Belafsky PC, Postma GN, Reulbach TR, Holland BW, Koufman JA (2002) Muscle tension dysphonia as a sign of underlying glottal insufficiency. Otolaryngol Head Neck Surg 127:448–451
9. Benninger MS, Ahuja AS, Gardner G, Grywalski C (1998) Assessing outcomes for dysphonic patients. J Voice 12:540–550
10. Bielamowicz S (2004) Aging voice or vocal fold paresis: What can I do about it? Arch Otolaryngol Head Neck Surg 130:1114–1118
11. Bielamowicz S, Berke GS, Gerratt BR (1995) A comparison of type I thyroplasty and arytenoid adduction. J Voice Dec 9:466–472
12. Billante CR, Clary J, Childs P, Netterville JL (2002) Voice gains following thyroplasty may improve over time. Clin Otolaryngol 27:89–94
13. Boone DR, McFarlane S (1988) The voice and voice therapy. Prentice-Hall, Englewood Cliffs, New Jersey
14. Brasnu DF, Hans S, Hartl DM, Riquet M, Vaissiere J (2001) Objective voice quality analysis before and after onset of unilateral vocal fold paralysis. J Voice 15:351–361
15. Carding PN, Steen IN, Webb A, MacKenzie K, Deary IJ, Wilson JA (2004) The reliability and sensitivity to change of acoustic measures of voice quality. Clin Otolaryngol 29:538–544
16. Casper JK (2000) Vocal fold paralysis–paresis–immobility. In: Freeman M, Fawcus M (eds) Voice disorders and their management, 3rd edn. Whurr, London
17. Casper JK (2001) Treatment outcomes in occupational voice disorders. In: DeJonckere PH (ed) Occupational voice: care and cure. Kugler Publications, The Hague, pp 187–199
18. Colton RH, Casper JK (1996) Understanding voice problems: a physiological perspective for diagnosis and treatment, 2nd edn. Williams and Wilkins, Baltimore
19. Cooper M (1984) Change your voice, change your life. Macmillan, New York
20. DeJonckere PH, Crevier-Buchman L, Marie JP, Moerman M, Remacle M, Woisard V (2003) Implementation of the European Laryngological Society (ELS) basic protocol for assessing voice treatment effect. Rev Laryngol Otol Rhinol (Bord) 124:279–283
21. Froeschels E, Kastein S, Weiss D (1955) A method of therapy for paralytic conditions of the mechanisms of phonation, resonation, and glutination. J Speech Hear Disord 20:365–370
22. Gliklich RE, Glovsky RM, Montgomery WW (1999) Validation of a voice outcome survey for unilateral vocal cord paralysis. Otolaryngol Head Neck Surg 120:153–158
23. Gray SD, Barkmeier J, Jones D, Titze I, Druker D (1992) Vocal evaluation of thyroplastic surgery in the treatment of unilateral vocal fold paralysis. Laryngoscope 102:415–421
24. Heuer RJ, Sataloff RT, Emerich K, Rulnick R, Baroody M, Spiegel JR, Durson G, Butler J (1997) Unilateral recurrent laryngeal nerve paralysis: the importance of «preoperative» voice therapy. J Voice 11:88–94
25. Hirano M (1981) Clinical examination of voice. Springer, Berlin, Heidelberg New York
26. Hirano M, Koike Y, Joyner J (1969) Style of phonation. An electromyographic investigation of some laryngeal muscles. Arch Otolaryngol 89:902–907
27. Hirano M, Hibi S, Yoshida T, Hirade Y, Kasuya H, Kikuchi Y (1988) Acoustic analysis of pathological voice. Some results of clinical application. Acta Otolaryngol 105:432–438
28. Hixon TJ (1987) Respiratory function in speech. In: Hixon TJ (ed) Respiration function in speech and song. College Hill Press, Boston, pp 1–54
29. Hogikyan ND, Sethuraman G (1999) Validation of an instrument to measure voice-related quality of life. J Voice 13:557–569
30. Huber JE, Stathopoulos ET (2003) Respiratory and laryngeal responses to an oral air pressure bleed during speech. J Speech Lang Hear Res 46:1207–1220
31. Isshiki N (1998) Mechanical and dynamic aspects of voice production as related to voice therapy and phonosurgery. J Voice 12:125–137
32. Jacobson BH, Johnson A, Grywalski C et al. (1997) The Voice Handicap Index (VHI): development and validation. Am J Speech Lang Pathol 6:66–70
33. Jonsdottir VI (2002) Cordless amplifying system in classrooms. A descriptive study of teachers' and students' opinions. Logoped Phoniatr Vocol 27:29–36

34. Jonsdottir V, Rantala L, Laukkanen AM, Vilkman E (2001) Effects of sound amplification on teachers' speech while teaching. Logoped Phoniatr Vocol 26:118–123
35. Kelchner LN, Lee L, Stemple JC (2003) Laryngeal function and vocal fatigue after prolonged reading in individuals with unilateral vocal fold paralysis. J Voice 17:513–528
36. Kent RD, Moll KL (1969) Vocal-tract characteristics of the stop cognates. Acoust Soc Am 46:1549–1555
37. Kreiman J, Gerratt BR, Kempster GB, Erman A, Berke GS (1993) Perceptual evaluation of voice quality: review, tutorial, and a framework for future research. J Speech Hear Res 36:21–40
38. Lubker J (1973) Transglottal airflow during stop consonant production. J Acoust Soc Am 53:212–215
39. MacKenzie K, Millar A, Wilson JA, Sellars C, Deary IJ (2001) Is voice therapy an effective treatment for dysphonia? A randomized controlled trial. Br Med J 323:658–661
40. MacLarnon AM, Hewitt GP (1999) The evolution of human speech: the role of enhanced breathing control. Am J Phys Anthropol 109:341–363
41. McFarlane SC, Holt-Romeo TL, Lavorato AS, Warner L (1991) Unilateral vocal fold paralysis: perceived vocal quality following three methods of treatment. Am J Speech Lang Pathol 1:45–48
42. McFarlane SC, Nelson W, Watterson TL (1998) Acoustic physiologic and aerodynamic effects of tongue protrusion /i/ in dysphonia. ASHA Leader 18:72
43. Miller S (2004) Voice therapy for vocal fold paralysis. Otolaryngol Clin North Am 37:105–119
44. Morrison MD, Rammage LA (1994) The management of voice disorders. Chapman and Hall, London
45. Murry T, Rosen CA, Sonbolian M, Zinn A, Zullo T (2000) Voice handicap index change following treatment of voice disorders. J Voice 14:619–623
46. Netter FH (1980) The CIBA collection of medical illustrations, vol 7, respiratory system. CIBA, West Caldwell, New Jersey
47. Paseman A, Casper J, Colton R, Kelley R (2004) The effect of head position on glottic closure in patients with unilateral vocal fold paralysis. J Voice 18:242–247
48. Perie S, Roubeau B, Liesenfelt I, Chaigneau-Debono G, Bruel M, Guily JL (2002) Role of medialization in the improvement of breath control in unilateral vocal fold paralysis. Ann Otol Rhinol Laryngol 111:1026–1033
49. Perkell J (1969) Physiology of speech production: results and implications of a quantitative cineradiographic study. MIT Press, Cambridge Massachusetts
50. Phillips P (1998) Voice range in superior laryngeal nerve paresis and paralysis. J Voice 12:340–348
51. Pinho SM, Pontes PA, Gadelha ME, Biasi N (1999) Vestibular vocal fold behavior during phonation in unilateral vocal fold paralysis. J Voice 13:36–42
52. Proctor DF (1980) Breathing, speech, and song. Springer, Berlin Heidelberg New York
53. Ramig LO, Verdolini K (1998) Treatment efficacy: voice disorders. J Speech Lang Hear Res 41:S101–S116
54. Rihkanen H, Reijonen P, Lehikoinen-Soderlund S, Lauri ER (2004) Videostroboscopic assessment of unilateral vocal fold paralysis after augmentation with autologous fascia. Eur Arch Otorhinolaryngol 261:177–183
55. Roy N, Gray SD, Simon M, Dove H, Corbin-Lewis K, Stemple JC (2001) An evaluation of the effects of two treatment approaches for teachers with voice disorders: a prospective randomized clinical trial. J Speech Lang Hear Res 44:286–296
56. Roy N, Weinrich B, Gray SD, Tanner K, Toledo SW, Dove H, Corbin-Lewis K, Stemple JC (2002) Voice amplification versus vocal hygiene instruction for teachers with voice disorders: a treatment outcomes study. J Speech Lang Hear Res 45:625–638
57. Roy N, Weinrich B, Gray SD, Tanner K, Stemple JC, Sapienza CM (2003) Three treatments for teachers with voice disorders: a randomized clinical trial. J Speech Lang Hear Res 46:670–688
58. Russell BA, Cerny FJ, Stathopoulos ET (1998) Effects of varied vocal intensity on ventilation and energy expenditure in women and men. J Speech Lang Hear Res 41:239–248
59. Sabol JW, Lee L, Stemple JC (1995) The value of vocal function exercises in the practice regimen of singers. J Voice 9:27–36
60. Sataloff RT (1991) Professional voice: the science and art of clinical care. Raven Press, New York
61. Schneider B, Schickinger-Fischer B, Zumtobel M, Mancusi G, Bigenzahn W, Klepetko W, End A (2003) Concept for diagnosis and therapy of unilateral recurrent laryngeal nerve paralysis following thoracic surgery. Thorac Cardiovasc Surg 51:327–331
62. Sellars C, Carding PN, Deary IJ, MacKenzie K, Wilson JA (2002) Characterization of effective primary voice therapy for dysphonia. J Laryngol Otol 116:1014–1018
63. Shulman S (2000) Symptom modification for chronic cough syndrome. In: Stemple J (ed) Voice therapy. Singular, San Diego, pp 341–349
64. Smith E, Verdolini K, Gray S, Nichols S, Lemke J, Barkmeier J, Dove H, Hoffman H (1996) Effect of voice disorders on quality of life. J Med Speech Lang Pathol 4:223–244

65. Speyer R, Wieneke GH, Dejonckere PH (2004) Self-assessment of voice therapy for chronic dysphonia. Clin Otolaryngol 29:66–74
66. Speyer R, Wieneke GH, Dejonckere PH (2004) Documentation of progress in voice therapy: perceptual, acoustic, and laryngostroboscopic findings pretherapy and posttherapy. J Voice 18:325–340
67. Stempel JC, Glaze LE, Klaben BG (2000) Clinical voice pathology: theory and management, 3rd edn. Singular, San Diego
68. Stemple JC, Lee L, D'Amico B, Pickup B (1994) Efficacy of vocal function exercises as a method of improving voice production. J Voice 8:271–278
69. Titze IR (2001) Acoustic interpretation of resonant voice. J Voice 15:519–528
70. Verdolini K, Druker DG, Palmer PM, Samawi H (1998) Laryngeal adduction in resonant voice. J Voice 12:315–327
71. van den Berg JW (1956) Direct and indirect determination of the mean subglottal pressure. Folia Phoniatrica 8:1–24
72. Watterson T, McFarlane SC, Menicucci AL (1990) Vibratory characteristics of Teflon-injected and noninjected paralyzed vocal folds. J Speech Hear Disord 55:61–66
73. White F (1946) Some causes of hoarseness in children. Ann Otol Rhinol Laryngol 55:537–542
74. Wilson DK (1987) Voice problems in children, 3rd edn. Williams and Wilkins, Baltimore
75. Yamaguchi H, Yotsukura Y, Sata H, Watanabe Y, Hirose H, Kobayashi N, Bless DM (1993) Pushing exercise program to correct glottal incompetence. J Voice 7:250–256

Chapter 8

Injection Augmentation

Karen Cooper, Charles N. Ford

Introduction

The essential goal of injection laryngoplasty is to implant a substance that can fill space and restore characteristics of the vocal fold favoring oscillation without inducing adverse tissue reaction. To this end, it is desirable to use a substance with characteristics of vocal fold lamina propria. The evolution of injection laryngoplasty began with a simple goal of filling space to achieve glottic competence with an inert substance that could be easily injected. Later clinical interest was directed at bio-implants because they more closely resembled tissues in the vocal fold lamina propria. Rather than posing a risk of granuloma or migration, the bio-implants (collagen, fat, fascia) tend to be assimilated and replaced with host tissue. Bovine and human-derived materials were introduced, including xenographs, homographs, and autogenous material. Although space-filling remains an essential goal, the current challenge is to provide a substance that matches the viscoelastic properties of lamina propria or promotes generation of substances favorable for normal vocal fold oscillation.

Indications

The most common indication for vocal fold injection augmentation is unilateral vocal fold paralysis. Other problems treated this way include traumatic and iatrogenic tissue loss, scarring, neurogenic atrophy, and presbylaryngis.

Glottic insufficiency, or failure of the glottis to close, impairs cough, airway protection, and phonation. Patients complain of difficulty projecting their voices, increased phonation effort, breathy dysphonia, vocal fatigue, painful phonation, choking, and aspiration. Measures to treat vocal fold paralysis seek to resolve glottic insufficiency, to improve swallowing and voice production, and to decrease aspiration. Specific voice goals include decrease in patient effort and improvement in perceptual and acoustic parameters of voice quality. Although it is unrealistic to expect patients to have a completely normal voice after therapeutic intervention, the goal of treatment should be achievement of glottic competence with improvement of voice. The most common immediate response to restoration of glottic competence is that the patient experiences less effortful phonation, a louder voice with greater frequency range, and improved glottic efficiency measures. Improved harmonics-to-noise ratio and reduced phonatory threshold pressure correlate well with restoration of effective glottic closure during phonation.

Among the various methods of treating vocal glottic insufficiency, injection augmentation has the advantage of simplicity. The procedure involves injection of a substance into the vocal fold that passively displaces the medial aspect of the affected vocal fold toward the midline. When this is successful, glottic closure is accomplished by active adduction of the contralateral vocal fold. Injection augmentation can be easily and quickly performed in an office setting and usually requires only topical anesthesia. It produces immediate results, with improved phonation and glottic competence, and it is generally well tolerated by patients.

Historical Note

Injection augmentation of the vocal fold dates back to 1911, when Brünings injected paraffin via indirect laryngoscopy to medialize the immobile vocal fold [1]. Although paraffin allowed for adequate medialization with improved voice, the injectate often caused secondary paraffinomas. Paraffin was replaced by other inorganic or alloplastic materials, including silicone, Teflon (polytetrafluoroethylene), and a less viscous variant (Bioplastique). Similar but apparently less reactive implants consisting of suspended hydroxyl apatite particles (Radiance, Bioform, Franksville, Wis., and San Mateo, Calif.) have recently been introduced [2]. Due to foreign body reaction and granulomas caused by alloplasts, alternatives were sought. Bovine collagen (Zyderm, Collagen Corp., Palo Alto, Calif.) was the first bio-implant tried [3]; the cross-linked form (Zyplast, Collagen Corp., Palo Alto, Calif.) offered decreased risk of allergic reaction but was perhaps not as suitable for very superficial use. Both materials appeared to soften scar tissue and seemed suitable for small glottic gaps, focal scars, and tissue defects. Autologous collagen proved effective and safe [4] but cumbersome and costly, so it was abandoned. Later bio-implants included autogenous fat and fascia, and more recently, substances such as freeze-dried irradiated human fascia (Fascian, Fascia Biosystems, LLC, Beverly Hills, Calif.) [5] and micronized homologous dermis (Cymetra, Life-Cell Corporation, The Woodlands, Texas) [6] have become available. The essential problem with currently available bio-implants is their unpredictable durability in tissue [7]. Extracellular matrix components, such as hyaluronic acid with varying levels of cross-linkage to enhance durability (e.g., double cross-linked hyaluronan – Hylan B), are also being investigated [8]. Ongoing research is addressing the role of active substances that might attract favorable extracellular matrix ingrowths and growth factors that might induce production of favorable substances in the lamina propria [9].

Alloplastic materials allow more permanent medialization, whereas bio-implants tend to resorb over time; however, alloplastic materials, such as Teflon, have been associated with complications including foreign body reaction, granulomas, and injectate migration. Bio-implants are better tolerated, and may become incorporated in host tissues to replace normal extracellular matrix with a substance possessing similar viscoelastic properties. They can provide a matrix for ingrowth of natural host tissues. In these cases, long-term correction of vocal fold position and function is more important than persistence of the graft material. Certain bio-implants have fallen out of favor or have limited use due to various concerns, principally regarding long-term efficacy. Concerns regarding allergic reaction initially limited use of bovine collagen, but some practitioners still find it useful as a temporary filler and for very superficial applications. Injected fat is difficult to contour, tends to backflow out of the injection site, and needs to be placed throughout the vocal fold tissues because of the size of the needle (18–19 G). This makes precise medialization in an adynamic segment difficult. Furthermore, fat has a tendency to resorb; overinjection is necessary, and the extent of resorption can be difficult to predict.

Timing of Intervention

Timing of injection augmentation depends on several factors, including etiology of the paralysis, prognosis for return of function, and degree of functional impairment. When prognosis for recovery is poor or functional impairment is severe, as in the case of aspiration or severe dysphonia, injection can be performed immediately. There is usually little harm in immediately using a bio-implant for injection, given that it tends to resorb and does not pose a problem in the event of complete recovery from paralysis. When prognosis is unclear, alloplasts should not be used immediately, as they lead to irreversible tissue changes and possible symptomatic granulomas. On the other hand, in patients with grave prognoses, it is often best to proceed with immediate medialization using Teflon or other durable alloplastic material. Injection should generally be delayed for patients with a minimal functional impairment or a good prognosis.

Technique

Injection can be performed via direct laryngoscopy, indirect laryngoscopy, or under telescopic guidance. Injection techniques originally employed either indirect or direct laryngoscopy without magnification. Vocal fold injection has been facilitated by the development of fiberoptic endoscopy, which has improved visualization and accuracy and thus decreased morbidity. In addition, the improved visualization has allowed injection to be performed more accurately in the awake patient under topical anesthesia.

Although direct microlaryngoscopy can provide optimal exposure without requiring patient cooperation, laryngeal anatomy is distorted both by suspension laryngoscopy and the endotracheal tube. In addition, the procedure requires general anesthesia with its associated risks, and immediate functional outcome, including voice characteristics and status of the mucosal wave, cannot be assessed. Indirect laryngoscopy obviates the risks of general anesthesia and can be done in the office, although visualization is relatively poor. Telescopic laryngoscopy under topical anesthesia performed on the awake patient obviates these disadvantages. Visualization and precision are optimized (Fig 8.1). With the patient awake, incremental placement of the injectate guided by immediate functional assessment of voice and videostroboscopic observations can be performed. Either transoral or transcutaneous injection can be performed using telescopes. Transcutaneous injection combined with flexible fiberoptic laryngoscopy may be useful in patients with difficult laryngeal exposure due to such factors as impaired neck extension, strong gag reflex, omega-shaped epiglottis, or movement disorder. In such cases, either a straight or curved needle is placed through the cricothyroid membrane or through the thyroid cartilage directed into the affected vocal fold, with care taken not to enter the lumen. Topical laryngeal anesthesia is then not necessary, although local anesthesia may be injected at the cutaneous site of needle insertion. Choice of approach for injection depends largely on patient factors. Each patient must be considered individually, as exposure and appropriate patient selection are critical to the success of injection augmentation.

Optimal results depend on restoring proper glottic contour and matching the contralateral vocal fold. Ideally, the injectate should provide smooth medial displacement of the membranous vocal fold. Essentially, it should displace the injected vocal fold to reproduce the structure of the contralateral vocal fold, not only at the level of the vibratory margin, but in vertical cross section as well. If only the superior surface of the membranous vocal fold is displaced, the vocal fold may appear adequately medialized but the voice will remain dysphonic. This is in part due to the importance of the infraglottic region in achieving the proper geometric configuration of the glottis for optimal aerodynamic function [10]. Efficacy of injection should be judged both by the distance the vocal fold moves to the midline as well as the location along the membranous vocal fold where the movement occurs. Typically, the greatest need for medialization is in the mid and posterior vocal fold. Medialization in the anterior one-third of the vocal fold tends to be excessive, causing early contact with the contralateral vocal fold, impeding oscillation and degrading the voice. Over-medialization anteriorly can also limit posterior glottic closure so the voice might remain breathy and dysphonic after injection. One may attempt to displace the cartilaginous component of the vocal fold, and thus correct posterior glottic insufficiency, by placing injectate lateral to the vocal process and medially rotating the vocal process. Overall, the injection should restore vocal fold contour and glottic closure without disturbing normal viscoelasticity.

Office-Based Procedure

When the procedure is performed in clinic, the patient is seated in the sniffing position (leaning forward with the neck extended). It is helpful to have an assistant present to assist with videostroboscopy which is performed before, during, and after the procedure. A small amount of topical benzocaine is initially sprayed onto the soft palate and posterior oropharyngeal wall. The patient then extends and grasps his/her tongue with a 4×4 gauze sponge. Topical 4% lidocaine is incrementally dripped onto the tongue base, the laryngeal surface of the epiglottis, the supraglottis, and the true vocal folds during phonation. Approximately 0.3 ml is used with each step for a total of 1.2 ml, and approximately 1 min is allowed to elapse between each application. Either a laryngeal mirror or the rigid telescope may be used to provide visualization for this step. Proper application should provide adequate anesthesia.

As a general guideline, injection of alloplastic compounds should be relatively deep in the thyroarytenoid muscle and paraglottic space. Bio-implants are more forgiving, and although a variety of preferred placements have been described, most can be effective at levels varying from the superficial lamina propria to the deep thyroarytenoid muscle. Superficial placement can introduce stiffness and should be placed with accuracy and care not to over-inject, whereas deeper injection requires larger amounts and can be effective with less precision and some over-filling. Further discussion of specific injection substances is found elsewhere in this volume.

A Brünings syringe (Storz, St. Louis) with an 18-G needle is used to inject most alloplastic compounds. Teflon, the most time-honored of these, is injected lateral to the vocal ligament, into the thyroarytenoid muscle and paraglottic space (Fig. 8.2). This prevents extrusion of the material, limits distortion of the vocal fold, and minimizes stiffness. Teflon provides excellent medialization and is effective in patients with large glottic gaps; therefore, initial underinjection is preferred, with continuous observation, and intermittent videostroboscopy and voice

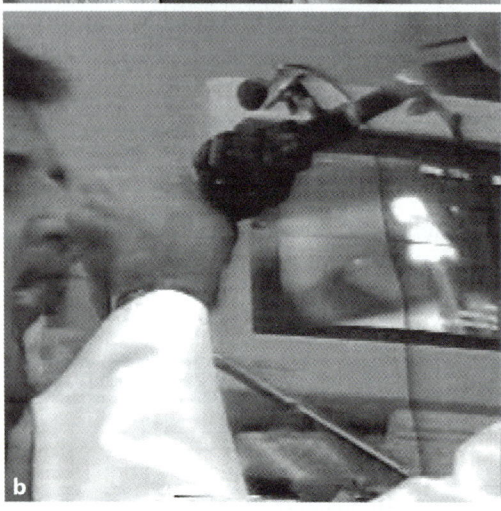

Fig. 8.1. a Telescopic guidance facilitates visualization of the vocal folds for injection. b Demonstration of transoral in-office injection with use of telescopic guidance

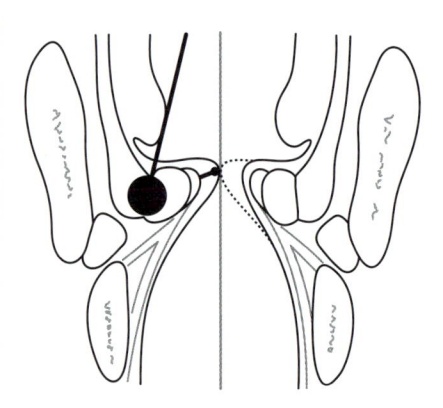

Fig. 8.2. Coronal section through vocal folds demonstrates alloplast injection into deep thyroarytenoid muscle on the left with resultant displacement of vocal fold to the midline. Dashed lines show projected motion of right vocal fold during phonation [13].

assessment. Injection begins just anterior and lateral to the tip of the vocal process of the arytenoid. If the glottic gap is not adequately corrected, more material may be injected into the mid-membranous vocal fold. Injection into the anterior one-third of the vocal fold as well as the subglottis should not be performed, so as to avoid the complications of worsened voice and even airway obstruction. Occasionally, Teflon may correct a posterior glottic gap by injection lateral to the vocal process of the arytenoids. If the patient has a large glottic gap with significant functional impairment, poor prognosis for recovery of vocal fold motion, and is elderly or has a terminal disease, an alloplast, such as Teflon, can be used. Its use should be limited to those patients in whom long-term voice outcome is not the primary concern. Extreme caution should be used if considering Teflon use in other patients given the significant side effects of granuloma formation, foreign body reaction, and implant migration.

For most bio-implants, superficial injection provides the best results and minimal absorption (Fig. 8.3). A curved laryngeal injector (Medtronics Xomed, Jacksonville, Fla.) with a disposable 27-G needle is ideal. Keeping in mind the anatomic goals outlined above, one should inject the material at the level of the deep lamina propria to prevent impaired vocal fold vibration. Superficial blebs should be avoided. Injection should begin at the posterior third of the membranous vocal fold. The needle is passed through the epithelium to the level of the vocal ligament, at which point injection commences. When the injection material is placed in the posterior one-third of the vocal fold, it should spread and fill the mid-membranous and anterior vocal fold. Approximately 0.3–0.8 cm^3 should adequately medialize the membranous vocal fold. The side of the needle can be used to shape the injected vocal fold and to facilitate injectate diffusion into surrounding tissues. If there are persistent focal gaps, further material may be placed into these areas, again with care being taken not to place much material directly into the anterior one-third of the vocal fold. The vocal fold should be slightly overmedialized given the resorption expected with bio-implants. Again, there will be more resorption with implants placed deeper in the thyroarytenoid muscle and paraglottic space than with more superficial placement. Considerable over-injection is often tolerated when injectate is placed in deeper planes. Overall, most bio-implants have proved forgiving over time. Bio-implants cannot effectively medialize a posterior glottic gap by injection lateral to the vocal process. One may have limited success in attempts to improve a posterior glottic gap by injection of material medial to the vocal process of the arytenoid, although if superficial blebs are raised in this area, they may lead to dyspnea and diplophonia. In general, bio-implants are best for treating smaller gaps and focal defects, and they are often useful as a temporizing measure while awaiting spontaneous recovery from paralysis.

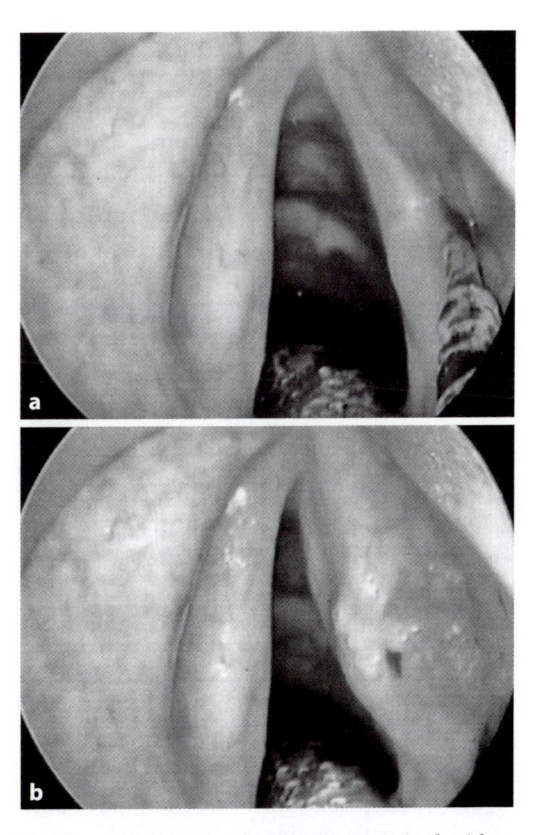

Fig. 8.3. a The minimal correction required with a bio-implant such as Cymetra. **b** The over-correction required for fat injection

Results

The most common immediate outcome of injection laryngoplasty is that the patient is able to produce a louder voice for a longer time with much less effort. More objective assessment of efficacy is facilitated by the use of videostroboscopy to assess vocal fold vibration, mucosal wave pattern, degree of glottic closure, vocal fold symmetry, and supraventricular hyperfunction. Acoustic measures may also allow objective analysis of voice. Specifically, one expects improvement in vocal intensity, increased signal-to-noise ratio and frequency range, and decreased pertubation measures. Aerodynamic changes to anticipate include increased phonation time and decreased transglottic airflow during phonation. Maximum phonation time is one simple test that can be used to assess the immediate effect of augmentation, although this may be altered by patient factors such as pulmonary reserve, practice, and instruction in the technique. Certainly, factors other than the augmentation alone may affect outcomes. The pliability or scarring of the contralateral vocal fold as well as the patient's neurologic and pulmonary status may also alter the expected result.

Complications

There are a variety of complications associated with injection augmentation of the vocal fold. Failure to displace the affected true vocal fold in the vertical plane of the contralateral vocal fold will not correct the symptoms of glottic insufficiency. Although examination may demonstrate apparent medialization, persistent breathy dysphonia will indicate that the injection is not in the proper plane. In addition, injection in the anterior one-third of the vocal fold may lead to stiffening of the injected site with resultant decrease in mucosal wave of the opposite vocal fold and possible worsening of the posterior glottic gap.

Use of alloplasts, such as Teflon, have been associated with significant foreign body reaction and granuloma formation as well as migration to distant sites. Virtually all injected Teflon results in a granuloma. The granuloma is asymptomatic when circumscribed in the paraglottic space but can significantly impede vocal fold function when placed – or when migrated – close to the superficial layers of the vocal fold. In such cases the voice result is poor and airway might be compromised. The key to correcting the problem is to remove the granuloma. Partial removal can be achieved by transoral direct laryngoscopic techniques, but in our experience the best results are obtained by total removal using an external approach as described by Netterville et al. [11]. This technique consists of removal of Teflon granulomas via a lateral laryngotomy and reconstruction of the vocal soft tissues by placement of an inferiorly based sternohyoid muscle flap.

Avoidance of complications requires a thorough understanding of the relevant anatomy. Injectates should not be placed in the false vocal folds, ventricles, subglottis, or anterior one-third of the vocal folds. The injected material should be tailored to the individual patient. Precise visualization and placement of the injected material as well as continual assessment via videostroboscopy and voice monitoring are necessary for a good outcome.

Current Status and Future Goals

Currently, there is a cornucopia of materials that can be applied to different specific clinical situations. For example, Teflon is an effective way to restore function in the terminal cancer patient with paralysis since migration and granuloma are of less concern. Various forms of collagen are useful for temporary corrections of glottic insufficiency and might give lasting benefit to patients with smaller gaps, focal defects, and minimal scar [12]. Bovine collagen (Zyderm and Zyplast) may still have a role in superficial corrections, whereas fat, fascia, and micronized human dermis (Cymetra) are more effective at multiple levels.

Future directions include development of a more universally effective injectable substance. Such an injectate should be capable of being precisely injected, non-allergenic, or carcinogenic, and provoke minimal inflammatory response. It should provide persistent and stable correction. It must be compatible with host tissue structure and mimic the viscoelastic properties of the vocal fold lamina propria. Fulfilling the ideals of a bio-implant, it would allow assimilation with in-growth of surrounding cellular and acellular tissue elements that reproduce the normal vocal fold lamina propria. Introduction of bioactive matrices and growth factors through tissue engineering might also lead to host deposition of extracellular substances favoring normal vocal fold oscillation. Ultimate rehabilitation of patients with vocal fold paralysis will depend on progress in restoring vocal fold structure and parallel developments in reinnervation.

References

1. Brunings W (1911) Uber eine neue Behandlungsmethode der Rekurrenslahmung. Verh Dtsch Laryngol 18:93–151
2. Chhetri DK, Jahan-Parwar B, Hart SD, Bhuta SM, Berke GS (2004) Injection laryngoplasty with calcium hydroxylapatite gel implant in an in vivo canine model. Ann Otol Rhinol Laryngol 113:259–264
3. Ford CN, Bless DM (1986) Injectable collagen in vocal cord augmentation: a preliminary clinical study. Otolaryngol Head Neck Surg 94:104–112
4. Ford CN, Staskowski PA, Bless DM (1995) Autologous collagen vocal fold injections: a preliminary clinical study. Laryngoscope 105:944–948
5. Rihkanen H, Lehikoinen-Soderlund S, Reijonen P (1999) Voice acoustics after autologous fascia injection for vocal fold paralysis. Laryngoscope 109:1854–1858
6. Lundy DS, Casiano RR, McClinto ME, Xue JW (2002) Early results of transcutaneous injection laryngoplasty with micronized acellular dermis versus type-I thyroplasty for glottic incompetence dysphonia due to unilateral vocal fold paralysis. J Voice 17:589–595
7. McCulloch TM, Andrews BT, Hoffman HT, Graham SM, Karnell MP, Minnick C (2002) Long-term follow-up of fat injection laryngoplasty for unilateral vocal cord paralysis. Laryngoscope 112:1235–1238
8. Hertegard S, Hallen L, Laurent C, Lindstrom E, Olofsson K, Testad P, Dahlqvist A (2002) Cross-linked hyaluronan used as augmentation substance for treatment of glottal insufficiency: safety aspects and vocal fold function. Laryngoscope 112:2211–2219
9. Hirano S, Bless D, Heisey D, Ford C (2003) Roles of hepatocyte growth factor and transforming growth factor beta-1 in production of extracellular matrix by canine vocal fold fibroblasts. Laryngoscope 113:144–148
10. Tayama N, Kaga K, Chan RW, Titze IR (2002) Functional definition of vocal fold geometry for laryngeal biomechanical modeling. Ann Otol Rhinol Laryngol 111:83–93
11. Netterville JL, Coleman JR Jr, Chang S, Rainey CL, Reinisch L, Ossoff RH (1998) Lateral laryngotomy for the removal of Teflon granuloma. Ann Otol Rhinol Laryngol 107:735–744
12. Ford CN, Bless DM, Loftus JM (1992) Role of injectable collagen in the treatment of glottic insufficiency: a study of 119 patients. Ann Otol Rhinol Laryngol 101:237–247
13. Ford CN, Bless DM (1991) Phonosurgical assessment and surgical management of voice disorders. Raven, New York

Autologous Fat for Vocal Fold Injection

Clark A. Rosen

Introduction

Vocal fold injection for global augmentation of the vocal fold is a successful way to treat glottal closure insufficiency [1]. Autologous fat is an excellent material for this type of vocal fold injection. This chapter discusses the patient selection, clinical aspects, and post-operative management issues related to vocal fold lipoinjection.

Rationale for Vocal Fold Lipoinjection

The distinct advantage of vocal fold lipoinjection is the use of an autologous material that is usually readily available. Furthermore, autologous fat has been found to have excellent biomechanical properties associated with vocal fold vibration when placed into the larynx [2]. No discernable stiffness or alteration of normal vibratory function has been seen by this author nor reported in the literature following lipoinjection of the vocal folds [3–8].

There are several important advantages of vocal fold injection vs laryngeal framework surgery; these include the ease of bilateral vocal fold injection (when clinically necessary) and the opportunity for direct visualization of the pathologic defect of the vocal fold(s) (paresis, atrophy, or scar) immediately before and during the vocal fold injection procedure. Laryngeal framework surgery, in contrast, involves augmenting the vocal fold from an "outside to inside" approach relying on fiberoptic imaging and perceptual feedback results to judge an endpoint [9]. A bilateral procedure requires a longer neck incision and more surgical dissection. Some surgeons are not willing to perform bilateral medialization laryngoplasty which results in suboptimal voice outcomes. This is common in patients with a unilateral vocal fold paralysis and contralateral age-related vocal fold atrophy who are treated only with a unilateral medialization laryngoplasty and experience partial improvement in their voice quality due to the failure to address the glottal insufficiency component from the atrophy.

Disadvantages of vocal fold lipoinjection include variable survival of the transplanted autologous fat and the consequent need for overinjection [10, 11]. Given that lipoinjection will involve some loss of the transplanted material in the first 6-week period, a slight to moderate overinjection of the vocal fold is required. This poses a problem clinically if there is an already borderline airway. Furthermore, overinjection can be problematic due to the resulting temporary dysphonia and delayed voice improvement for as long as 4–6 weeks postoperatively.

Another consideration is the labor required and method used to harvest the fat, a disadvantage of lipoinjection compared with an injection using an "off-the-shelf" product. Typically, fat harvest in preparation for lipoinjection is performed as an open removal of subcutaneous fat or liposuction.

Patient Selection

Vocal fold lipoinjection is best used to treat insufficiency of glottal closure when the gap is small to medium in size. This is often the case in patients with vocal fold paralysis, paresis, atrophy, and scar. For patients with glottal gaps greater than ~4 mm, as well as patients with a shortened or "slack" vocal fold sometimes associated with vocal fold paralysis, lipoinjection is not an optimal treatment method. In the vocal fold paralysis patient, the contralateral vocal fold should be carefully observed preoperatively to identify (a) patients who have relatively poor abduction of their contralateral vocal fold, and (b) patients with loss of bulk of the contralateral vocal fold. The first group of patients are a relative contraindication for VFL due to the temporary reduction of the airway associated with the overinjection required. In contrast, patients with contralateral loss of vocal fold bulk are excellent candidates for bilateral vocal fold lipoinjection. Patients that have significant concerns regarding open neck surgery and/or foreign substance implantation are also excellent candidates for autologous vocal fold augmentation.

The amount of subcutaneous fat available for harvest should be evaluated prior to VFL. For patients who have an extremely small amount of subcutaneous fat, liposuction is not a reasonable harvest technique, and in fact, even open fat harvest can be problematic. In this specific patient group, subcutaneous open fat harvest will most likely be more involved and may have an increased complication rate than in patients with generous subcutaneous fat deposits. Furthermore, in the extremely lean patient, surgical harvest of subcutaneous fat may not yield adequate amounts of fat for successful VFL.

Given that lipoinjection involves a "deep" or "lateral" vocal fold injection, patients selected should be those with a "global" glottal insufficiency and not those with small, focal lamina propria defects. This contraindication does not apply to patients with a substantive "cookie cutter defect" of the vocal fold following cancer excision. These patients can in fact be quite successfully treated with VFL when performed carefully and properly [12].

Technical Aspects of Vocal Fold Lipoinjection

Fat Harvest

Fat harvest for lipoinjection can be done either via an open, subcutaneous fat harvest or via liposuction. Liposuction is the preferred technique because it is expedient, less invasive and provides perfect-sized injection material. For patients with only modest amounts of subcutaneous fat, open harvest is recommended. The most reasonable location for open harvest is in the infra-umbilical region or through a pre-existing abdominal scar. The former area of the body typically has a plentiful amount of material and an incision immediately underneath the umbilicus can be easily hidden. Fat harvest can be done under local or general anesthesia.

The patient's abdomen is prepped and draped in a sterile fashion. If not performed under a general anesthetic, local injection is done as for a regional block (and in the proposed incision site for hemostasis). A curvilinear incision is made at the junction of the umbilicus and the infra-umbilical region, approximately from 4 o'clock to 8 o'clock position. Subcutaneous elevation of the dermis proceeds in an inferior direction, releasing the subcutaneous fat off the subdermal plane. The fat is sharply dissected out with cold steel instruments, taking care to not violate the skin above or the peritoneum below. Hemostasis can be obtained with electric cautery as needed. Tacking sutures are placed from the deeper aspect of the wound to the subdermal base to minimize the dead space and the cutaneous incision is closed with absorbable sutures. The harvested fat is then carefully cut into small pieces with scissors, approximately $1 \times 2 \times 1$ mm. This aspect of the procedure is time-consuming and laborious but important. If the fat graft material is not properly prepared, it will not flow smoothly through the injection needle. These small pieces of fat are then handled in a similar fashion as the liposuction harvested material, described below.

Liposuction should be done using a large-bore, low-pressure liposuction technique. Small-gauge and high-pressure liposuction devices should be avoided to minimize the trauma to the fat during the harvest process. The author uses a 4.6-mm single-hole liposuction cannula (Tulip Products, San Diego, Calif.).

Liposuction from the subcutaneous abdominal space can be done under general or local anesthesia; the latter requires local anesthesia to be injected in the area of the intended liposuction. After the abdominal skin is prepped and draped in a sterile fashion, a small skin incision (~ 5 mm) is made in the right upper quadrant of the abdomen. The liposuction cannula is passed through the skin and into the subcutaneous space. Negative pressure is applied from the liposuction device and the cannula is then moved through the subcutaneous plane in a controlled but expedient fashion (Fig. 8.1.1). This results in adequate amounts of fat for vocal fold lipoinjection after approximately 30–90 s of vigorous movement of the liposuction cannula in the subcutaneous plane.

Fat harvested by any method is covered with free fatty acids, blood, and serum (Fig. 8.1.2) [13]. The free fatty acids are from ruptured lipocytes and induce an intense inflammatory response if not removed. The fat must be carefully and atraumatically cleaned prior to lipoinjection to maximize graft survival. Fat is placed in a sterile funnel that is lined by strips of Merocel (Medtronics/Xomed, Jacksonville, Fla.). Suction tubing is applied to the down spout of the funnel and 2 liter of saline is used to rinse and irrigate blood and fatty acids from the surface of the harvested fat (Fig. 8.1.3) The fat is soaked in a small dish with 100 units of regular insulin for 5 min. The insulin is theorized to stabilize the lipocyte cell membranes and thus improve cell survival during the transplantation process. To remove excessive moisture, the fat is then placed on a dry Merocel sponge and partially dried by the air. It can then be loaded into the injection device in preparation for a VFL. Figure 8.1.4 demonstrates the "cleaned" fat af-

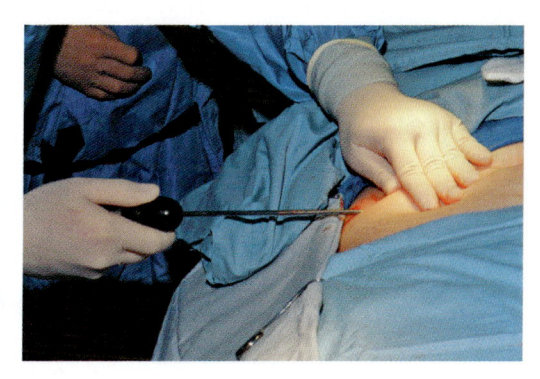

Fig. 8.1.1. Liposuction from subcutaneous area of the abdomen

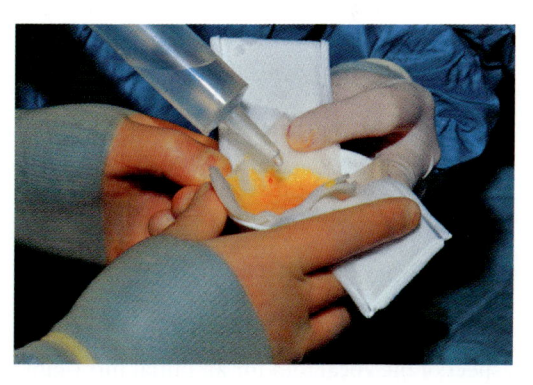

Fig. 8.1.3. Saline irrigation to clean the harvested fat in funnel lined with a Merocel sponge

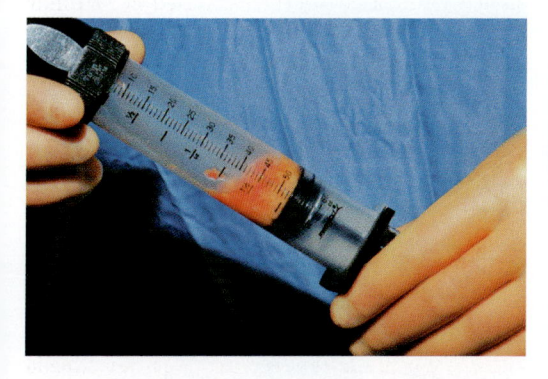

Fig. 8.1.2. Fat harvested from liposuction. Note mixture of fatty acid-based liquid, serum, and graft material

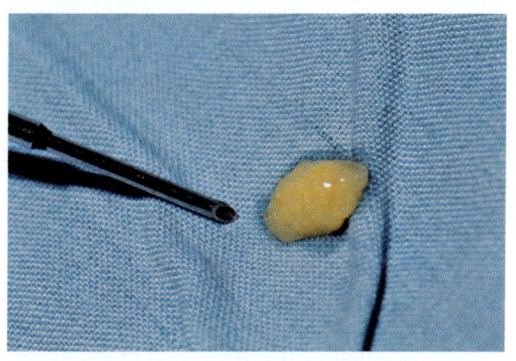

Fig. 8.1.4. Fat material following "cleaning"

ter passing through the injection device. Note the absence of a "greasy" sheen (free fatty acids) and minimal moisture.

Lipoinjection

Lipoinjection of the vocal folds may be performed through an 18- or 19-G needle. Using any smaller needle is likely to disrupt the injection material and compromise graft survival. Lipoinjection is designed for a deep/lateral vocal fold injection and can be done either via an endoscopically guided direct laryngoscopic approach or suspension microlaryngoscopy approach [1, 14]. Given the viscous nature of the fat, a pressurized injection device such as a Brünings syringe (Storz, St. Louis, Mo.) or a lipoinjection device designed by Instrumentarium (Montreal, Canada) is required. The optimal location for the initial site for lipoinjection is at the junction of a horizontal line drawn through the tip of the vocal process and the superior arcuate line. The approximate depth of this injection should be 5 ± 2 mm. The angle of the needle should be directed in a slightly posterior and lateral direction to ensure that the injection is not placed inferior to the vocal fold nor in a too superficial/medial a plane. The ideal location for deep vocal fold injection is identified by careful observation of the infra-glottic aspect of the vocal fold for an initial infra-glottic "bulge" or appearance of augmentation in the immediate infra-glottic region at the start of the injection. As additional fat is injected into the vocal fold, the vocal fold augmentation will proceed in a cephalad fashion. If this does not occur spontaneously, the needle should be slightly adjusted to find the proper location. The surgeon should perform approximately 30% overinjection of the vocal fold to compensate for expected fat loss in the transplantation process. (Figs. 8.1.5, 8.1.6) Often, a second injection site is placed in the mid-membranous vocal fold at the level of the superior arcuate line. Care should be taken to avoid injection anterior to this point because excessive augmentation of the anterior half of the vocal fold typically results in a strained voice quality. Often bilateral VFL in patients with mobile vocal folds will be done to the extent that at immediate completion of the procedure the membranous vocal folds will be in complete approximation.

Post-operative Care Following Lipoinjection

Patients are placed on strict voice rest for 6 days following VFL. Routine use of prophylactic antibiotics is not indicated. Both intravenous (peri-operative) and oral steroids (post-operative) are typically used to minimize peri-operative swelling. The patient should be counseled to avoid throat clearing if possible and beware of any signs of breathing difficulties.

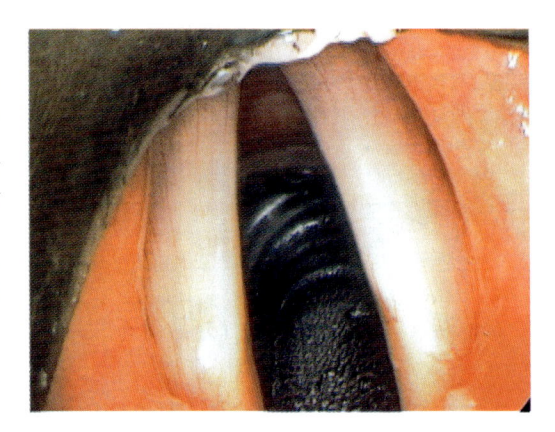

Fig. 8.1.5. Pre-Lipoinjection

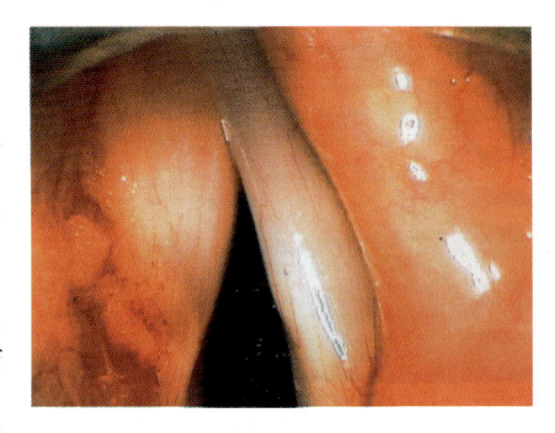

Fig. 8.1.6. Post-Lipoinjection (immediate)

Duration of Benefit

Vocal fold lipoinjection involves over injection because of partial loss of some of the transplanted material over the 4–6 weeks following the procedure. Although there are no studies comparing different practices, survival of the graft material is thought to be optimized with strict voice rest for the 6 days following surgery, proper harvesting in as non-traumatic a fashion as possible, and proper handling of the fat following harvest. Patients should be warned that their voice may remain dysphonic or actually deteriorate while the swelling and over correction of the vocal fold slowly resolves for as long as 6 weeks following lipoinjection; however, patients typically report that their voice dramatically improves 3–4 weeks following VFL. The degree and nature of the vocal fold augmentation that exists at 6 weeks following lipoinjection has been found by the author to be permanent. If a patient has a significant voice improvement prior to 6 weeks or no immediate post-operative dysphonia, then it is likely that injection will be inadequate to yield adequate medialization in the long term.

Recent review of the vocal fold lipoinjection results at the University of Pittsburgh Voice Center found 27 patients available for long-term follow-up (mean 11.3 months, range 3.0–28.9 months). Twelve of these patients had vocal fold atrophy, 14 had vocal fold paralysis, and 1 patient had both unilateral recurrent laryngeal nerve paresis and bilateral superior laryngeal nerve paralysis. Eleven of the 27 patients were male. Five of the patients in the study group required further laryngeal surgery, as follows: 1 patient experienced a lipogranuloma which was excised 2 months following lipoinjection; 1 patient required medialization laryngoplasty (to further enhance glottic closure following vocal fold lipoinjection); and 3 patients required repeat vocal fold lipoinjection, due to under-augmentation by the initial VFL.

Pre- and post-operative VHI results showed statistically significant difference ($p=0.0001$). Pre-operative mean VHI was 69.5 and post-operative was 38.2 with a mean follow up of 12 months. Mean flow rate differences pre- and post-VFL also showed statistically significant improvement from a pre-operative mean flow rate of 490 ml/s to a post-operative result of 283 ml/s ($p=0.01$).

Complications of Lipoinjection of the Vocal Folds

Airway

Approximately 1–3% of lipoinjection patients may experience some airway compromise, given that a moderate amount of overinjection of the vocal fold is required and that significant post-operative edema or infection can occur following injection. Airway difficulty following lipoinjection should be managed using the same principles as in other upper airway difficulties, specifically, careful observation, steroids (i.v. or oral) and mechanical intervention for re-establishment of the airway, if needed. Clinicians who are concerned about the patient's airway following bilateral lipoinjection may elect to stage the injections. This allows the surgeon to maximally overinject the vocal fold and minimize the risk of airway difficulties in the post-operative period.

Suboptimal Voice Improvement

Under-medialization can occur in approximately 5–10% of patients undergoing lipoinjection. This problem most likely represents an inadequate amount of fat material survival and/or an insufficient amount of fat injected into the vocal fold, but can also occur from suboptimal injection location. This can be corrected with a repeat lipoinjection, vocal fold injection with an alternative material, or laryngeal framework surgery.

Overinjection

In rare instances, an excessive amount of fat following lipoinjection can persist, resulting in persistent post-operative dysphonia. When this is suspected, the patient should be observed for the first 2 or 3 months. This allows localized edema to resolve. If after several months it is clear that persistent post-operative dysphonia is due to overinjection, then injected material can be removed via a lateral cordotomy using the principles of phonomicrosurgery. This is done through an incision through the superior surface of the vocal fold at approximately the superior arcuate line. Dissection proceeds down to the deeper aspect of the vocal fold until the injected fat material is identified and removed with cup forceps until an appropriate amount of vocal fold augmentation is still present. In the present author's experience, this has happened only once in over 300 cases.

References

1. Bouchayer M et al. (1985) Epidermoid cysts, sulci, and mucosal bridges of the true vocal cord: a report of 157 cases. Laryngoscope 95:1087–1094
2. Chan RW, Titze IR (1999) Hyaluronic acid (with fibronectin) as a bioimplant for vocal fold mucosa. Laryngoscope 109:1142–1149
3. Hsiung MW et al. (2003) Eur Arch Otorhinolaryngol, series online
4. Hsiung MW et al. (2000) Fat augmentation for glottic insufficiency. Laryngoscope 110:1026–1033
5. Laccourreye O et al. (1998) Recovery of function after intracordal autologous fat injection for unilateral recurrent laryngeal nerve paralysis. J Laryngol Otol 112:1082–1084
6. Laccourreye O et al. (2003) Intracordal injection of autologous fat in patients with unilateral laryngeal nerve paralysis, long-term results from the patient's perspective. Laryngoscope 113:541–545
7. Mikaelian DO, Lowry LD, Sataloff RT (1991) Lipoinjection for unilateral vocal cord paralysis. Laryngoscope 101:465–468
8. Shaw GY et al. (1997) Autologous fat injection into the vocal folds: technical considerations and long-term follow-up. Laryngoscope 107:177–186
9. Netterville JL et al. (1993) Silastic medialization and arytenoid adduction: the Vanderbilt experience. A review of 116 phonosurgical procedures. Ann Otol Rhinol Laryngol 102:413–424
10. Shindo ML, Zaaretsky LS, Rice DH (1996) Autologous fat injection for unilateral vocal fold paralysis. Ann Otol Rhinol Laryngol 105:602–606
11. Saccogna PW et al. (1997) Lipoinjection in the paralyzed feline vocal fold: study of graft survival. Otolaryngol Head Neck Surg 117:465–470
12. Zeitels SM, Mauri M, Dailey SH (2003) Medialization laryngoplasty with Gore-Tex for voice restoration secondary to glottal incompetence: indications and observations. Ann Otol Rhinol Laryngol 112:180–184
13. Mikus JL, Koufman JA, Kilpatrick SE (1995) Fate of liposuctioned and purified autologous fat injection in the canine vocal fold. Laryngoscope 105:17–22
14. Alper C et al. (2001) Vocal fold paralysis: unilateral. In: Alper C, Myers EN, Eibling DE (eds) Decision making in ear, nose and throat disorders. Saunders, Philadelphia

Chapter 8

Collagen in Vocal Fold Injection   8.2

Mark S. Courey

Physiologic Considerations

In order to produce efficient normal voice, the vocal folds must be able to achieve a nearly closed, parallel prephonatory position. This ability is regulated by neurologic input to the intrinsic laryngeal muscles, the bulk or mass of the vocal fold body and cover, and the structural and functional integrity of the cricoarytenoid joints. If any one of these systems is impaired, the prephonatory position is less than ideal and vibratory efficiency is compromised. Neurologic input to the thyroarytenoid muscles and the cricothyroid muscles also controls vocal fold tone. Efficiency of vibration is best when the vocal folds are matched in terms of this tone or tension.

If an adequate prephonatory position can be achieved, and the vocal fold mass and tone are nearly symmetric, then the vocal fold cover, the epithelium, and superficial layer of the lamina propria must be of sufficient viscosity to allow vibration. If the cover is stiff or deficient from scarring, air pressures required to initiate and sustain vibration will be increased. Patients will not be able to finely modulate vocal fold tone, their dynamic range will be compromised, and they will complain of increased phonatory effort.

Injection laryngoplasty with collagen, or most currently available substances for that matter, can increase vocal fold bulk, but will not restore the neurologic function required to balance vocal fold tone and cannot reduce the viscosity of the cover to improve its vibratory function. It is important for the surgeon to understand these limitations of injection laryngoplasty to allow better patient selection and better understanding of surgical outcomes.

Historical Considerations

Collagen was first reported for the management of glottic closure defects during the early 1980s [1]. In these original animal models and clinical reports surgeons used available forms of bovine collagen as a xenograft to reshape the vocal fold [2–4]. The reports were innovative and encouraging, but scientific evidence supporting the use of bovine collagen in this manner was scant and other surgeons were not able to achieve the same results.

The original forms of solubilized collagen were produced from bovine species and were intended for use in the management of dermal deficiencies [5]. Specifically for cosmetic dermal application, collagen was isolated from animal dermal material, purified, and then processed for injection into humans in the form of a xenograft. These bovine collagen compounds, with and without glutaraldehyde cross-linkages, were developed to be placed in the region of the mid-reticular dermis known to be deficient in aging skin. The collagen graft was designed to replace the natural deficiency with similar tissue. The addition of the specific concentration of glutaraldehyde cross-linkages to the collagen implant was hypothesized to increase host fibroblast invasion and neovascularization of the graft [6]. Multiple reports emphasized ease of placement and the relatively stable results in skin augmentation [7–11]. After clinical trials, collagen compounds received approval of the U.S. Food and Drug Administration (FDA) for use in the correction of skin defects.

Despite the ease of injection and relative tolerance, the main objection to the use of bovine collagen products remained the potential host-vs-graft reaction to the xenograft protein material. A localized reaction to the xenograft was shown to occur in 3.5% of patients. In addition, delayed hypersensitivity was demonstrated in 1.3% of patients [3, 12–14]. These reactions resulted in localized erythema and induration. While less than desirable in dermal applications, this type of reaction could have potentially devastating results in the larynx or airway, an off-label use of bovine collagen products; therefore, it is recommended that patients have a small test dose planted in the forearm and be observed for 6 weeks prior to clinical use. This problem has always tempered the use of bovine collagen products, particularly in the larynx [14]. A comparison of collagen products is given in Table 8.2.1.

To address these concerns and eliminate the main objection to the use of bovine collagen – the unpredictable host/graft reaction – work with purified human forms of collagen was undertaken. During the early 1990s, the initial work was performed for dermal applications and recipients served as their own donors. Skin was harvested and collagen isolated from the dermal tissue. Reinjection into the same patient at another intradermal site revealed the autologous implants to be well tolerated and of 6-month duration [16, 17]. Histologic evaluation of implants showed a minimal inflammatory reaction with ingrowth of native fibroblasts. With repeated application to the same region over a 6-month period, skin augmentation for the elimination of fine wrinkles was demonstrated to persist for up to 4 years in limited case reports [18, 19].

This same process for preparing autologous collagen was then evaluated for use in human vocal folds. Initial and subsequent clinical reports were encouraging, both in terms of tolerance and persistence of graft materials. Evaluation of vocal changes with perceptual, aerodynamic, and acoustical measures demonstrated limited improvements over a 6-month follow-up period [20–22]. In addition, limited numbers of animal studies demonstrated persistence of graft material with minimal foreign body reaction and ingrowth of host fibroblasts into the implanted material [23].

Despite promise for dermal and vocal fold augmentation, clinically, objections to the use of allograft material arose from donor site morbidity, the required delay in implant availability due to processing time, and the increased cost associated with individual graft preparation. To overcome these objections, purified forms of human collagen from cadaveric skin were developed during the 1990s [24, 25]. Homologous collagen compounds are currently available in both glutaraldehyde cross-linked forms and non-glutaraldehyde cross-linked forms. In addition, micronized dermis containing both collagen and elastin particles is also available for use [26]. While these substances have been given FDA approval for dermal augmentation, laryngeal application is still regarded as an off-label application due to the lack of controlled clinical trials.

Technical Considerations

Due to the relative success of collagen for the management of dermal deficiencies, the rela-

Table 8.2.1 Comparison of collagen products

Substance	Source	Glutaraldehyde cross-linkages	Characteristics
Zyderm	Bovine	No	Superficial injection, relatively more rapid resorption
Zyplast	Bovine	Yes	Deeper injection, potentially longer lasting
Cosmoderm	Human	No	Superficial injection, relative rapid resorption
Cosmoplast	Human	Yes	Deeper injection, potentially longer lasting
Micronized alloderm, Cymetra	Human	No	Powdered form, reconstituted in clinic or OR. Contains elastin fibers

tively low risk of adverse reactions, particularly if human preparations are utilized, and the continued difficulty with other substances for the management of glottal insufficiency, otolaryngologists have continued to experiment with collagen as a substance for laryngeal augmentation by injection. For cosmetic applications, collagen preparations are injected into the midreticular dermis under direct visualization through a 27-G needle. By expanding the volume of the intradermal region, superficial wrinkles are filled in. Unlike the skin, however, laryngeal mucosal tissue must be supple to vibrate during voice production. In addition, vocal fold mucosa does not have a region analogous to the midreticular dermis. Due to these two technical problems, intramucosal laryngeal injection is different from intradermal injection. The simple addition of a filler substance to augment the vocal fold, while it may result in improved glottic closure, does not result in significant improvements in the viscosity of the mucosal membrane for voicing [27].

The original investigators of collagen for laryngeal augmentation suggested that placement of the collagen graft material within specific layers of the vocal fold significantly affected the results and longevity of the injection. They specified that the attempt should be made to place the collagen graft into the deeper layers of the vocal fold lamina propria, which they termed a superficial injection [4]. This was consistent with the concept for skin injections in which the goal was to place the collagen graft within the midreticular dermis. The vocal fold submucosa is roughly divided into three layers by variations in the concentration of the extracellular matrix proteins. The two deeper layers, termed the intermediate and deep layer, form the vocal ligament and are composed of primarily elastin fibers and collagen fibers, respectively. Morphometric evaluation from cadaver specimens in multiple studies reveals that the combined thickness of the intermediate and deep layers is less than 1 mm [28–30]. Injecting a region that is only 1 mm thick or less is technically challenging under any circumstances. The region can only be reached with a 400-mm needle placed transorally or a shorter needle inserted percutaneously through or under the thyroid cartilage, and this restricted access to a small site further complicates accurate placement.

Cadaver vocal folds were injected with collagen under direct visualization using 27-G needles to evaluate the ability to accurately place the collagen graft [31]. The goal was to place the collagen within the plane of the vocal ligament as had been suggested. Manufacturers' standards indicate that these needles are produced with a 400- to 600-µm-long bevel which represents roughly 50% of the size of the region to be injected. Histologic analysis revealed that the collagen material flowed either into the superficial layer of the lamina propria above the vocal ligament or between the thyroarytenoid muscle bundles just below the vocal ligament. In several cases, a tract of collagen could be seen extending through the vocal ligament. Reviewing these results and comparing the needle size and bevel configuration with the actual sizes of the vocal ligament region, one can appreciate the difficulty in exact placement of the graft into the vocal ligament. The vocal ligament itself is relatively dense with increased numbers of cross-linkages between the collagen fibers in comparison with the other surrounding tissues. If the needle is only slightly outside of the desired region, the injected material will flow more readily into the less viscous tissue found in the superficial region of the lamina propria or between the thyroarytenoid muscle bundles. In addition, if the target region is composed primarily of scar tissue, it is equally unlikely that the injection will dissect between scar bundles rather than flow into the less viscous surrounding tissue; therefore, it is unlikely that injected material can be placed into "the plane of the vocal ligament."

With regard to influencing viscosity of the vocal fold vibratory membrane, the initial experience with bovine collagen in both skin and vocal folds suggested that the xenograft collagen fibers stimulated activity of host fibroblasts. This host fibroblast activity was theorized to increase both native collagen production and host collagenase activity to remodel the existing scar and decrease its viscosity. The laboratory evidence in support of this hypothesis consisted of the study of small numbers of animals in a few models. No rheologic evaluation of tissue after injection was undertaken. In addition, in the 1990s, when otolaryngologists switched to using mostly human forms of collagen, this theory about the xenograft stimulation of collagenase activity was abandoned.

In vitro measurements of available collagen preparations have shown that these preparations are significantly more viscous than the normal superficial layer of the lamina propria. Cadaver models demonstrate that if the collagen preparation is injected into the deep region of the superficial layer of the lamina propria, vibration of the membrane cannot be produced. If, however, the collagen substance is placed just beneath the vocal ligament into the superficial portion of the thyroarytenoid muscle, the forces required to adduct the vocal folds into a position for phonation are significantly reduced and the vibratory patterns are relatively unchanged [31]. Finally, injecting the collagen substance into the lateral portion of the thyroarytenoid muscles, as advocated for Teflon and other substances in the original descriptions of injection laryngoplasty, allows the development of normal vibratory patterns but requires significantly more substance to medialize the vocal fold than injection into the medial or superficial portion of the thyroarytenoid muscle.

Clinical Applications

Most surgeons agree that collagen-containing substances produce temporary medialization of the vocal fold through a mass effect. For the reasons stated above, the injection should be placed into the thyroarytenoid muscle. In this position, the collagen substances last for 2–6 months before resorption. The clinical indications for collagen injection include the management of unilateral vocal fold paralysis, unilateral or bilateral vocal fold paresis, presbyphonia, or glottal insufficiency secondary to scarring of the mucosal membrane [32].

For the management of unilateral vocal fold paralysis, collagen injections usually produce only temporary benefit and are resorbed without significant adverse reactions. For this reason collagen can be used in the acute situation for patients who cannot tolerate the dysphonia, need an improved cough for pulmonary toilet, or are having significant dysphagia with aspiration. The injection can be performed either percutaneously or transorally in the clinic or in the operating room. The percutaneous injection route can either be accomplished by passing the needle under the thyroid cartilage through the cricothyroid membrane or transcartilaginously directly through the thyroid lamina. Cadaver models have demonstrated that if the collagen is deposited into the lateral portion of the thyroarytenoid muscle, approximately 0.7 ml of substance will be required to move the vocal fold to midline. Injection into the medial portion of the thyroarytenoid muscle requires about 0.2 ml to bring the vocal fold medial surface to midline. This difference is statistically significant [31]. When determining the amount of over-injection, the surgeon must consider the concentration of the collagen in the solution that is being injected and the rate of resorption of the carrier vehicle. The vehicle is either saline or glycerine. Usually saline is resorbed within the first 48 h [31]. Glycerine resorption, however, may take longer and is dependent on the compounds with which it is injected. Micronized alloderm (Cymetra) is usually mixed into a 50% solution with injectable xylocaine or saline; therefore, a 50% over injection is indicated to produce significant vocal improvements. In clinical experience, the over-injection is somewhat less with the glycerine-based compounds due to the longer resorption time of the carrier.

For the management of paresis or presbyphonia, injections can be accomplished with the same techniques. The injection can be performed bilaterally during the same intervention if needed. Airway obstruction has not been reported as a significant problem if caution is used in the amount of over-medialization.

Scar tissue on the vibratory surface of the vocal fold does not respond well to injection laryngoplasty. This is due to the fact that the injected material usually flows around the dense/viscous scar tissue into the less viscous surrounding tissue. In addition, the scarred epithelial surface does not hold the injected material well as it tends to be friable and easily disrupted.

Conclusion

Collagen-based compounds have been used over the past 25 years for treatment of glottal insufficiency. These compounds were originally developed for augmentation of skin and were intended to be injected into the midreticular dermis. Through distention of the dermal tissues, the implant decreased small wrinkles. Repeated applications into the skin have been shown to produce stable reductions in facial lines. Due to the lack of a vocal fold structure comparable to the midreticular dermis and the need for the vocal fold mucosa to be supple to vibrate, vocal fold augmentation results with collagen compounds have been less than ideal. The collagen can be used as a filler substance to increase the bulk of the vocal fold. If the collagen is placed above the vocal ligament, it will result in increased viscosity of the mucosal membrane and loss of the normal vibratory characteristics. The collagen compounds, therefore, need to be injected below the vocal ligament. In this position they increase the bulk of the vocal fold and lessen the forces required to produce vocal fold adduction. When injected into the thyroarytenoid muscle, either medially or laterally, the collagen compounds are most likely resorbed by the host. There are only scant reports of long-term vocal improvements after collagen injection and most surgeons regard collagen compounds as a temporary method of vocal fold medialization.

References

1. Ford CN, Martin DW, Warner TF (1984) Injectable collagen in laryngeal rehabilitation. Laryngoscope 94:513–518
2. Ford CN (1986) Histological studies on the fate of soluble collagen injected into canine vocal folds. Laryngoscope 96:1248–1257
3. Ford CN, Bless DM (1986) A preliminary study of injectable collagen in human vocal fold augmentation. Otolaryngol Head Neck Surg 94:104–112
4. Ford CN, Bless DM (1986) Clinical experience with injectable collagen for vocal fold augmentation. Laryngoscope 96:863–869
5. Knapp, TR, Luck E, Daniels JR (1977) Behavior of solubilized collagen as a bioimplant. J Surg Res 23:96–105
6. McPherson JM, Saamura S, Armstrong R (1986) An examination of the biologic response to injectable, glutaraldehyde cross-linked collagen implants. J Biomed Mater Res 20:93–107
7. Kamer FM, Churukian MM (1984) Clinical use of injectable collagen. A 3-year restropsective review. Arch Otolaryngol 110:93–98
8. Castrow FF 2nd, Krull EA (1983) Injectable collagen implant-update. J Am Acad Dermatol 9:889–893
9. Klein AW (1983) Implantation technics for injectable collagen. Two and one-half years of personal clinical experience. J Am Acad Dermatol 9:224–228
10. Cooperman LS, Mackinnon V, Bechler G, Pharriss BB (1985) Injectable collagen: a 6-year clinical investigation. Aesthetic Plast Surg 9:145–151
11. Watson W, Kaye RL, Klein A, Stegman S (1983) Injectable collagen: a clinical overview. Cutis 31:543–546
12. Swanson NA, Stoner JG, Siegle RJ, Solomon AR (1983) Treatment site reactions to Zyderm collagen implantation. J Dermatol Surg Oncol 9:377–380
13. Labow TA, Silvers DN (1985) Late reaction at Zyderm skin test sites. Cutis 35:154–156, 158
14. Charriere G, Bejot M, Schnitzler L, Ville G, Hartmann D (1989) Reactions to a bovine collagen implant. J Am Acad Dermatol 21:1203–1208
15. Takayama E, Ikeda M, Tsuru S, Ogura M, Kitahara S, Inouye T et al. (1992) Is injectable collagen truly safe? J Laryngol Otol 106:704–708
16. Valigra L (1997) In the business of saving one's skin. The Boston Globe, 15 January
17. DeVore DP, Kelman CD, Fagien S, Casson P (1996) Autologen: autologous, injectable dermal collagen. In: Bosniak SL (ed) Principles and practice of ophthalmic plastic and reconstructive surgery, vol 1. Saunders, Philadelphia, pp 670–675
18. DeVore DP, Hughes E, Scott JB (1994) Effectiveness of injectable filler materials for smoothing wrinkle lines and depressed scars. Med Progr Technol 20:243–250
19. Fagien S, Elson ML (2001) Facial soft-tissue augmentation with allogeneic human tissue collagen matric (Dermalogen and Dermaplant). Clin Plast Surg 28:63–81
20. Sakai N, Takizawa M, Furuta Y, Kumagai M, Anadolu YR, Inuyama Y (1991) Histological study of atelocollagen infused into the human vocal cords. Auris Nasus Larynx 18:61–65

21. Ford CN, Staskowski PA, Bless DM (1995) Autologous collagen vocal fold injection: a preliminary clinical study. Laryngoscope 105:944–948
22. Remacle M, Lawson G, Keghian J, Jamart J (1999) Use of injectable autologous collagen for correcting glottic gaps: initial results. J Voice 13:280–288
23. Remacle M, Lawson G, Delos M, Jamart J (1999) Correcting vocal fold immobility by autologous collagen injection for voice rehabilitation. A short-term study. Ann Otol Rhinol Laryngol 108:788–793
24. Scalafani AP, Romo T III, Jacono AA, McCormick S, Cocker R, Parker A (2000) Evaluation of Acellular dermal graft in sheet (Alloderm) and injectable (micronized Alloderm) forms for soft tissue augmentation. Clinical observations and histological analysis. Arch Facial Plast Surg 2:130–136
25. Scalafani AP, Romo T III, Parker A, McCormick SA, Cocker R, Jacono AA (2002) Mologous collagen dispersion (dermalogen) as a dermal filler, persistence and histology compared with bovine collagen. Ann Plast Surg 49:181–188
26. Hotta T (2004) Dermal fillers. The next generation. Plast Surg Nurs 24:14–19
27. Kriesel KJ, Thiebault SL, Chan RW, Suzuki T, Van Groll PJ, Bless DM, Ford CN (2002) Treatment of vocal fold scarring: rheologic and histological measures of homologous collagen matrix. Ann Otol Rhinol Laryngol 111:884–889
28. Garrett CG, Coleman JR, Reinisch L (2000) Comparative histology and vibration of the vocal folds: implications for experimental studies in microlaryngeal surgery. Laryngoscope 110:814–824
29. Gray SD, Chan KJ, Turner B (2000) Dissection plane of the human vocal fold lamina propria and elastin fiber concentration. Acta Otolaryngol 120:87–91
30. Hammond TH, Gray SD, Butler J, Zhou R, Hammond E (1998) Age- and gender-related elastin distribution changes in human vocal fold. Otolaryngol Head Neck Surg 119:314–322
31. Courey MS (2001) Homologous collagen substances from vocal fold augmentation. Laryngoscope 111:747–758
32. Courey MS (2004) Injection laryngoplasty. Otolaryngol Clin North Am 37:121–138

Chapter 8

Treatment of Glottal Insufficiency Using Micronized Human Acellular Dermis (Cymetra)

8.3

Albert L. Merati

Introduction

Micronized acellular dermis (Cymetra) is an important material for all practitioners managing glottic insufficiency because of its overall safety and availability for immediate use. When used for vocal augmentation, the duration of clinical benefit from micronized acellular dermis is not well established scientifically. Although it appears to last about 3 months, this may not be predictable in all cases.

Cymetra (LifeCell Corporation, Branchburg, N.J.) is a preparation of dried, micronized human acellular dermis. It has been commercially available since 2000, coming to market 6 years after LifeCell introduced Alloderm, the product from which Cymetra is derived. The vast majority of patients receiving these products are treated for rhytids, burns, and other plastic/reconstructive purposes. Though the portion of the "market" using micronized acellular dermis for injection laryngoplasty as opposed to soft tissue augmentation elsewhere in the body is exceedingly small, there is a fair amount of supporting information with which the practitioner should become familiar. This chapter reviews fundamental information about the product itself, its use and characteristics which define its role in laryngology, and provides an overview of the existing literature regarding its use. Logistical aspects of reconstitution are presented, though the specifics related to the technique of injection are detailed elsewhere in this book.

Background

Micronized acellular dermis is unique among glottic injectables in that it is a product of human organ donation. The dermis that comprises it is harvested from the torso and legs of cadavers in accordance with the standards and practices of local and national organ procurement agencies. The World Health Organization has categorized it as a level-IV human allograft, i.e., with no detectable infectious properties [1]. To prepare the material, the dermis is harvested in a thickness ranging from 0.005 to 0.907 in., depending on the characteristics of the donor skin/site [2]. The donors undergo extensive screening, including assays for bacterial, fungal, and viral pathogens (Table 8.3.1). Prions and other atypical agents are not able to be detected. It is noteworthy that the product insert provides the following caveat:

> "The process includes a step in which donor tissue is incubated in a solution demonstrated to inactivate HIV-I (>99.9% reduction of virus titer). However, this model cannot absolutely preclude the possibility of viral contamination of the processed human tissue with yet-to-be identified strains of HIV or guarantee that the tissue is absolutely virus-free. Therefore, Cymetra may transmit infectious agents."

Nonetheless, the manufacturer states that there have been no reported allergic reactions or evidence of viral transmission in over 100,000 uses of its human dermal products, micronized or not.

Once obtained, the donated skin tissue is rendered acellular, leaving the remaining proteins: collagen; elastins; and proteoglycans. In its structurally unaltered form, this product is sold as Alloderm, or human acellular dermis. It has many uses in reconstructive surgery [3–5] and has found a place in management of many surgical challenges, including slings for facial

Table 8.3.1. Infectious agents screened for in the procurement of dermis for micronized acellular dermis

Hepatitis B
Hepatitis C
Human immunodeficiency virus I
Human immunodeficiency virus II
HTLV-I
HTLV-II
Syphilis

paralysis, abdominal hernia repair, and post-parotidectomy rehabilitation, to name a few.

By design, the structure of the acellular dermis is to provide a "scaffold" upon which ingrowth of tissue and neovascularity occurs. This has been demonstrated in the rabbit abdominal wall model [6]. Little histological information about the fate of the micronized material is available, however. It has been concluded from a randomized prospective clinical trial studying lip augmentation that the cumulative volume enhancement in the micronized acellular dermis group was found to be greater than that in a group receiving bovine collagen [7]. While this is promising, the parallel study in laryngology has not been executed. The histological fate of injected micronized dermis has been evaluated as part of Courey's study [8] using a rabbit model. Neither ingrowth nor persistence of the injectate, however, was demonstrated in the killed animals. It is not known what the impact of paralysis on implant persistence would be.

Klemuk and Titze[9] recently published a study investigating the rheological properties of micronized acellular dermis in comparison with bovine collagen as well as to a hyaluronic acid derivative. The viscoelastic properties observed in the study revealed similarities between the bovine and human dermis preparations, though the hyaluronic acid derivative used had a better "match" to vocal fold mucosa. Further investigations will likely be forthcoming to determine the ideal use for each of the material available for soft tissue replacement in the vocal fold.

Advantages and Disadvantages of Micronized Acellular Dermis for Clinical Use

Advantages and Disadvantages of Micronized Acellular Dermis for Clinical UseThe principal advantage of micronized acellular human dermis reflects its origin as human tissue. It is not believed to be allergenic and therefore requires no pre-testing prior to its use. This allows it to be used in nearly all clinical scenarios on short notice. This is in contrast to bovine collagen preparations, such as Zyplast/Zyderm (Inamed, Santa Barbara, Calif.), which do require allergy testing. The testing process itself is not an obstacle, but it can delay the treatment process up to 4 weeks, which has been the recommended observation period following skin test prior to injection for bovine collagen. It is noteworthy that many practitioners, including the present author, choose to wait only 1 week following skin testing for bovine collagen injection laryngoplasty. The advantage remains with micronized acellular dermis, however, as the patient with aspiration or difficulties with travel cannot wait or is inconvenienced by the return trip to clinic necessitated by the skin test.

One modest disadvantage of micronized acellular dermis relates to the preparation process. It does require some time and features several steps which are prone to error. There have been several modifications in response to concerns from users, including providing a larger amount of substrate and the option to use saline instead of plain lidocaine (1%) as the mixing agent (see below). Its short half-life once reconstituted is a drawback compared with the available bovine collagen preparations, which may be held in a refrigerator for several years.

While some may describe the impermanent nature of injected micronized acellular dermis as a limitation, the clinical scenarios in which a practitioner treats glottic insufficiency are varied enough that there are many, if not the majority of, cases in which transience is an asset rather than a liability. Though cumulative, lasting effects have been described for lip augmentation using micronized acellular dermis [7], no similar study has been reported in humans.

Micronized Human Acellular Dermis in Clinical Laryngology

Early reports of success using micronized acellular dermis have been promising. Pearl et al. [1], published a series of injections performed under general anesthesia with excellent results over a 3-month period. Their patients experienced significant improvement in phonation time, reduction in airflow, and improvement in the voice handicap index (Fig. 8.3.1). This initial study was followed by a comprehensive evaluation of a series of 10 patients reported by Karpenko et al. [10]. While many of the same parameters were improved following augmentation with micronized acellular dermis at 1 month, they felt that it was limited as a material for vocal injection because of the lack of persistence in clinical benefit at the 3-month follow-up period. The authors also stated that these findings «have strengthened our beliefs that patients with irreversible vocal paralysis may receive the best long-term symptom resolution with from medialization thyroplasty.» While this is likely true, the role of micronized acellular dermis as a temporary augmentation material for vocal paralysis is becoming better established. It should not be compared to open thyroplasty for long-term results.

Recently, a promising study from the Cleveland Clinic [11] was published in which 20 patients having undergone injection laryngoplasty using micronized human dermis were reviewed. 75% of patients had significant benefit past 6 months; 8 of the 20 patients had long term (greater than 12 months) improvement. One of the key strengths of the study, in addition to prospectively acquired subjective and objective voice quality data demonstrating benefit in many parameters, was that all of the treated patients had well-established paralysis, making the likelihood of spontaneous neural recovery unlikely as a confounding variable.

Beyond vocal paralysis, injection laryngoplasty is often the treatment of choice for vocal paralysis and non-paralytic glottic insufficiency. Though no published study to date has focused on this, Woo has recently presented a series [12] of injections performed for reasons other than paralysis. Based upon the results of his study, he concluded that «micronized dermis injection laryngoplasty is a viable soft tissue replacement in membranous glottal defects due to bowing, scar, and sulcus vocalis. The success rates when treating sequelae of laryngeal fracture, partial laryngectomy defects, and intubation injury was limited, with only 8 of 21 (38%) of their patients experiencing improvement in his early report. This parallels the present author's experience. Not surprisingly, Woo [12] also found that smaller defects were more readily managed than large defects. Further

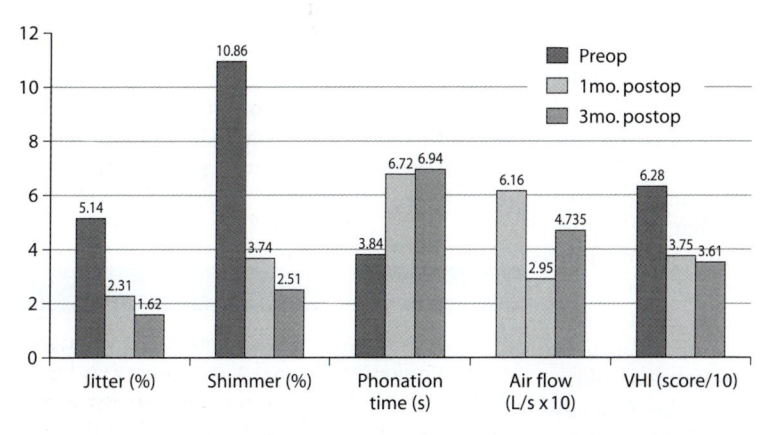

Fig. 8.3.1. Preoperative and postoperative (at 1 and 3 months) acoustic parameters and voice handicap index data. Jitter and shimmer are reported in percent, phonation time in seconds, airflow in l/sec × 10, and the Voice Handicap Index as the total score divided by 10, so that it fits the graph's y axis scale. (From [1])

studies in this area, along with comparisons of paresis and paralysis injections, may help clarify the role of micronized acellular dermis in injection laryngoplasty.

Complications

There are few reports regarding complications specific to this material. While the expected concerns for airway, hemorrhage, and exacerbation of dysphonia can accompany any injection laryngoplasty, none appear to be unique to micronized acellular dermis. Zapanta and Bielamowicz [13] did present a case of laryngeal abscess 4 days after trans-oral injection under general anesthesia. The patient recovered and maintained glottic closure following intensive treatment with intravenous steroids and antibiotics. To date, there are no reports of infection or abscess following percutaneous injection.

Technical Aspects for Using Micronized Acellular Human Dermis

The package insert for Cymetra, the commercially available form of micronized acellular dermis, comes with step-by-step instructions for preparation and use. The technical aspects of injection laryngoplasty, either in the awake setting or under general anesthesia, are presented elsewhere in this book. Some key points in the reconstitution of the micronized dermis include the following:

1. It is imperative that the syringe containing the powdered dermis be "declumped" and separated within the provided 5-cc syringe prior to mixing.
2. The most error-prone step is in the initial mix. The user must assure that the liquid, be it lidocaine or sterile saline, blend thoroughly with the micronized dermis prior to pushing the mix back and forth across the syringe adaptor. If a clump of product is not in the mix, the administered solution will be relatively thin, and theoretically more transient. Several experienced laryngologists have advocated retrograde manipulation of the "clump" with a sterile needle through the distal end of the syringe so that it can blend better.
3. It is possible to intentionally use more liquid for reconstitution, thus making a more easily injected material. For the 2-cc syringe of micronized dermis, it is possible to use 1.9 cc instead of 1.7 cc.
4. Care must be taken to expel air pockets from the syringes prior to transfer to the final syringe. Air mixed into the final product may be responsible for what appears to be "rapid absorption", i.e., a technically well-injected vocal fold may appear nearly empty within a matter of days if the volume of injectate contained air.
5. Use a Luer-Lok style syringe/needle for percutaneous injections to prevent the needle from becoming a projectile due to the force occasionally necessary to pass the material through a small lumen.

Conclusion

Micronized acellular dermis (Cymetra) is an important material for all practitioners managing glottic insufficiency because of its overall safety and availability for immediate use. This latter point is a key advantage over bovine collagen. With the advent of other materials, such as non-donor human collagen protein (Cosmoplast, Inamed Corp., Santa Barbara, Calif.), this feature may no longer be unique. There are several technical issues with preparation that must be mastered to have predictable results. When used for vocal augmentation, the duration of clinical benefit from micronized acellular dermis is not well established scientifically. While it appears last about 3 months, this may not be true in all cases.

References

1. Pearl AW, Woo P, Ostrowski R, Mojica J, Mandell DL, Costantino P (2002) A preliminary report on micronized AlloDerm injection laryngoplasty. Laryngoscope 112:990–996

2. LifeCell corporation package insert from company website, accessed 10 January 2005. www.lifecell.com
3. Morgan AS, McIff T, Park DL, Tsue TT, Kriet JD (2004) Biomechanical properties of materials used in static facial suspension. Arch Facial Plast Surg. 6:308–310
4. Buinewicz B, Rosen B (2004) Acellular cadaveric dermis (AlloDerm): a new alternative for abdominal hernia repair. Ann Plast Surg 52:188–194
5. Sinha UK, Saadat D, Doherty CM, Rice DH (2003) Use of AlloDerm implant to prevent frey syndrome after parotidectomy. Arch Facial Plast Surg. 5:109–112
6. Menon NG, Rodriguez ED, Byrnes CK, Girotto JA, Goldberg NH, Silverman RP (2003) Revascularization of human acellular dermis in full-thickness abdominal wall reconstruction in the rabbit model. Ann Plast Surg 50:523–527
7. Scalfani AP, Romo T III, Jacomo AA (2002) Rejuvenation of the aging lip with an injectable acellular dermal graft (Cymetra). Arch Facial Plast Surg. 4:252–257
8. Courey MS (2001) Homologous collagen substances for vocal fold augmentation. Laryngoscope 111:747–758
9. Klemuk SA, Titze IR (2004) Viscoelastic properties of three vocal-fold injectable biomaterials at low audio frequencies. Laryngoscope 114:1597–1603
10. Karpenko AN, Dworkin JP, Meleca RJ, Stachler RJ (2003) Cymetra injection for unilateral vocal fold paralysis. Ann Otol Rhinol Laryngol 112:927–934
11. Milstein CF, Akst LM, Hicks MD, Abelson TI, Strom M (2005) Long-term effects of micronized alloderm injection for unilateral vocal fold paralysis. Laryngoscope. Sep; 115(9):1681-6
12. Woo P (2004) Presented at the 2004 annual meeting of the American Broncho-Esophagological Association, Scottsdale, Arizona, 1 May
13. Zapanta PE, Bielamowicz SA (2004) Laryngeal abscess after injection laryngoplasty with micronized AlloDerm. Laryngoscope 114:1522–1524

Vocal Fold Augmentation with Calcium Hydroxylapatite

8.4

Peter C. Belafsky, Gregory N. Postma

Introduction

Synthetic calcium hydroxylapatite (CaHA; Radiesse, BioForm, Franksville, Wis.) was approved for vocal fold augmentation by the United States Food and Drug Administration (FDA) Center for Devices and Radiological Health in January 2002. Calcium hydroxylapatite is the primary mineral constituent of bone and teeth. The substance has a proven track record of being highly biocompatible [1–6]. The laryngeal implant is created by suspending CaHA spherules in a gel carrier composed primarily of glycerin and water. The gel is reabsorbed and eventually replaced by soft tissue in-growth. The CaHA remains at the site of injection and has the potential for long-standing augmentation. Since its approval by the FDA, we have injected over 100 vocal folds with CaHA and have achieved excellent results [7]. Theoretical complications include implant migration, granuloma formation, vocal fold mucosal wave irregularities, allergic reaction, infection, and ectopic calcification. None of these complications have been reported as a consequence of vocal fold CaHA injection [7–10]. This chapter reviews the concepts necessary for successful vocal fold augmentation with CaHA.

Indications for Vocal Fold Augmentation with CaHA

Injection augmentation is best reserved for persons with a small (1 mm) or medium-sized (2–3 mm) glottal gap. Individuals with a large gap (>4 mm) may be better served with a medialization laryngoplasty and arytenoid repositioning if indicated. The majority of the vocal folds that we have injected with CaHA (61%) have been mobile (e.g., vocal fold paresis/senile atrophy). We routinely inject both vocal folds at the same time, if necessary. Even when injecting a paralyzed vocal fold, we often inject a mobile contralateral vocal fold if it is bowed and atrophic. Our indications for injection augmentation with CaHA are presented in Table 8.4.1. We have performed bilateral injections in 13 individuals with glottal insufficiency secondary to Parkinson's hypophonia. Our results have been extremely positive and appear to be similar to the degree of improvement reported by other investigators with collagen augmentation [11, 12].

Table 8.4.1. Indications for injection augmentation with calcium hydroxylapatite

Indication	%
Unilateral vocal fold paralysis	39
Unilateral vocal fold paresis	22
Bilateral vocal fold paresis	9
Presbylarynx	13
Parkinson's disease	13
Abductor spasmodic dysphonia	4

Technique of Injection Augmentation with CaHA

Each package of Radiesse includes 1 cc of implant in a Luer-Lok syringe (Fig. 8.4.1). A 25-G laryngeal injection needle is now available (BioForm, Franksville, Wis.). The needle is 25 cm long and has a laser marked band 5 mm from the tip to help gauge injection depth. There are several possible techniques of CaHA injection. These techniques are categorized into in-office and operating-room-based procedures.

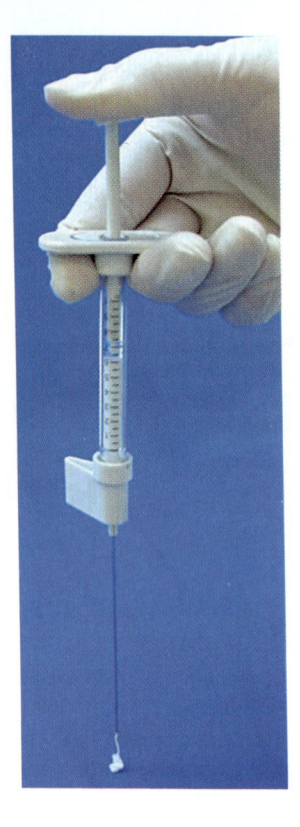

Fig. 8.4.1. Each package of Radiesse contains 1 cc of implant in a Luer-Lok syringe

In-Office Injection of CaHA

Radiesse can be injected percutaneously either through the cricothyroid membrane or directly through the thyroid cartilage under transnasal fiberoptic laryngoscopy (TFL) guidance. The CaHA can also be injected in the office setting per-orally through a curved laryngeal needle. Anesthesia can be achieved with a combination of superior laryngeal nerve blocks and an instillation of 2 cc of 1% lidocaine into the trachea as described by Sulica and Blitzer [13]. We have found that injecting lidocaine at the site of skin puncture is also beneficial. The CaHA can be injected through a 25-G needle or larger. The disadvantage of injection through the thyroid cartilage is that the needle can become blocked with cartilage or bone. The disadvantage of injection through the cricothyroid membrane or per-orally is that these procedures are technically difficult for most otolaryngologists. Because of the potential for permanent augmentation, and our uncertainty of how the implant would perform if injected into a suboptimal location in the vocal fold, i.e., superficially, we choose to do the majority of our injections in the operating room under more controlled circumstances.

Injection of CaHA in the Operating Room

Although CaHA can be injected in the operating room through a rigid laryngoscope in an awake but adequately sedated and anesthetized patient, we choose to do the majority of our injections in paralyzed patients under general anesthesia. This technique provides maximal control for the most precise injection possible. We must reiterate our concern for the potential of long-term sequelae from inaccurate CaHA injection and for the uncertain risks of inadvertently injecting the implant into the airway.

The patient's eyes and teeth are protected and microlaryngoscopy is performed. We use a Hunsaker Mono-Jet subglottic ventilation tube (Xomed Surgical Products, Jacksonville, Fla.) or intermittent Venturi jet ventilation from above the vocal folds [14]. Use of the Hunsaker tube affords an unobstructed view of both vocal folds while providing continuous ventilation (Fig. 8.4.2). The 25-G laryngeal injection needle (BioForm, Franksville, Wis.) is fastened to the Luer-Lok syringe and per-oral injection is then performed. The first author (P.C.B.) prefers to use a Brünings-type laryngeal injector that allows for precise implant delivery (Karl Storz, Tuttlingen, Germany; Fig. 8.4.3). Each click of this injector delivers 0.04 cc of implant. This helps prevent over-injection. The second author prefers to use the syringe that is packaged with the product (Fig. 8.4.1).

The location of CaHA injection is crucial. The implant must be delivered deep to the thyroarytenoid (TA) muscle. A superficial injection could severely compromise mucosal vibration and is to be avoided. Placing a hand on the neck from the outside and pushing the thyroid cartilage medially toward the tip of the needle assists with injection deep to the TA muscle against the inner perichondrium of the thyroid cartilage. The anterior aspect of the vocal process is a useful landmark. We inject just anterior and lateral to the vocal process (Fig. 8.4.4). The amount of CaHA to inject depends on the degree of vocal fold mobility, the need for a bilateral injection, the degree of atrophy, and the position of the vocal fold if immobile. The gel carrier constitutes approximately 30% of the implant by volume and will eventually be absorbed. We have noticed absorption of the gel carrier in some individuals at 3 months post-implantation. We take this 30% absorption into consideration when injecting the CaHA. Because the individual is under general anesthesia and the surgeon is unable to titrate the amount of CaHA injected by improvement in the patients' voice, we err on the side of undercorrection for fear of the consequences of over-

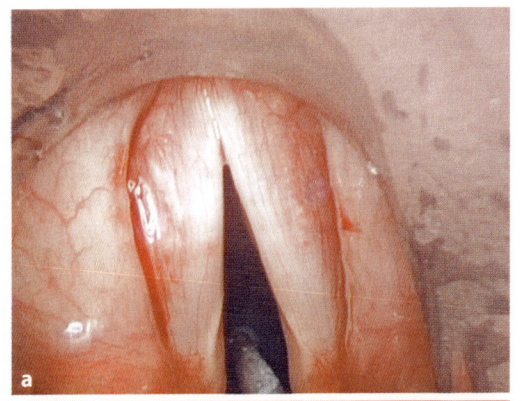

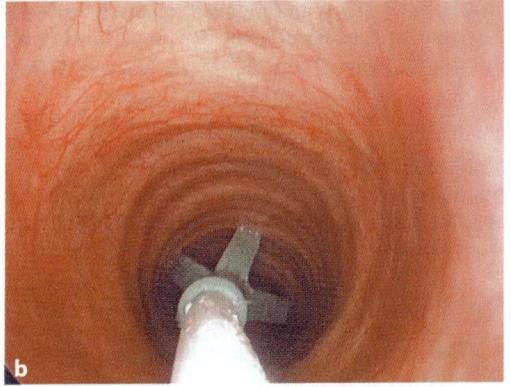

Fig. 8.4.2. a Surgical view for injection augmentation of the vocal folds. Hunsaker Mono-Jet subglottic ventilation tube can be visualized inferiorly. b Subglottic view of Hunsaker tube

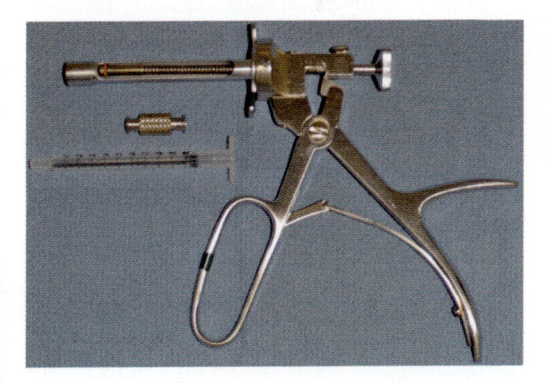

Fig. 8.4.3. Storz viscous fluid injector. The Radiesse implant must be transferred from the Luer-Lok syringe in which it is packaged into a 1-cc non-Luer-Lok tuberculin syringe in order to utilize the injector

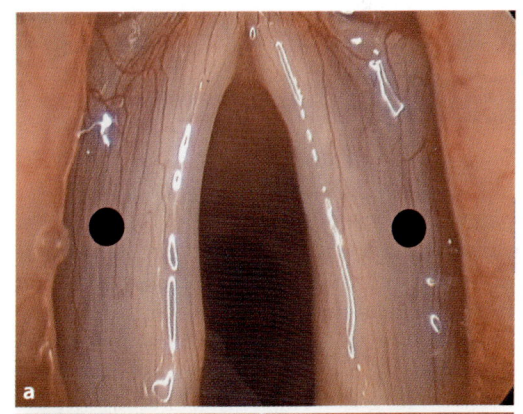

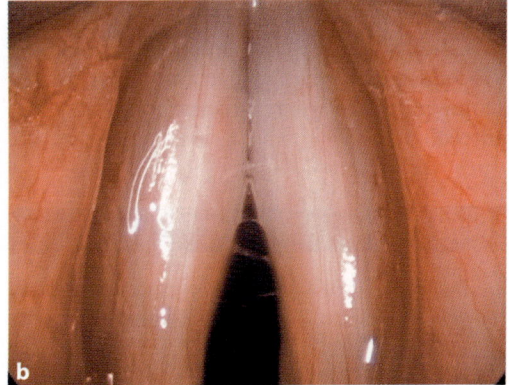

Fig. 8.4.4. a Pre- and b post-injection images. The black circles represent the optimal site for injection just anterior and lateral to the anterior extent of the vocal process of the arytenoid

correction. We inform all patients of this limitation preoperatively and prepare them for the possibility of a second injection at some point in the future.

Removing the needle slowly from the vocal fold helps seal the injection site and limit implant extrusion. We previously utilized the CO_2 laser on a defocused setting to "spot-weld" the injection site closed. Since the introduction of the 25-G laryngeal injection needles, extrusion has not been problematic, and we have stopped using the laser. Postoperatively the patient is observed in the post-anesthesia care unit room for 45 min. If the patient emerges from anesthesia with no evidence of airway compromise, he or she is sent home directly from the recovery room. Perioperative steroids and antibiotics have not been necessary. We currently recommend 3 days of postoperative voice rest along with avoidance of strenuous activity.

Conclusion

Injection augmentation with CaHA is an exciting new addition to the laryngologist's therapeutic armamentarium in the treatment of glottal insufficiency. The implant is safe, efficacious, and initial experience suggests that it is extremely durable. Vocal fold augmentation with Radiesse can be performed in the office under local anesthesia or in the operating room under general anesthesia. Because we are uncertain about the adverse effects of inaccurate CaHA injections, we prefer to perform the procedure in the operating room under microscopic guidance where precision can be guaranteed.

References

1. Jarcho M (1981) Calcium phosphate ceramics as hard tissue prosthetics. Clin Orthop 157:259–278
2. Constantino PD, Friedman CD, Jones K et al. (1992) Experimental hydroxyapatite cement cranioplasty. Plast Reconstr Surg 90:174–185
3. Constantino PD, Friedman CD, Jones K et al. (1991) Hydroxyapatite cement: I. Basic chemistry and histologic properties. Arch Otolaryngol Head Neck Surg 117:379–384
4. Friedman CD, Constantino PD, Jones K et al. (1991) Hydroxyapatite cement: II. Obliteration and reconstruction of the cat frontal sinus. Arch Otolaryngol Head Neck Surg 117: 385–389
5. Jarcho M (1986) Biomaterial aspects of calcium phosphates: properties and applications. Dent Clin North Am 30:25–47
6. Holmes RE, Hagler HK (1988) Porous hydroxyapatite as a bonegraft substitute in cranial reconstruction: a histometric study. Plast Reconstr Surg 81:662–671
7. Belafsky PC, Postma GN (2004) Vocal fold augmentation with calcium hydroxylapatite. Otolaryngol Head Neck Surg 131:351–354
8. Chhetri DK, Jahan-Parwar B, Hart SD, Bhuta SM, Berke GS (2004) Injection laryngoplasty with calcium hydroxylapatite gel implant in an in vivo canine model. Ann Otol Rhinol Laryngol 113:259–264
9. Lee B, Woo P (2004) Use of injectable hydroxyapatite in the secondary setting to restore glottic competence after partial laryngectomy with arytenoidectomy. Ann Otol Rhinol Laryngol 113:618–622
10. Rosen CA, Thekdi AA (2004) Focal fold augmentation with injectable calcium hydroxylapatite: short-term results. J Voice 18:387–391
11. Berke GS, Gerratt B, Kreiman J, Jackson K (1999) Treatment of Parkinson hypophonia with percutaneous collagen augmentation. Laryngoscope 109:1295–1299
12. Kim SH, Kearney JJ, Atkins JP (2002) Percutaneous laryngeal collagen augmentation for treatment of parkinsonian hypophonia. Otolaryngol Head Neck Surg126:653–656
13. Sulica L, Blitzer A (2000) Anesthesia for laryngeal surgery in the office. Laryngoscope 110:1777–1779
14. Orloff LA, Parhizkar N, Ortiz E (2002) The Hunsaker Mon-Jet ventilation tube for microlaryngeal surgery: optimal laryngeal exposure. Ear Nose Throat J 81:390–394

Chapter 8

Treatment of Glottal Insufficiency Using Hyaluronan

8.5

Stellan Hertegård, Åke Dahlqvist, Lars Hallén, Claude Laurent

Introduction and Core Messages

The main things to be understood about hyaluronan are as follows:
- Hyaluronan (hyaluronic acid, HA) is a linear polysaccharide ubiquitous in all mammals which is naturally present in tissues, including the vocal folds.
- Hyaluronan is non-toxic, non-antigenic, non-inflammatory and is involved in many biological actions, such as wound healing and anti-adhesion.
- Hyaluronan binds water, regulates tissue osmosis and exerts viscoelasticity.
- Experiments in animals and clinical research have shown minimal inflammation and no long-term side effects after injection of HA into the vocal folds. Rabbit vocal folds injected with HA derivatives showed favourable viscoelastic properties comparable to non-injected vocal folds.
- Resorption of HA can be decreased through cross-linking of the molecule with preserved favourable viscoelasticity. Cross-linked HA can easily be injected through a fine-diameter cannula.
- Several commercial preparations of HA have good long-term effects (lasting 2 years) in the treatment of glottal insufficiency due to unilateral paresis or vocal fold atrophy.
- Preliminary findings from animal experiments and injections in humans indicate that HA seems to be advantageous in the treatment of vocal fold scarring and sulcus vocalis.

Rationale

Hyaluronan (hyaluronic acid, HA) is a high molecular weight glycosaminoglycan, present in the extracellular matrix, including the vocal fold lamina propria [2]. Hyaluronan is present in virtually all tissues, but the highest concentrations in humans are found in the umbilical cord, synovial fluid, vitreous body and skin [18]. The molecule is ubiquitous in all mammals and consists of a repetitive disaccharide chain of D-glucuronic acid and N-acetyl-D-glycosamine (Fig. 8.5.1). This chain is free from amino acids and proteins and is therefore non-antigenic. Hyaluronan is hydrophilic and highly soluble

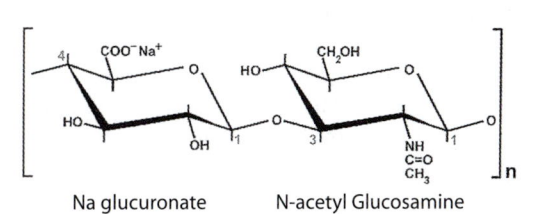

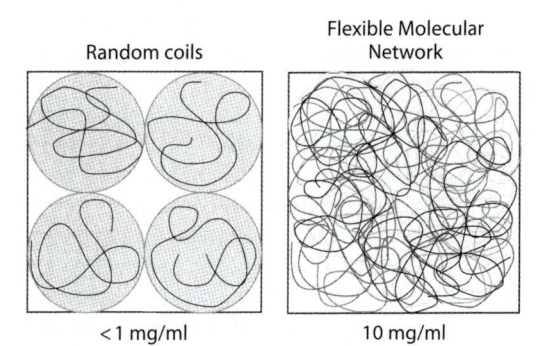

Fig. 8.5.1. Hyaluronan (HA) chemical structure. Top left D-glucuronic acid; top right N-acetyl-D-glycosamine forms the basic disaccharide unit; bottom coils of HA at different concentration <1 mg/ml and at 10 mg/ml

in water forming a network at higher concentrations. The molecular weight of native HA in tissues varies between 10,000 and 20,000 Da (low molecular HA) up of 5–10 million Da (high molecular HA) [24]. The synthesis takes place in the cell membrane of fibroblasts and other connective tissue cells, and HA is then extruded to the extracellular space. Most of the HA is degraded in lymph nodes and in the liver. The total amount of native HA has been estimated to be 15 g, with a half-life in the skin of less than 24 h [22, 23].

Hyaluronan has viscoelastic properties, binds water and regulates hydration of the soft tissue matrix. It is a multi-functional extracellular structural component with lubricating and shock-absorbing action and has important biological functions in, for example, wound healing [16, 18].

Hyaluronan is present in normal vocal folds in the lamina propria (LP). Its properties to regulate water content and viscosity are probably very important in the ability to initiate and maintain vocal fold oscillation. Chan et al. [3] found that removal of HA from the superficial LP resulted in a decreased elasticity and increased viscosity generating increased stiffness.

It is possible that the wound-healing properties of HA play a role in repairing damage caused by repetitive collision forces between the vocal folds during phonation. Interestingly, there is a gender difference concerning HA with a higher concentration and a more even distribution in the LP in men. Women have the highest concentration in the deeper part of LP, which also vibrates less during phonation [2]. Females are overrepresented among patients with vocal nodules and other benign lesions, and it is possible that differences in HA concentration between the sexes contributes to this fact. Furthermore, there seems to be a decrease of HA in the LP with advancing age, particularly in males [9]. Recent studies [5, 9] have found that age-related vocal fold atrophy is caused mainly by reduced thickness of the LP, and that both the HA and collagen content is decreased in the LP of the aged larynx.

Hyaluronan has many desirable characteristics of an augmentation substance for reconstruction or improvement of vocal fold biomechanics; however, exogenous HA solution, extracted from biological tissues or synthesized, does not have the necessary rheological properties to be used for augmentation [16]; therefore, exogenous derivatives have been developed in order to improve the characteristics. These can be made by alteration of concentration or modification of the molecules (e.g. by cross-linking) rendering different molecular gel bead sizes. In this way the viscoelasticity and durability can be improved [17, 20]. Hyaluronan derivatives are widely used in dermatology and plastic surgery for skin augmentation, as a augmentative substance in paediatric vesicoureteral reflux treatment and in gynaecology for incontinence. Hyaluronan has also proved to have positive effects in orthopaedics for joint injections, and it has revolutionised ophthalmological surgery.

Several HA derivatives have been studied in animal experiments for vocal fold injections. Favourable viscoelastic properties of vocal folds injected with HA derivatives, both in short-term and long-term perspective (6 months), have been found [4, 11]. Minimal inflammation is seen and the durability in tissue is at least 1 year (Hylan B gel, DiHA) [6, 7]. Furthermore, experiments in rabbit vocal folds indicate that injections of a HA derivative may be beneficial to the viscoelasticity of scarred vocal folds [13].

Indications

Currently (2005) HA derivatives for laryngological practice have been used mostly in Europe, but several products have now also been approved in the U.S. for non-laryngological indications. To our knowledge, there is no HA substance which presently is specifically marketed for laryngological indications. They are, however, used off-label by some laryngologists.

Studies in humans have shown positive results (improved glottal closure and mucosal vibration, and subjective voice improvements) in the treatment of glottal insufficiency by injection of HA derivatives (Hylan B gel, a divinyl cross-linked HA and DiHA, dextranomers in HA solution). Hyaluronan also seems to improve vocal fold viscoelasticity. The follow-up time of these studies was between 12 and 24 months [8, 11, 14].

The indications with proven positive treatment effect of HA injections are (Fig. 8.5.2):
1. Glottal insufficiency due to unilateral vocal fold paresis.
2. Glottal insufficiency due to uni- or bilateral vocal fold atrophy (bowing)

Indication Under Investigation

The primary indication under investigation is anti-adhesion and augmentation after intracordal dissection, e.g. sulcus vocalis and treatment of vocal fold scarring.

Table 8.5.1 shows a summary of derivatives used in humans thus far.

Patient Selection

Patients with unilateral idiopathic or iatrogenic vocal fold paresis with voice symptoms for at least 3–6 months are candidates for treatment. Because of the favourable effects of HA and lack of side effects, we do not think it is necessary to wait for reinnervation 1 year into vocal fold paresis. Unilateral paresis due to extralaryngeal malignancy can be treated promptly. To address remaining compensatory voice habits, such as pressed voice, suboptimal breath support and abnormal phonation frequency, we recommend that the patients be examined by a speech pathologist before injection, and that the appropriate amount of voice therapy be offered. Usually, postoperative voice therapy also ensures optimal long-term voice habits.

Anticoagulant therapy is no contraindication, provided that the medication is optimized. We do not recommend injections to be performed when a patient has an upper respiratory tract infection or a general infection. Patients with airway obstructions (e.g. due to inflammation, oedema or bilateral vocal fold paresis) should not be injected.

In patients with glottic insufficiency due to unilateral or bilateral vocal fold atrophy or focal defects, one or both vocal folds can be injected at the same time.

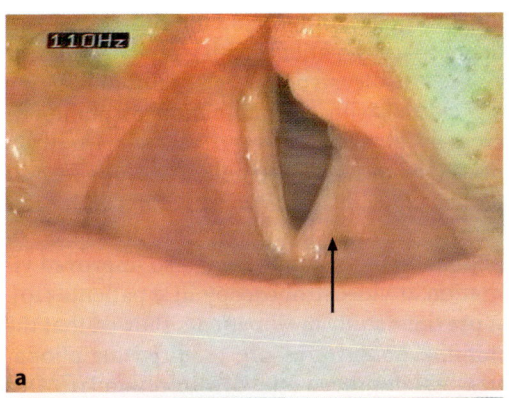

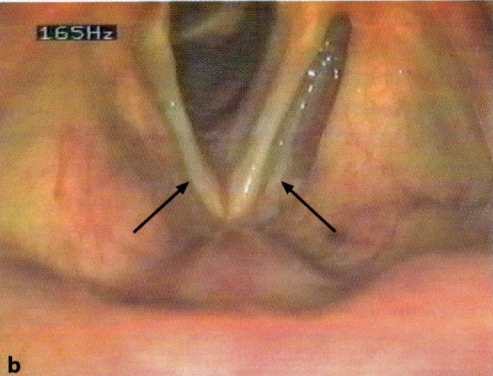

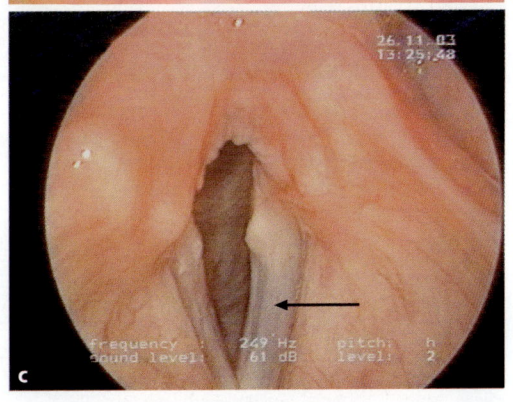

Fig. 8.5.2. Disorders where currently injections of HA derivatives are used or evaluated for treatment. a unilateral vocal fold paresis of left side; b bilateral vocal fold atrophy; c sulcus vocalis. Arrows mark the vocal fold changes

Depending on the HA derivative used, it may be necessary to perform a re-injection 1–2 months after the first to ensure long-term benefit in patients with either vocal fold paresis or atrophy (see Table 8.5.1).

Sulcus Vocalis and Vocal Fold Scarring. In an ongoing study, patients with glottal insufficiency due to sulcus vocalis or vocal fold scarring are treated with a combination of phonomicrosurgical dissection and several HA injections (Hylan B gel). Preliminary results from 11 patients (7 with sulcus vocalis and 4 with scarring) show subjective improvements in ease of phonation in 10 patients and also improved vibration at videostroboscopy in 9 patients [10]. A previous study in GI patients showed that the minimal sound pressure required for phonation was improved after HA injection [11]. Our hypothesis is that this parameter was also improved in the patients with sulcus and scarring. The mechanism is not clear, but it is known that HA has anti-adhesive properties [1]. Many questions remain regarding the treatment of sulcus vocalis and scarring with HA, particularly with respect to timing of treatment, optimal HA derivative and other complementary treatment.

Advantages

The advantages of using hyaluronan are as follows:
- The HA derivatives are easy to inject through a fine-diameter cannula (see Table 8.5.1).
- Injections of HA derivatives with relatively small particle size (e.g. Hylan B gel and Restylane) can be performed into the LP including the Reinke's space without disturbing the vibratory properties (see Table 8.5.1 and below).
- Hyaluronan does not have antigenic properties, and allergic testing is therefore not necessary before injection.

Table 8.5.1. Characteristics of different hyaluronan (*HA*) derivatives used for vocal fold injections. *LP* lamina propria, *TA* thyroarytenoid muscle

HA derivative	Composition	HA concentration	Recommended minimum cannula diameter	Recommended injection site in vocal fold	Residence time
Hylan B Gel (Hylaform)[a]	HA from rooster combs, double cross-linked	5.5 mg/ml, 250-μm molecule gel bead size	27–30 G	In LP, including Reinke's space, initially two injections	12 months 1/2 time in skin[b], >25% of patients need repeat treatment after a year[b]
Restylane[b]	Non-animal stabilized HA (NASHA, from bacterial fermentation)	20 mg/ml, 250-μm molecule gel bead size	27–30 G	In TA muscle or in LP, initially one to two injections	Effect 6–2 months in skin[c], resorption in vocal folds unknown
DiHA (Deflux)	Mixture of NASHA and dextranomers	50 mg/ml dextranomere + 20 mg/ml NASHA	23 G (≥ 0.6 mm)	In TA muscle, one or two injections over a year[b]	Effect ≥ 4 years in urinary tractb, effect ≥ 1 year in vocal fold[b]

[a] Also marketed as Hylaform plus, with a higher particle size (700-μm gel bead) which is the equivalent to Perlane. [Perlane is another NASHA gel (see Restylane) with particle size 1000 μm. We have limited experience with Perlane, but this should probably be injected in the TA]. Our experience in vocal folds injections of this is limited
[b] See Reference List
[c] NASHA monograph (see Reference List)

Disadvantages

Resorption has been noted after vocal fold injections with HA derivatives [11, 13]: The extent of resorption in the human vocal fold is unknown for several of the existing preparations. It is possible that DiHA and HA derivatives with higher particle size (e.g. Perlane) show less resorption (H. Svanholm, personal communication). According to the documentation of DiHA (Deflux), this substance remains at least 3–5 years after treatment of vesicourethral reflux in the urinary tract [19, 21].

Complications

Complications of hyaluronan use are as follows:
- A slight inflammation or bleeding at the injection site has been noted in less than 4% of the injections [12]. Usually this inflammation resolves without treatment within a week. We have seen a few patients who had laryngitis after injection. This resolved with broad-spectrum antibiotics within a week. No long-term inflammation or granuloma formation has been noted after HA injections.
- A temporary decrease in mucosal wave pliability is sometimes noted after injections of Hylan B Gel or Restylane in the superficial LP (including Reinke's space). This is normalized within a few weeks. We are, however, aware of 1 patient with long-lasting vocal fold stiffness, reduced mucosal wave and a rough voice quality after superficial injection of DiHA. This substance is known to induce new soft tissue formation (mainly collagen) in the injected area [6], and it is possible that DiHA may induce some stiffness when injected into the superficial LP. On the other hand, animal experiments have shown positive viscoelastic properties in injected rabbit vocal folds after 6 months using this compound [4]; however, we caution against injection of DiHA or other HA derivatives with larger particle size (e.g. Perlane, Q-med Inc.) superficially in the LP until the effect of them has been studied more in detail. If these HA derivatives are used, the injections should be made into the thyroarytenoid muscle.

Technique

There are four techniques for injection [11, 15], as illustrated in Fig. 8.5.3.
1. Under local anaesthesia through a transoral route using a curved cannula under with a rigid endoscope guidance. Cannula diameter is usually 27 G. Most often we use the Medtronic Xomed Oro-Tracheal laryngeal Injector.
2. Under local anaesthesia with a transcutaneous needle passed through the cricothyroid membrane under transnasal fiberscope guidance. This us usually performed with an intramuscular injection needle.
3. Under local anaesthesia transnasally via the working channel of a fiberscope (cannula size 23 G). At present, we use a specially designed catheter from Sugimed Inc.
4. Under general anaesthesia via a laryngoscope using a straight-injection cannula (diameter between 23 and 27 G). Several injection cannulas are available (e.g. the Medtronic Xomed Oro-Tracheal laryngeal Injector).

Methods 1–3 are usually performed as an in-office procedure. In our previous studies, 67% of the injections were performed as an out-patient procedure [11], and currently this figure is even higher. Methods 2 and 3 require an assistant performing the fibrescopic examination while the surgeon injects. As topical anaesthetic we use lidocaine 2 or 4% given as spray or inhalation in the oral cavity, pharynx and larynx. Sometimes 10% lidocaine spray is added. In the transcutaneous method (no. 2) the local anaesthetic can be injected through the cricothyroid membrane prior to insertion of the intramuscular injection needle. It is important that the laryngeal reflexes be completely abolished during the injection and that it be performed with optimal vision of the glottic area. The amount of substance injected is determined on-line and glottal closure can be tested by asking the

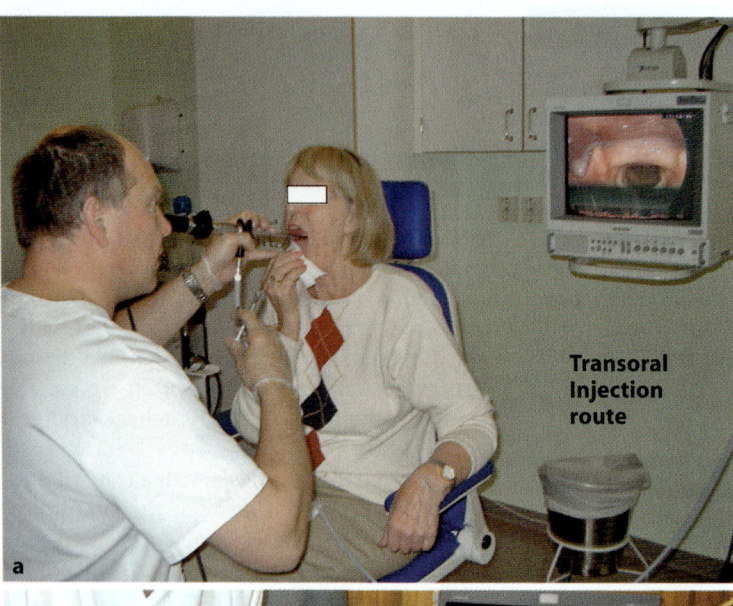

Fig. 8.5.3. Injection techniques: **a** transoral route; **b** transcutaneous route

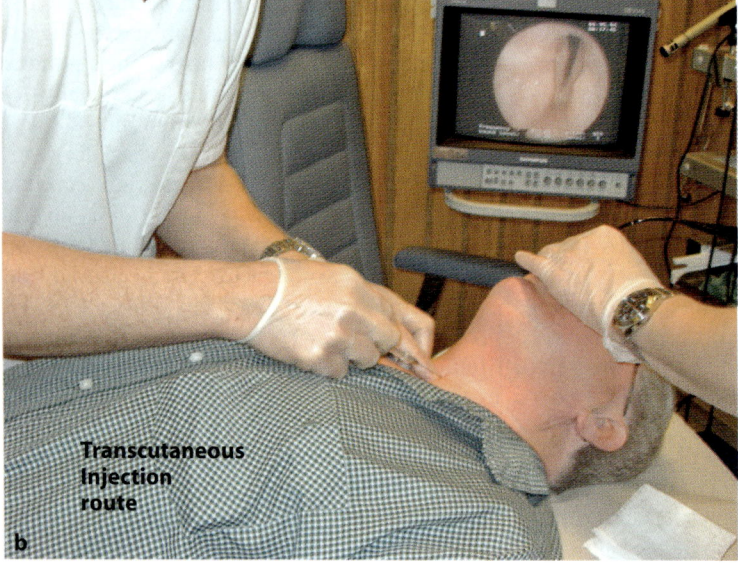

Transoral Injection route

Transcutaneous Injection route

patient to phonate during the procedure. It is also possible to perform a stroboscopy directly after the injection. Normally we do not overinject, except for Hylan B gel, which is injected to achieve a slightly convex vocal fold edge. Usually the total amount of HA injected ranges between 0.15 up to maximum 1 ml depending on the cause and severity of GI. Patients with a large glottal gap due to unilateral paresis often receive larger amount of HA. The duration of the procedure is usually only a few minutes. In the local procedures, the patients are observed for about 1 h after the procedure and then discharged. One or 2 days voice rest is recommended after treatment.

Injections under general anaesthesia include all phonomicrosurgical procedures with dissection of sulcus vocalis and vocal fold scarring.

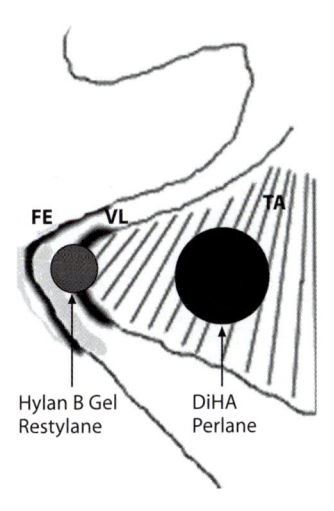

Fig. 8.5.4. Recommended placement of different HA derivatives during injection treatment. Coronal plane of a vocal fold. *FE* free edge of vocal fold, *VL* vocal ligament, *TA* thyroarytenoid muscle

This is necessary to ensure optimal placement of the HA in the treated vocal fold (Fig. 8.5.4). Patients who do not tolerate a local procedure are also included in this group. The operations are usually same-day procedures. For the sulcus operations, a week of absolute voice rest is recommended.

References

1. Becker JM, Dayton MT, Fazio VW et al. (1996) Prevention of postoperative abdominal adhesions by a sodium hyaluronate-based bioresorbable membrane: a prospective, randomized, double-blind multicenter study. J Am Coll Surg 183:297–306
2. Butler JE, Hammond TH, Gray SD (2001) Gender related differences of hyaluronic acid distribution in the human vocal fold. Laryngoscope 111:907–911
3. Chan RW, Gray SD, Titze IR (2001) The importance of hyaluronic acid in vocal fold biomechnics. Otolaryngol Head Neck Surg 124:607–614
4. Dahlqvist Å, Gärskog O, Laurent C, Hertegård S, Ambrosio L, Borzacchiello A (2004) Viscoelasticity of rabbit vocal folds after injection augmentation. Laryngoscope 114:138–142
5. Filho J, Tsuji D, Nascimento P, Sennes L (2003) Histological changes in human vocal folds correlated with aging: a histomorphometric study. Ann Otol Rhinol Laryngol 112:894–898
6. Hallén L, Dahlqvist Å, Laurent C (1998) Dextranomeres in hyaluronan DiHA): a promising substance in treating vocal cord insufficiency. Laryngoscope 108:393–397
7. Hallén L, Johansson C, Laurent C (1999) Cross-linked hyaluronan (Hylan B gel): a new injectable remedy for treatment of vocal fold insufficiency – an animal study. Acta Otolaryngol (Stockh) 119:107–111
8. Hallén L, Testad P, Sederholm E, Dahlqvist A, Laurent C (2001) DiHA (dextranomeres in hyaluronan) injections for treatment of insufficient closure of the vocal folds. Early clinical experiences. Laryngoscope 111:1063–1067
9. Hammond TH, Gray SD, Butler JE (2000) Age- and gender related collagen distribution in human vocal folds. Ann Otol Rhinol Laryngol 109:913–920
10. Hertegård S (2003) Hyaluronan vid fonokirurgisk behandling av sulcus vokalis samt ärrbildning i stämbanden. Poster presentation at the Annual Swedish Medical Association Conference, Stockholm, November 2003 [in Swedish]
11. Hertegård S, Dahlqvist Å, Laurent C, Olofsson K, Sederholm E, Hallén L, Testad P (2002) Cross-linked hyaluronan (hylan B gel) and bovine collagen used as augmentation substances for treatment of patients with glottal insufficiency – evaluation of safety and vocal fold function. Laryngoscope 112:2211–2219
12. Hertegård S, Dahlqvist Å, Laurent C, Borzacchiello A, Ambrosio L (2003) Viscoelastic properties of rabbit vocal folds after augmentation. Otolaryngol Head Neck Surg 128:401–406
13. Hertegård S, Dahlqvist Å, Goodyer E, Maurer F (2004) Viscoelasticity in scarred rabbit vocal folds after hyaluronan injection: short term results. Abstract. Report presented at the Annual American Academy of Otolaryngology Head and Neck Surgery Conference, New York, September 2004
14. Hertegård S, Dahlqvist Å, Laurent C, Olofsson K, Sederholm E, Hallén L, Testad P (2004) Cross-linked hyaluronan for injection treatment of glottal insufficiency: 2-year follow-up. Acta Otolaryngol (Stockholm) 124:1208–1214
15. Hirano M, Tanaka S, Tanaka Y, Hibi S (1990) Transcutaneous intrafold injection for unilateral vocal fold paralysis: functional results. Ann Otol Rhinol Laryngol 99:598–604
16. Lapcik L, De Smedt S, Demester J, Chabrecek P (1998) Hyaluronan: preparation, structure, properties, and applications. Chem Rev 98:2663–2684
17. Larsen NE, Leshchiner E, Pollak CT, Balazs EA, Piacquadio D (1995) Evaluation of Hylan b (hylan gel) as soft tissue dermal implants. In: Mikos AG, Leong KW, Radomsky ML, Tamada JA, Yaszem-

ski MJ (eds) Polymers in medicine and pharmacy. Proc Materials Research Society. Spring meeting, April 1995. Materials Research Society, Pittsburgh, pp 193–197
18. Laurent T (1987) Biochemistry of hyaluronan. Acta Otolaryngol (Stockh) Suppl 442:7–24
19. Läckgren G, Wahlin N, Skoldenberg E, Stenberg A (2001) Long-term follow-up of children treated with dextranomer/hyaluronic acid copolymer for vesicoureteral reflux. J Urol 166:1887–1892
20. Manna F, Dentini M, Desideri P, Pita O de, Mortilla E, Maras B (1999) Comparative chemical evaluation of two commercially available derivatives of hyaluronic acid (hylaform from rooster combs and restylane from streptococcus) used for soft tissue augmentation. J Eur Acad Dermatol Venereol 13:183–192
21. Ågerup B, Wik Y (2001) NASHA. The monograph. Q-med AB. Uppsala, Sweden
22. Reed RK, Lilja K, Laurent T (1988) Hyaluronan in the rat with special reference to the skin. Acta Physiol Scand 13:405–411
23. Reed RK, Laurent UBG, Fraser JRE, Laurent T (1990) Removal rate of [^{3}H] hyaluronan injected subcutaneously in rabbits. Am J Physiol 259:H532–H535
24. Ward PD, Thibeault SL, Gray SD (2002) Hyaluronic acid: its role in voice. J Voice 16:303–309

Chapter 9

Principles of Medialization Laryngoplasty

C. Blake Simpson, Lucian Sulica

Introduction

Medialization for vocal fold paralysis by means of alteration of the laryngeal cartilaginous framework was first described by Payr in 1915 [1], not long after Brünings achieved the same end by vocal fold injection [2]. Both of these initial approaches had shortcomings that prevented their widespread adoption. Brünings used paraffin as the injectable material, which provoked a florid inflammatory response. Payr, on the other hand, created an anteriorly based cartilage flap from the thyroid ala overlying vocal fold which was displaced medially. Not only did it prove difficult to "greenstick" a thyroid cartilage flap in this way, but subsequent experience showed that cartilage tended to be difficult to stabilize and to resorb over time. Subsequent efforts by Meurman [3] and Waltner [4] using costal cartilage, and Opheim using thyroid cartilage [5], encountered some of the same difficulties, but remain important precursors to modern medialization laryngoplasty. The introduction of polytetrafluoroethylene polymer (Teflon; Polytef) as an injectate in the 1960s [6, 7] convinced many otolaryngologists that injection was the rehabilitation procedure of choice until the description of Silastic block medialization laryngoplasty by Isshiki et al. [8], initially performed in combination with cartilage. The increased precision and finesse of framework surgery, as well as its reversibility, were clear advantages over injection augmentation, including Teflon techniques. Fine-tuning of the voice result could be achieved in the awake patient under local anesthesia without undue risk. In contrast to Teflon, there was a less hazardous learning curve: residents and practitioners could learn the technique without risk of an irreversible adverse outcome. Additionally, the occasional adverse tissue response to Teflon was avoided.

The general goal of framework surgery is to improve phonatory glottal closure by altering vocal fold position. Medialization laryngoplasty, also called thyroplasty, is the most commonly performed framework surgery, typically used to correct glottic insufficiency from several causes, but most often from unilateral vocal fold paralysis. Whereas injection augmentation techniques principally improve glottal closure by expansion of the thyroarytenoid muscle, laryngoplasty repositions the affected vocal fold(s) medially into a more favorable phonatory position. Alternative medialization materials in addition to the Silastic block have been described since Isshiki et al.'s [8] work; these include pre-molded Silastic and hydroxylapatite implants, polytetrafluoroethylene ribbon (Gore-Tex), and titanium, each discussed in detail elsewhere in this volume. Medialization laryngoplasty may be used in conjunction with an arytenoid repositioning procedure, an adjunctive technique that can be used to alter vocal fold height and tension by manipulating the arytenoid along its physiologic axis of rotation.

Indications and contraindications for medialization laryngoplasty are given in Table 9.1.

Indications for Surgery

The primary indication for medialization laryngoplasty is symptomatic glottic insufficiency. The goals of the surgery are to improve voice quality and protect the airway by achieving complete glottic closure during phonation and swallowing.

Table 9.1. Indications and contraindications for medialization laryngoplasty

Indications
— Symptomatic (dysphonia, aspiration) glottic insufficiency, especially if there is little chance of return of normal neurologic function. Glottic insufficiency can be due to: — Unilateral vocal fold paralysis — Unilateral or bilateral vocal fold paresis[a] — Vocal fold atrophy, including age-related atrophy

Contraindication
— Malignant disease overlying the laryngotracheal complex — Poor abduction of the contralateral vocal fold (due to airway concerns)[a] — Previous history of radiation therapy to the larynx (relative contraindication)

[a]Because medialization inevitably leads to some narrowing of the airway, patients with moderate to severe bilateral vocal fold paresis may not be candidates for medialization. At least one vocal fold should have intact inspiratory vocal fold abduction for a medialization procedure to be considered

Breathy dysphonia is the hallmark symptom of glottic insufficiency, but voice symptoms are not always so self-evident. More subtle cases of glottic insufficiency may present as limitations in volume and/or in vocal stamina which are not readily apparent during the patient interview, but which present difficulties in "real-word" environments which feature background noise, such as industrial or outdoor workplaces, or demand projection, such as classroom teaching, or sustained voice use, such as in customer-relation tasks.

Evidence suggests that laryngeal penetration and aspiration occurs in up to one-third of patients with vocal fold paralysis [9, 10], a figure which may be even higher in selected subgroups with cranial nerve injuries beyond the recurrent nerve. From a medical point of view, complaints of dysphagia usually supersede dysphonia in considering whether to perform medialization, and Netterville and Civantos [11] have observed that airway protection benefits may even occasionally exceed voice results. Nevertheless, it is important to understand that vocal fold medialization does not always provide a sure remedy. In the presence of other motor or sensory deficits, as in a vagal nerve lesion at the base of skull, the ability to close the glottis does not necessarily mean that this will occur appropriately during deglutition. Medialization is indeed likely to help, and may even spare the patient a tracheostomy, but some patients continue to have medically significant aspiration, despite satisfactory voice results [12]. Due caution is warranted in making feeding recommendations after medialization in such individuals, and a complete re-evaluation of swallowing function is prudent.

A symptom which can prove misleading in cases of vocal fold paralysis is the complaint of dyspnea with exertion. This is sometimes taken as a symptom of pulmonary dysfunction or even of obstruction from the paralyzed vocal fold, the latter case typically after a pulmonary function test has revealed a fixed extrathoracic obstruction. In most cases of vocal fold paralysis, this breathlessness is more likely to represent a compromise of thoracic fixation during the Valsalva maneuver, which aids in a wide variety of physical tasks, such as lifting weights, climbing stairs, and rising from a sitting or lying position. Unfamiliarity with laryngeal biomechanics may lead the physician directly away from steps necessary to restore glottic competence, thoracic fixation, and normal phonation.

Medialization laryngoplasty has been advocated by some as a treatment for glottic insufficiency due to soft tissue loss in the layers of the vocal fold superficial to the thyroarytenoid muscle (the "vocal fold cover") such as is found in post-surgical scarring or sulcus vocalis. However, it is not well suited for these conditions, as it in no way addresses the lack of tissue pliability and may not yield significant voice improvement. It is noteworthy that there is considerable evidence to suggest that at least part of the so-called bowing which has been accepted as the clinical correlate of vocal fold aging may also be due to changes in the lamina propria, and thus medialization may represent only a partial solution.

Arytenoid Adduction

Arytenoid adduction or other arytenoid repositioning procedure is an important adjunctive measure in selected cases of vocal fold paralysis. Although some debate continues regarding the physiologic effects of arytenoid adduction, there is general consensus concerning the following basic premises [13, 14]: arytenoid adduction (a) rotates the arytenoid cartilage, (b) displaces the vocal process medially and caudally, and (c) stabilizes the vocal process.

In patients with vocal fold paralysis who have a lack of vocal process contact during phonation (posterior gap) and those with vocal folds at different levels, arytenoid adduction should be considered in addition to medialization laryngoplasty. Videostroboscopy often provides valuable information about vocal process contact and vocal fold height, and therefore is useful preoperatively in assessing which patients may need an arytenoid adduction. A maximum phonation time of less than 5 seconds has also been identified as a predictor of the need for arytenoid adduction in cases of vocal fold paralysis [15]. A more complete discussion of the rationale and technique of arytenoid repositioning procedure follows later in this volume.

Procedure Selection: Framework Surgery vs Injection Augmentation

The scarcity of comparative trials among procedures for glottic insufficiency has resulted in a lack of evidence on which to base treatment decisions. The choice of procedure is often a reflection of the surgeon's own preference and bias. In general, injection augmentation has been used for temporary correction of unilateral vocal fold paralysis, when the prognosis for recovery is uncertain. Injection results in improvement of voice and/or swallowing, while allowing a period for recovery of vocal fold function. After a period of weeks to months, the injected substance is typically resorbed. Should recovery not take place, such resorption becomes the primary disadvantage of injection. There are currently no safe injection materials for consistent and permanent correction of glottal closure problems, although calcium hydroxylapatite paste (Radiesse) is being investigated as a long-term injectable substance at the time of this writing.

In addition, severe degrees of glottic incompetence appear to be more difficult to correct with injection augmentation. Koufman has observed that a glottic gap of 2–3 mm or greater during phonation is better treated with thyroplasty rather than with lipoinjection (J. Koufman, personal communication).

Most injection augmentation procedures require over-injection to allow for reabsorption, rendering fine adjustments to vocal fold position difficult, if not impossible. The vocal outcome is rendered even more approximate in those patients who require a general anesthetic for injection, and whose voice result cannot be immediately assessed. Compared with injection techniques, thyroplasty can achieve fine, graduated adjustments in the degree of medialization of the vocal fold. In addition, thyroplasty can be used to focally medialize a segment of the affected vocal fold by means of the shape of the implant. Injection techniques are less likely to achieve this due to the tendency of most materials to spread through tissue planes somewhat unpredictably. Lastly, framework surgery is performed under local anesthesia, which gives the surgeon immediate feedback on the most important outcome measure of all: the patient's voice.

Patient Selection

Although any patient with symptomatic glottic insufficiency is technically a candidate for framework surgery, medialization laryngoplasty is not necessarily the best approach in every case. The ideal candidate for medialization laryngoplasty is a patient with moderate to severe glottic insufficiency (2- to 3-mm or greater glottic gap on phonation) manifested by weak, breathy dysphonia and/or dysphagia. Conversely, patients with minor degrees of glottic insufficiency (<1-mm glottic gap on phonation) who have minimal voice symptoms (e.g., vocal fatigue) may be better suited for injection augmentation and/or voice therapy.

As medialization laryngoplasty is performed under local anesthesia, anxious/uncooperative patients and pediatric patients are not ideally suited for this technique.

Timing of Medialization Laryngoplasty

Many otolaryngologists prefer to defer medialization laryngoplasty 6–12 months. This is thought to represent the time required for spontaneous recovery of the vocal fold to take place, although there is little clinical evidence to support a specific time interval. Most likely, this period varies depending on location and degree of injury. There is nothing to suggest that the surgery compromises the chances of recovery, and in any case, medialization laryngoplasty is entirely reversible.

A sound reason for delay has to do with the dynamic nature of vocal fold paralysis, despite immobility of the vocal fold proper. On the one hand, severely denervated vocal folds tend to atrophy over time, increasing glottal gap; on the other, the tendency for vocal fold reinnervation is robust, as demonstrated by experimental and clinical evidence [16], even in the absence of recovery of motion. Such reinnervation frequently serves to maintain bulk and tone, and may provide the primary mechanism by which certain individuals with vocal fold paralysis may achieve good glottic function without any intervention by the physician [17]. Experience with nerve section for spasmodic dysphonia has shown that some nerve regrowth, be it from the recurrent nerve or from some other nearby source, may occur even in cases of avulsion of significant segments of recurrent laryngeal nerve [18, 19]. Since a medialization implant provides a stable degree of vocal fold displacement, it follows that it is best to perform such a procedure in a patient in whom the vocal fold position, bulk and tone is not likely to change (or at least, to atrophy) over time.

Just as in recovery of vocal fold motion, there is no unequivocal evidence regarding the time needed for the neuromuscular status of the vocal fold to reach a stable state, but obviously, the longer the time from the paralysis, the likelier it is that there will be little further change. The circumstances of the paralysis and laryngeal electromyography may provide relevant information.

Immediate medialization laryngoplasty has been advocated for those patients undergoing sacrifice of the tenth cranial nerve during skull base procedures. More recently, this technique has fallen into disfavor for two principal reasons: precise medialization is difficult to achieve in a patient under general anesthetic due to lack of vocal feedback; and beneficial results may be short lived, due to progressive atrophy of the vocal fold from ongoing nerve degeneration, which results in a return of glottal insufficiency. Most surgeons advocate waiting at least 3 months after a known vagal or recurrent nerve transection before performing medialization laryngoplasty. Concerns regarding swallowing safety may supersede such considerations.

In select cases, early (<6 months post-injury) laryngoplasty can be considered, especially if electromyography shows severe neuronal degeneration without evidence of neural recovery or the history strongly suggests nerve transection. In these cases, the patient should be counseled that the implant may need to be removed if vocal fold function returns. It is noteworthy that in the very rare cases of recovery of vocal fold motion after laryngoplasty that have been observed by the authors, the implant does not appear to interfere with function, and has not required removal.

If the status of the nerve injury is unknown or LEMG data are equivocal or favorable, medialization surgery is best delayed until 9–12 months after nerve injury to allow for spontaneous recovery. The patient with troublesome symptoms may be treated by any of a number of temporary measures in the meantime.

Technical Notes and Pertinent Anatomic Landmarks

Although many different implant materials and variations in technique for medialization laryngoplasty exist, certain general principles of laryngeal anatomy can be universally applied. The central and critical anatomic task is to identify the level of the vocal fold in relation to the thyroid lamina so that the cartilage window can be appropriately placed. The window is the primary determinant of implant location, particularly when pre-formed implants are used. No single method of vocal fold localization is guaranteed to work in every patient, and inevitably, fenestration is occasionally made in a suboptimal location. It is important for the surgeon to plan for this contingency and have a means of correcting it should it occur, most typically by altering the implant. Many implant "kits" have built-in degrees of freedom to allow for this; others can be reshaped.

The level of the vocal fold lies closer to the lower border of the thyroid cartilage lamina than is generally believed, and not at its midpoint, as is frequently (and erroneously) stated. It is important to place the thyroplasty window at the most inferior location possible to encompass the level of the vocal fold and permit successful medialization with appropriate implant positioning. The inferior limit of placement is determined by the integrity of the cartilaginous strut below the window, which should be at least 3 mm tall to prevent fracture. Such a complication destabilizes the implant in a way that usually prevents effective medialization. As a result of this limit, the implant often needs to be carved or positioned such that medialization occurs at the inferior limit of the window to avoid displacement of the ventricle or ventricular fold.

Another important anatomic consideration is the gender-related difference in the configuration of the thyroid cartilage. In males, the vocal folds are longer, and the thyroid alae form a more acute angle when compared with the female larynx. These anatomic differences require a more posterior location of the cartilaginous window in the male larynx to avoid excessive or disproportionate displacement of the anterior third of the vocal fold, which will result in strained or "pressed" voice. In general, the leading edge of the window is placed 7 mm back from the midline of the thyroid cartilage in males and 5 mm in females. The soft tissue covering inside the thyroid cartilage is markedly thinner anteriorly and thus more prone to perforation from excessive medial pressure, either from a dissecting instrument or implant material.

Many implants are shaped to medialize tissue in a plane exactly parallel to the long axis of the thyroplasty window; its orientation is thus another important factor for surgical success. The inferior border of the thyroid lamina is the most reliable guide to this, once the irregularity of the inferior tubercle has been identified and visually excluded from the estimate of its direction. Failure to do this will skew the cartilage window downwards posteriorly. On the other hand, the leading edge of the thyroid cartilage is canted forward, especially in men. Orienting the anterior margin of the window perpendicular to this will cause it to shift upwards posteriorly.

As is evident, preserving some flexibility in medialization laryngoplasty technique to allow for individual variations in laryngeal anatomy

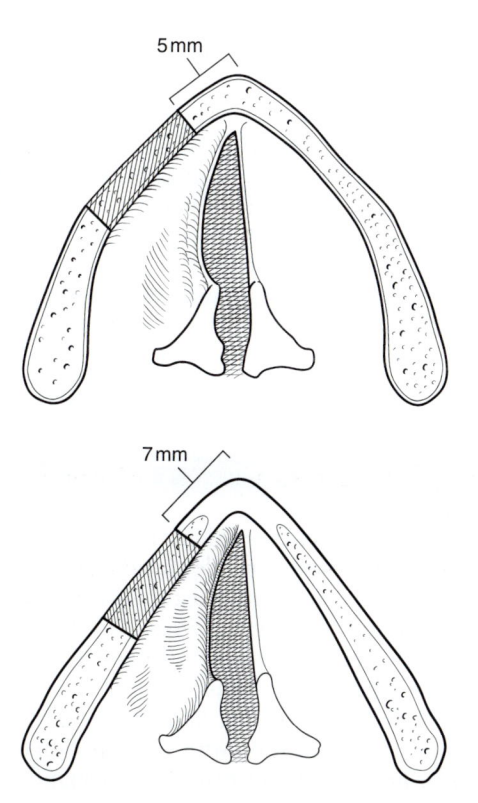

Fig. 9.1. Coronal section of the female (top) and male (bottom) larynx. There is less soft tissue cover anteriorly for a medialization implant in the male.

is necessary to achieve consistently satisfactory surgical results. Being able to check on the result of medialization intraoperatively by means of flexible fiberoptic laryngoscopy is essential to understanding the reason for a poor phonatory result in time to correct it. An endoscope, its light source, a camera, and a monitor should be available in the operating room for every case, even if they are not used throughout the operation.

Conflicting advice regarding the inner perichondrium has appeared in the literature. Maintaining the perichondrium intact effectively prevents medial migration and extrusion of the implant, and may minimize the possibility of endolaryngeal bleeding. Isshiki [20] continues to advise its preservation when using Silastic and a cartilage island, as do McCullough and Hoffman [31] when using expanded polytetrafluoroethylene ribbon; however, the marked medial projection of many pre-formed implants makes their insertion impossible unless the internal perichondrium is opened, at the same time that their fixation to the thyroid cartilage makes medial extrusion unlikely. Opening the perichondrium not only permits medialization in a more precise plane, but also requires a larger ("deeper") implant to achieve effective results.

Details of technique specific to various implant materials and steps and modifications required to perform arytenoid repositioning surgery in conjunction with medialization laryngoplasty are covered elsewhere in this text.

Complications

The principal complications specific to medialization laryngoplasty include airway obstruction and implant extrusion. The results of a survey of American otolaryngologists performed in 1998 [21] reveal incidences generally in line with those reported in various series.

Medialization necessarily narrows the glottic airway. In combination with post-operative edema or hematoma, this can result in significant airway obstruction, the most dangerous postoperative complication of medialization laryngoplasty. Surveyed surgeons reported some airway compromise in 13.8% of cases. Usually, this was minor and tended to occur more often after medialization laryngoplasty and arytenoid adduction rather than medialization laryngoplasty alone; however, approximately 0.6% of patients undergoing medialization laryngoplasty and 2.2% of patients undergoing medialization with arytenoid adduction required intubation or tracheostomy. Weinman and Maragos reported tracheostomy rates of 1.1 and 3.5% in these same patient groups [22].

Extrusion was extremely rare (0.8%) and predominantly into the airway rather than transcutaneous, as one would expect upon comparison of internal and external tissue covering of the implant. It is likely that at least some of these, particularly those that occur within a few weeks of surgery, are the result of perforations through the mucosa. If perforation goes unrecognized at the time of surgery, the implant is at risk for exposure and contamination. The implant then acts as a foreign body and may extrude, potentially precipitating an airway foreign body emergency. The delicate ventricular mucosa is often located in close proximity to the inner aspect of the anterior thyroid ala, and can be easily torn when working at the anterior aspect of the window. The key to preventing airway entry is to avoid undermining of the paraglottic space anterior to the window, and to use care when removing the anterior portion of the cartilaginous window. Mucosal tears are not always obvious, but blood seen via the flexible fiberoptic laryngoscope should prompt a careful inspection. One can also test for a mucosal perforation by flooding the operative field with irrigation and looking for air bubbles during a Valsalva maneuver

If accidental mucosal violation does occur, the tear can be closed with absorbable sutures, once again testing for the integrity of the repair by means of a Valsalva maneuver. If the tear is successfully closed, an implant can be safely placed in select cases. Securing the implant to the cartilage with sutures significantly reduces the risk of airway foreign body.

Suboptimal Results / Surgical Errors

The most common cause for revision medialization surgery is not an airway problem or implant extrusion, but rather an unsatisfactory voice result. Revision rates, reported to be 5.4% in the survey of complications, can reach 14% [23]. When secondary procedures, such as fat injection, are included, revision rates have been reported to be as high as 33% [24]. Certain causes of poor voice results occur regularly and with greater frequency than others in most published series, as well as in the authors' experience. These causes include:
- Persistent posterior glottic gap
- Undermedialization
- Superior implant malposition
- Anterior implant malposition

Persistent posterior glottic gap can account for up to 50% of revisions in cases in which arytenoid adduction has not been performed [25]. There is some doubt as to whether the vocal process of the arytenoid can be effectively and consistently medialized by a posterior projection of the medialization implant. Furthermore, the vocal process of a denervated vocal fold commonly rests at a different vertical position from that of its functioning pair [26, 27]. In fact, with muscle traction diminished or even absent, it may even lie outside of its normal trajectory, as in the case of a so-called prolapsed arytenoid, when the vocal process may lie below the plane of glottic closure. Simple medialization cannot remedy a height mismatch, nor can it readily correct the commonly associated mismatch in vocal fold tension, which may be an important cause of residual dysphonia.

Undercorrection is another relatively frequent cause of poor results [28]. This is especially likely to occur in cases that last longer than usual and thus allow normal intraoperative vocal fold edema to accumulate. Even mild edema can create enough medial displacement of the vibratory margin of the vocal fold to cause the surgeon to underestimate of the degree of medialization required. In these cases the patient will report good voice immediately after surgery, only to fade 1–2 weeks later, when the edema begins to resolve. The key to avoiding this complication is to keep the time from intralaryngeal elevation until final implant placement as brief as possible, which is a principal argument in favor of pre-formed implants. Many surgeons make it standard practice to administer intravenous steroids immediately before medialization surgery in order to minimize edema, both for reasons of airway safety and in order to better assess the voice result.

A subset of patients may be noted to have voice deterioration months to years after surgery. If a cartilage implant has not been used, this is probably best explained by continued atrophy of the vocal fold musculature from prolonged denervation.

Implant malposition generally accounts for the balance of revisions. Netterville and Billante [29] have identified placing the implant too far superior, which results in medialization of the ventricular mucosa or the false vocal fold, as the most common overall cause for revision. This can be avoided by placing the window no more than 3 mm above the inferior border of the thyroid ala, or as low as possible while maintaining a stable inferior frame of cartilage below the window. Also, one should carefully probe within the window to confirm the plane of the true vocal fold prior to using any depth-measuring devices. The image from an indwelling fiberoptic laryngoscope is extremely useful to confirm the correct medialization plane; a bulging ventricular fold or everted ventricular mucosa (or, more rarely, subglottis) indicates an incorrect medialization plane.

Over-medialization of the anterior vocal fold, caused by too anterior a placement of the implant, results in a distinctive pressed or strained vocal quality from early contact and "overclosure" of the anterior part of the membranous vocal fold during phonation. To prevent this, glottic tissues overlying the anterior third of the window are generally not medialized. This is especially true in men, in whom the extremely thin glottic tissue overlying this area is prone to overmedialization from even small amounts of medial displacement. It is not uncommon for even a well-carved implant to cause a slight amount of unintended anterior medial displacement. If a pressed voice is noted after implant placement, forceps can be used to pull the anterior portion of the implant partially out of the window, and re-test the voice. If the voice improves with this maneuver, trimming of the anterior portion of the implant is recommended.

Should the reason for an unsatisfactory result not be apparent after careful laryngoscopic evaluation using both flexible and rigid instruments, including stroboscopy if necessary, spiral CT or MRI may be helpful in identifying implant malposition or significant asymmetries between the vocal folds [25, 30].

Revision Surgery

The approach for revision surgery does not deviate much from that taken with primary surgery. The location of the cartilaginous window from the previous surgery is not taken into consideration when planning the location of the revision window. The same meticulous exposure of the thyroid ala and precise measurements should be used to establish the "new" window location, even if there is some overlap between this and the original window. In some cases this may result in a larger window, or one with an eccentric shape. As long as the revision implant is well seated in the new window location, and is secured within this space, the unusual window dimensions do not present a problem.

Most implants can be removed easily as the new window is opened, using two single-prong hooks. Once the revised window is created, the fibrous capsule that has formed medial to the implant must be incised. This fibrous tissue creates tethering of the thyroarytenoid muscle, and must be released to permit unencumbered medial displacement of the vocal fold, much as the internal perichondrium must usually be opened in primary surgery. The remainder of the surgical case proceeds in a similar fashion to primary medialization laryngoplasty.

Long-Term Surgical Issues

Patients who have undergone successful medialization laryngoplasty, with or without arytenoid adduction, often express concerns about the safety of endotracheal intubation for surgical procedures in the future. A waiting period of 6 months post-medialization (if the proposed surgery is elective) is advised. The anesthesiologist should place the smallest endotracheal tube that he or she feels is safe – ideally, size 6.0 or smaller – principally to avoid inducing laryngeal edema from a slightly constricted glottic aperture. Implants have proved quite stable in this situation, and implant displacement is rarely a problem.

Conclusion

Medialization laryngoplasty is designed to address problems of glottic insufficiency by shifting the vocal fold towards the midline. Its principal advantages include intraoperative flexibility to tailor implant size and position to the particulars of each patient's glottic insufficiency, guided by the immediate assessment of the effect of each change on the voice. The result is durable and generally satisfactory, although certain pitfalls of technique and strategy exist. A thorough knowledge of relevant laryngeal anatomy and phonatory physiology is necessary to navigate these and avoid the unsatisfactory voice result and other complications, regardless of the specific technique and medialization substance used.

References

1. Payr E (1915) Plastik am Schildknorpel zur Behebung der Folgen einseitiger Stimmbandlähmung. Dtsche Med Wochenshr 41:1265
2. Brünings W (1911) Über eine neue Behandlungsmethode der Rekurrenslähmung. Verhandl Deutsch Laryngol 18:93
3. Meurman Y (1952) Operative mediofixation of the vocal cord in complete unilateral paralysis. Arch Otolaryngol 55:544–553
4. Waltner JG (1958) Surgical rehabilitation of the voice following laryngofissure. Arch Otolaryngol 67:99–101
5. Opheim O (1955) Unilateral paralysis of the vocal cord. Operative treatment. Acta Otolaryngol 145:226–230
6. Arnold GE (1962) Vocal rehabilitation of paralytic dysphonia. Arch Otolaryngol 76:358–368

7. Lewy RB (1963) Glottic reformation with rehabilitation in vocal fold paralysis: the injection of Teflon and tantalum. Laryngoscope 73:547–555
8. Isshiki N, Morita H, Okamura H, Hiramoto M (1974) Thyroplasty as a new phonosurgical technique. Acta Otolaryngol 78:451–457
9. Bhattacharyya N, Kotz T, Shapiro J (2002) Dysphagia and aspiration with unilateral vocal cord immobility: incidence, characterization and response to surgical treatment. Ann Otol Rhinol Laryngol 111:672–679
10. Flint PW, Purcell LL, Cummings CW (1999) Pathophysiology and indications for medialization thyroplasty in patients with dysphagia and aspiration. Otolaryngol Head Neck Surg 349–354
11. Netterville JL, Civantos FJ (1993) Rehabilitation of cranial nerve deficits after neurotologic skull base surgery. Laryngoscope 103:45–54
12. Bielamowicz S, Gupta A, Sekhar LN (2000) Early arytenoid adduction for vagal paralysis after skull base surgery. Laryngoscope 110:346–351
13. Woodson GE, Rosen CA, Yeung D (1997) Changes in length and spatial orientation of the vocal fold with arytenoid adduction in cadaver larynges. Ann Otol Rhinol Laryngol 106:552–555
14. Woodson GE, Picerno R, Yeung D, Hengesteg A (2000) Arytenoid adduction: controlling vertical position. Ann Otol Rhinol Laryngol 109:360–364
15. Woo P (2000) Arytenoid adduction and medialization laryngoplasty. Otolaryngol Clin N Am 33:817–839
16. Zealear DL, Billante CR (2004) Neurophysiology of vocal fold paralysis. Otolaryngol Clin N Am 37:1–24
17. Blitzer A, Jahn AF, Keidar A (1996) Semon's law revisited: an electrophysiologic analysis of laryngeal synkinesis. Ann Otol Rhinol Laryngol 105:764–769
18. Netterville JL, Stone RE, Rainey C et al. (1991) Recurrent nerve avulsion for treatment of spastic dysphonia. Ann Otol Rhinol Laryngol 100:10–14
19. Aronson AE, De Santo LW (1983) Adductor spastic dysphonia: three years after recurrent laryngeal nerve section. Laryngoscope 93:1–8
20. Isshiki N (2000) Progress in laryngeal framework surgery. Acta Otolaryngol 120:120–127
21. Rosen CA (1998) Complications of phonosurgery: results of a national survey. Laryngoscope 108:1697–1703
22. Weinman EC, Maragos NE (2000) Airway compromise in thyroplasty surgery. Laryngoscope 110:1082–1085
23. Netterville JL, Stone RE, Luken ES, Civantos FJ, Ossoff RH (1993) Silastic medialization and arytenoid adduction: The Vanderbilt experience. A review of 116 phonosurgical procedures. Ann Otol Rhinol Laryngol 102:413–424
24. Anderson TD, Spiegel JR, Sataloff RT (2003) Thyroplasty revision: frequency and predictive factors. J Voice 17:442–448
25. Woo P, Pearl AW, Hsiung MW, Som P (2001) Failed medialization laryngoplasty: management by revision surgery. Otolaryngol Head Neck Surg 124:615–621
26. Yumoto E, Nakano K, Hyodo M (1999) Three dimensional endoscopic images of vocal fold paralysis by computed tomography. Arch Otolaryngol Head Neck Surg 125:883–890
27. Hong KH, Jung KS (2001) Arytenoid appearance and vertical height difference between the paralyzed and innervated vocal folds. Laryngoscope 111:227–232
28. Cohen JT, Bates DD, Postma GN (2004) Revision Gore-Tex medialization laryngoplasty. Otolaryngol Head Neck Surg 131:236–240
29. Netterville JL, Billante CR (2004) The immobile vocal fold. In: Ossoff RH, Shapshay SM, Woodson GE, Netterville JL (eds) The larynx. Lippincott, Williams and Wilkins, Philadelphia, pp 269–305
30. Bielamowicz S (2004) Perspectives on medialization laryngoplasty. Otolaryngol Clin N Am 37:139–160
31. McCullough TM, Hoffman HT (1998) Medialization laryngoplasty with expanded polytetrafluoroethylene. Surgical technique and preliminary results. Ann Otol Rhinol Laryngol 107:427–432

Chapter 9

Silastic Medialization Laryngoplasty

C. Blake Simpson

Introduction

Silicone elastomer, commonly referred to as "Silastic," is a polymerized form of silicone gel. Silastic is inert material which is well tolerated when implanted into the human body. A long track record of Silastic use exists (mostly in the orthopedic literature), and approximately 25 years of experience have accumulated for its use in the larynx [1]. Silastic can be used successfully as a long-term material for glottic insufficiency in both immobile and mobile vocal folds. Type-I allergic reactions and granuloma formation/long-term complications are almost non-existent [2].

This chapter describes medialization laryngoplasty using the surgical technique described by Netterville et al. [3] and Wanamaker et al. [4] which utilizes a hand-carved medium-grade Silastic block.

Procedure

Preparation

The patient is given 10 mg of decadron, as well as 1 g of ancef (or 900 mg clindamycin if PCN allergic) intravenously upon entering the OR. Intravenous sedation and monitoring by anesthesia is provided throughout the procedure. In general, light IV sedation is advocated, using benzodiazepam instead of propofol in most cases. Oversedation can lead to lack of patient cooperation, disinhibition/combativeness, and sometimes snoring. In the best of settings these side effects of oversedation make the case very difficult to perform, and in the worst of conditions may lead to an inability to complete the procedure; however, additional sedation at the beginning of the procedure, and after implant placement, is generally acceptable, and may be preferred.

The surgical region is liberally infiltrated with 1% lidocaine with 1:100,000 epinephrine from the hyoid down to the cricoid cartilage on the side of the intended surgery. Typically 15 cc are used. Four percent lidocaine and oxymetazoline nasal spray is applied to the most patent nasal cavity. A nasolaryngeal fiberoptic scope is inserted and positioned for videomonitoring of the larynx during the entire surgical procedure. Visual feedback from the larynx is invaluable when performing this surgery.

Surgical Approach

After sterile prep of the neck and fiberoptic scope, a horizontal incision is placed in a skin crease at the level of the mid-thyroid cartilage, typically 5–6 cm in length. Subplatysmal flaps are raised to the hyoid superiorly and the upper portion of the cricoid inferiorly; retention hooks are used to secure the flaps out of the way. The midline raphe of the strap muscles is divided with cautery, exposing the laryngeal cartilage. A single prong hook is placed through the cartilage under the thyroid notch, and the larynx is rotated to the side opposite the paralysis, bringing the entire thyroid ala of the side of the paralysis into view.

The outer perichondrium of the thyroid cartilage is incised with a no. 15 blade at the anterior midline and a posteriorly based flap is raised with a Cottle or Freer elevator. The inferior border of the thyroid ala is usually obscured by muscle fibers from the cricothyroid muscle inserting onto it, so these must be divided, typically with bipolar cautery followed by a no. 15

blade. The exposure of the inferior border is essential for the correct orientation of the medialization window. The exposure must extend posterior to the muscular tubercle (an inferior projection of the thyroid ala), as the angulation of this process can mislead the surgeon as to the proper orientation of the medialization window.

A 6×13-mm window is outlined in the thyroid cartilage using the window size gauge instrument. The window is placed 3 mm above the inferior border of the thyroid cartilage. Placement of the window any higher may result in medialization of the false vocal fold or ventricular mucosa, with poor voice results. The leading edge of the window is "set back" from the midline of the thyroid cartilage by a distance of 5 mm in women and 7 mm in men. This helps avoid medialization of the anterior vocal fold, which may result in "pressed" voice.

The window of cartilage is removed with a no. 15 blade, Kerrison rongeur, or drill as necessary depending on laryngeal calcification. In younger patients, the cartilage is soft, and can be removed with a no. 15 blade, provided caution is used to avoid penetration of the perichondrium with resultant paraglottic bleeding. Once the full thickness of cartilage is removed at a given point, a Kerrison rongeur can be used to complete the window.

Endolaryngeal/Paraglottic Manipulation

The inner perichondrium that lies deep to the window is removed, exposing the thyroarytenoid muscle fascia. Often this inner perichondrium has already been removed piecemeal with the Kerrison rongeur; however, if it remains intact, it can be incised superiorly, posteriorly, and inferiorly. A surgical plane is then developed with the "long elevator" (a right-angled soft tissue elevator) in the paraglottic space, just superficial (lateral) to the thyroarytenoid (TA) fascia. The plane is extended beyond the borders of the window in all directions except anteriorly. Dissection anterior to the window may result in perforation into the airway through the very thin and closely adherent ventricular mucosa, and should be avoided. The inferior paraglottic surgical plane should extend below the inferior strut of the thyroid ala. This can be achieved by undermining from below the strut, using the long elevator (Fig. 9.1.1).

Incising the inner perichondrium and establishing the surgical plane in the paraglottic space is important for successful medialization. An intact perichondrium remains tightly bound to the thyroid cartilage (even with undermining) and often provides great resistance to medialization. It is analogous to trying to displace a trampoline. In contrast, a plane in the paraglottic space allows for unencumbered medialization.

The TA muscle is then displaced at various points within the window using a small elevator such as a Woodson. This helps establish the correct plane of medialization (at the free edge of the vocal fold, usually at the posterior aspect of the membranous vocal fold). A depth gauge is used to displace the TA muscle medially, while the patient counts to 10. A combination

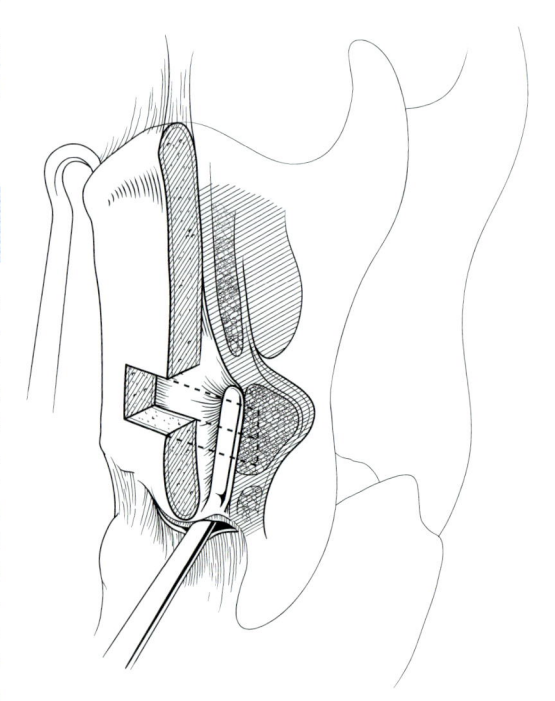

Fig. 9.1.1. Dissection of the paraglottic space

of visual feedback from the videolaryngoscopy monitor and the patient's vocal quality are used to judge the correct amount of medialization needed. Ideally, the vocal fold will assume a straight contour in the midline, allowing for complete glottic closure and significant voice improvement. Typically, 5–7 mm of medialization are needed at the posterior aspect of the window, and 0–2 mm are needed anteriorly. This depth of medialization is measured from the *inner* cartilage edge within the window.

Once the appropriate measurements are made, 3×1/2 cotton pledgets soaked in 1:10,000 epinephrine are placed inside the window to aid in hemostasis while the implant is carved.

Carving the Silastic Implant

The implant can be carved from a medium-grade Silastic block to meet the specifications provided by the depth gauge measurements. A preformed 20-mm wedge blank (Medtronic Xomed, Jacksonville, Fla.) simplifies this task and shortens surgical time (Fig. 9.1.2). This section describes its proper preparation for implantation.

The distance from the anterior edge of the window to the point of maximal medialization (typically 11–13 mm in males and 6–10 mm in females) is measured along the block (measurement "A" on the diagram), and a dot is placed with a marking pen (Fig. 9.1.3 a,b).

From the dot, a line is extended into the substance of the block (measurement "B" in the diagram) which corresponds to the depth of medialization. This measurement was obtained using the depth gauge and is typically 5–7 mm in most patients (Fig. 9.1.4 a,b). Lines are then drawn connecting the tip of line B with both the anterior and posterior portions of the block (measurements "C" and "D," respectively). This creates a characteristic triangular shape of the implant, with the edge "C" corresponding to the portion of the implant which displaces the vocalis muscle medially, and segment "D" corresponding to the posterior extension of the implant which helps to hold it in place (Fig. 9.1.5).

A no. 10 blade is used to cut along lines C and D, removing the excess portion of the block. One must be careful to make these cuts at 90° angles to maintain the integrity of the depth of the implant (Fig. 9.1.6). The implant is placed in a customized implant holder for further shaping (Fig. 9.1.7). The plane of medialization (lower, middle, or upper portion of the window) which corresponds to the plane of the true vocal fold is marked with a line along the implant border (Fig. 9.1.8). In general, this is the inferior or lower border of the window space. The line must be drawn along the medialization "zone" in the middle of the implant, not on the upper or lower "flange" portions of the implant. Using a no. 15 blade, the excess Silastic is removed superior and inferior to the plane of medialization, preserving an approximately 3-mm strip of material along the indicated line (Fig. 9.1.9). The extreme upper and lower edges of the implant must be thinned considerably to make the flanges flexible (Fig. 9.1.10 a,b). This facilitates easier placement of a large implant through the window. The A and B measurements are re-checked for accuracy.

Finally, the implant is removed from the holder, and the posterior 7 mm of the "slot" is removed from the implant. The implant is then ready for placement.

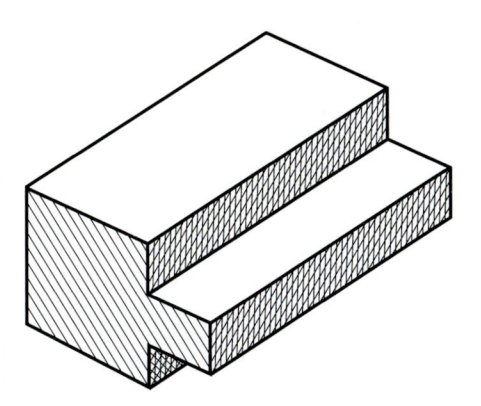

Fig. 9.1.2. Silastic implant block (Medtronic Xomed, Jacksonville, FL)

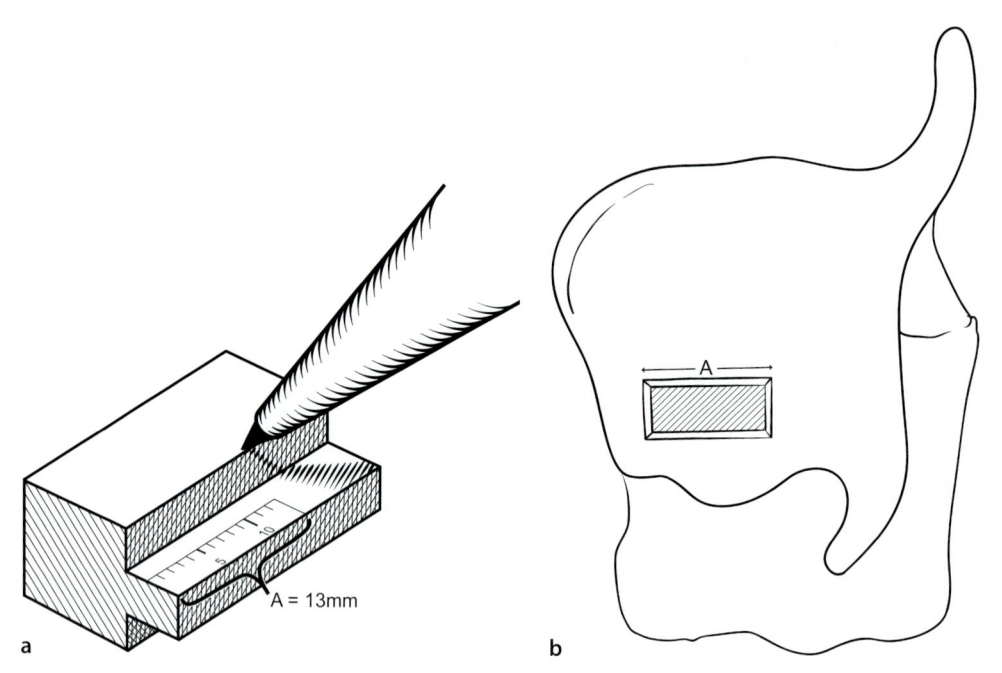

Fig. 9.1.3 a,b. Measurement *A*: Anterior edge of the thyrotomy window to the point of maximum medialization

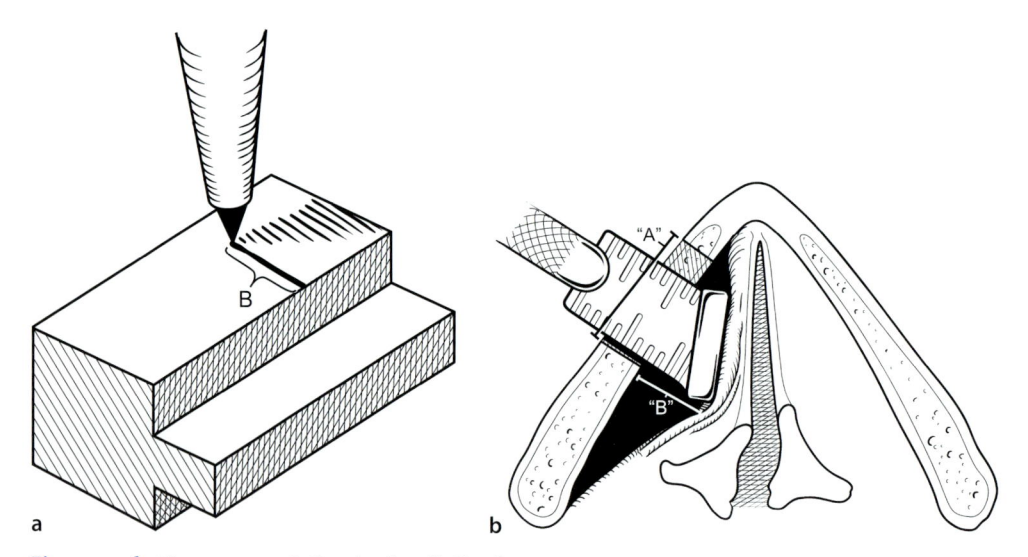

Fig. 9.1.4 a,b. Measurement *B*: Depth of medialization

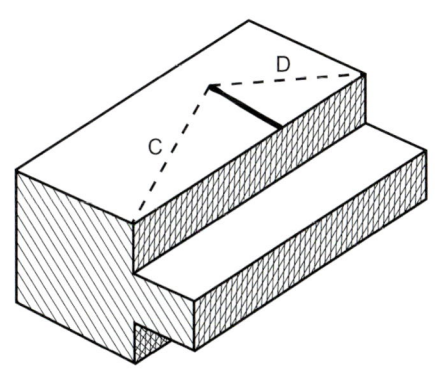

Silastic Medialization Laryngoplasty   Chapter 9.1   149

Fig. 9.1.5. Lines **c** & **d**: Creating a triangular implant

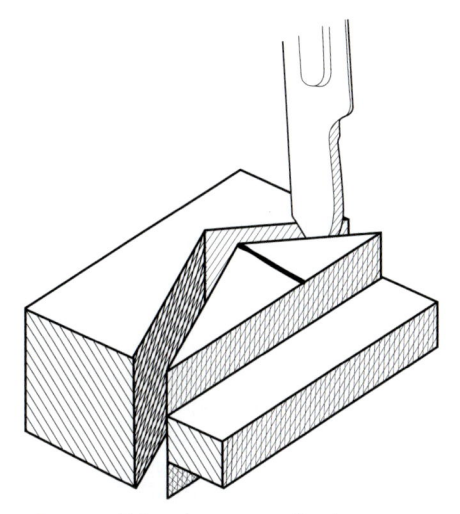

Fig. 9.1.6. Trimming excess silastic

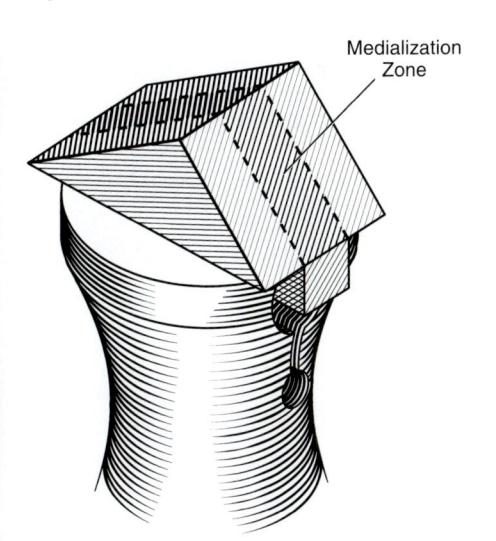

Fig. 9.1.7. Implant holder for further shaping

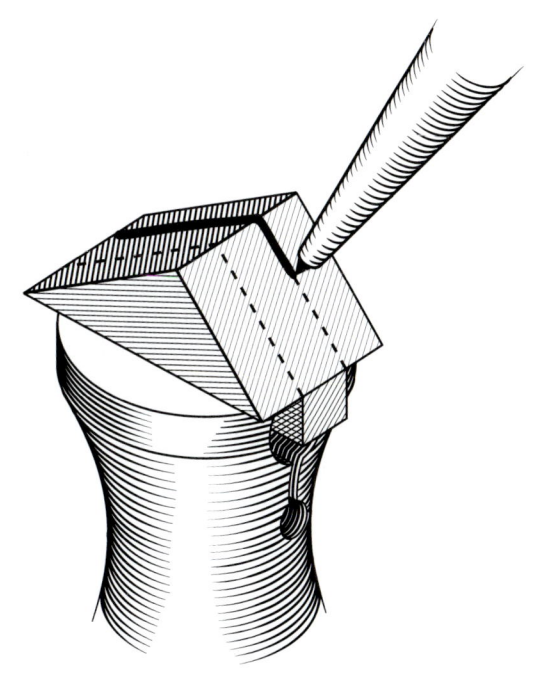

Fig. 9.1.8. Marking the plane of maximum medialization

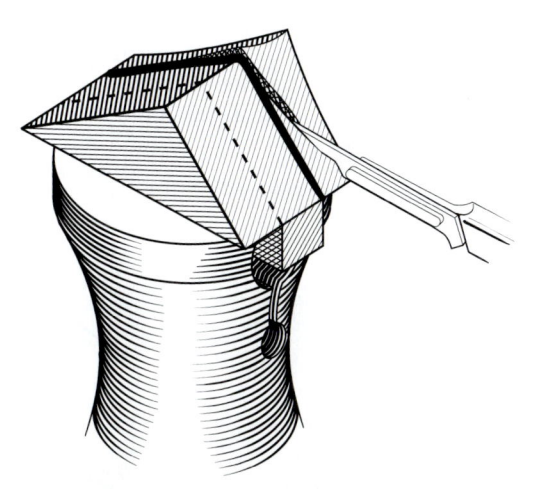

Fig. 9.1.9. Further removal of excess silastic

Implant Insertion

The implant is placed through the medialization window using two Adson forceps with teeth. The posterior inferior part of the implant should be advanced into the paraglottic space first. The implant is "locked" into position by the flanges.

Once the implant is in place, the patient's voice should be re-checked, and the videolaryngoscopic image should be observed to ensure that the medialization recreates what was achieved with the depth gauge. If the voice sounds "pressed" or "strained," the anterior portion of the implant should be pulled out of the window slightly. If this improves the voice, there is too much medialization anteriorly, and the implant should be removed and trimmed an appropriate amount. On the other hand, if the voice sounds breathy, the implant can be displaced posteriorly. One must be patient enough to try a variety of maneuvers to ensure that the optimal voice result is achieved.

Once the implant is definitively placed, the excess implant lateral to the thyroid ala is trimmed flush with the cartilage surface. The implant is secured to the thyroid cartilage with permanent sutures (4.0 monofilament) around the inferior "strut" of cartilage.

Closure

After a final check for hemostasis, all layers are closed sequentially, including outer perichondrium, strap muscles, platysma, and skin. In general, a drain is not necessary but may be placed depending on the surgeon's preference.

Postoperative Care

Because postoperative vocal fold edema may have a marked effect on voice quality and prolong recovery of normal voice, intravenous decadron (10 mg) is given preoperatively, followed by two additional doses at 8 and 16 h postoperatively.

Postoperative Issues and Expected Vocal Recovery

All cases are admitted for overnight observation, because of concern for airway edema. Patients may be fed the evening of surgery, with the diet advanced to regular as tolerated. If a drain has been placed, it is typically removed the next morning before discharge.

Most patients have good to excellent voicing intraoperatively but develop varying degrees of postoperative dysphonia as a result of edema or submucosal hemorrhage. Within hours, a

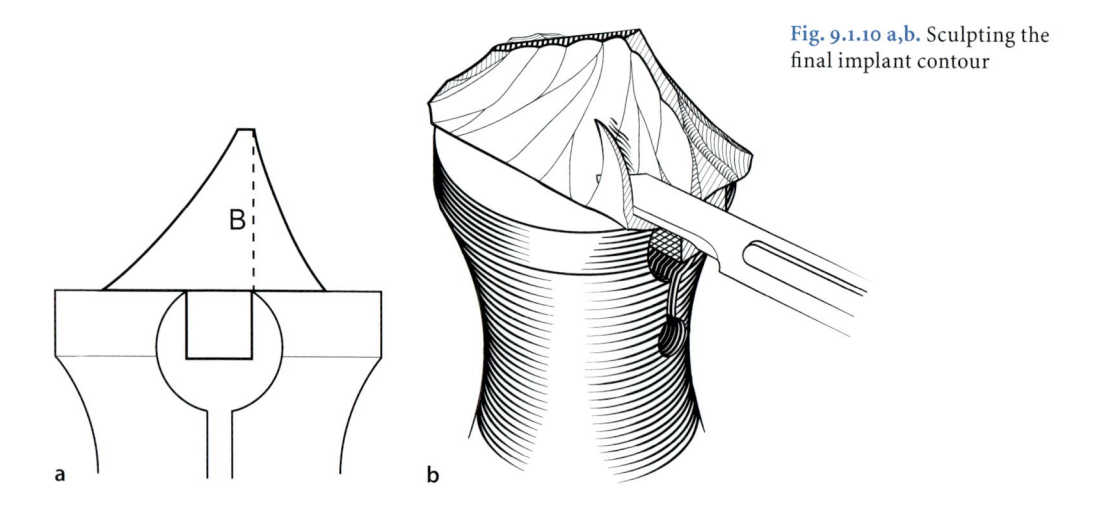

Fig. 9.1.10 a,b. Sculpting the final implant contour

good postoperative voice will become rough and hoarse. The patient should be warned of this before the surgery. To minimize this problem preoperative IV decadron is routinely given (10 mg), followed by two additional doses at 8 and 16 h postoperatively. The period of postoperative dysphonia is variable but may last between 2 and 6 weeks [5]. Rare cases may persist up to 3 months. Voice conservation is advocated. Total voice rest is unnecessary.

References

1. Koufman JA (1986) Laryngoplasty for vocal cord medialization: an alternative to Teflon. Laryngoscope 96:726–731
2. Hunsaker DH, Martin PJ (1995) Allergic reaction to solid silicone implant in medial thyroplasty. Otolaryngol Head Neck Surg 113:782–784
3. Netterville JL, Stone RE, Luken ES, Civantos FJ, Ossoff RH (1993) Silastic medialization and arytenoid adduction: the Vanderbilt experience. A review of 116 phonosurgical procedures. Ann Otol Rhinol Laryngol 102:413–424
4. Wanamaker JR, Netterville JL, Ossoff RH (1993) Phonosurgery: silastic medialization for unilateral vocal fold paralysis. Oper Techniques Otolaryngol Head Neck Surg 4:207–217
5. Gorham MM, Avidano MA, Crary MA, Cotter CS, Cassisi NJ (1998) Laryngeal recovery following type 1 thyroplasty. Arch Otolaryngol Head Neck Surg 124:739–742

Chapter 9

Medialization Thyroplasty Using the Montgomery Thyroplasty System

9.2

Mark A. Varvares, Rebecca M. Brandsted

Introduction

The Montgomery Thyroplasty Implant System was developed in order to simplify the implant technique while providing both anterior and posterior vocal cord medialization [1, 2]. Its design advantages include:

- A readily available implant in varying sizes, thus bypassing the necessity to fashion or alter the implant material
- Specially designed measuring tools to facilitate localization of the thyroid window
- The use of an implant measuring device, so that the correct size can easily be determined intraoperatively by laryngoscopic inspection and phonatory function
- An implant construction that snaps into place requiring no sutures and little risk of displacement
- An implant that can be easily removed if indicated
- An implant design that will medialize the vocal process

Design of Thyroplasty Prosthesis

The prosthesis is composed of two specially designed parts (Fig. 9.2.1). The outer, or lateral, portion serves to lock the prosthesis in the window made in the thyroid lamina (Fig. 9.2.1A). This lateral portion is constructed of three rectangular plates of firm material. The most lateral plate remains on the outer surface of the thyroid lamina and prevents medial displacement of the prosthesis. The middle portion (Fig. 9.2.1B), which is the same size as the thyroid lamina window, stabilizes the implant against movement. The inner plate (Fig. 9.2.1C) remains against the inner surface of the thyroid lamina and serves to prevent lateral displacement of the prosthesis. This outer portion of the implant remains constant for both the male and female larynges.

The inner, or medial, portion of the prosthesis serves to medialize the vocal cord and the vocal process of the arytenoid (Fig. 9.2.1D). It is triangular in shape and is softer in consistency. The hypotenuse of this triangle is designed to correspond to the long axis of the vocal cord when it is in the medial position. The base of

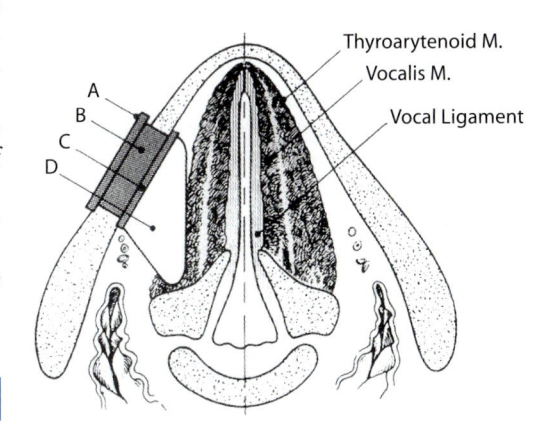

Fig. 9.2.1. Thyroplasty implant. Outer portion of implant consists of three tiers. **A** Lateral plate remains outside thyroid cartilage on its surface and prevents lateral displacement. **B** Middle plate stabilizes implant and is the same dimension as thyroid lamina window. **C** Medial plate secures inside thyroid lamina and prevents outward displacement. Outer portion of implant is of constant size for all male and all female implants. **D** Triangular intralaryngeal portion of implant designed to medialize vocal fold. The height of this portion varies depending on size of implant (females 6, 7, 8, 9, 10 mm, and males 8, 9, 10, 11, 12 mm). Tip of the implant projects posteriorly to reach vocal process of arytenoid, providing posterior medialization. (From [2])

the triangle is adherent to the inner plate of the prosthesis fixed to the thyroid lamina. The third side of the triangle makes a 116° angle to the plane of the base. Its apex projects posteriorly in order to medialize the vocal process of the arytenoid, thus closing the posterior commissure.

Extensive research was necessary to determine the type of polymer and density thereof for the prosthesis. It was concluded that a biocompatible, medical-grade silicone polymer was the ideal material. The implant is also radio opaque. There are five sizes each for the male and female larynx.

Patient Selection

The Montgomery Thyroplasty Implant System for vocal cord medialization is indicated for patients with unilateral vocal cord paralysis, resulting in dysphonia or aspiration due to glottic insufficiency. Patients known to have a wide gap at the posterior commissure may especially benefit. Medialization may be done for permanent or temporary vocal cord paralysis, due to the ease of implant removal if vocal cord function should recover.

Preoperatively, the larynx is evaluated by videolaryngoscopy and videolaryngostroboscopy. Voice evaluation including amplitude, range, fundamental frequency, jitter, and maximal phonation time (MPT) may also be useful. Evaluation is repeated 4–6 weeks after the operation, and again 6 months and 1 year postoperatively.

Anesthesia

A skilled anesthetist or anesthesiologist is essential for the success of this operation. The correct balance between sedation and responsiveness must be maintained during the entire operation. The suggested anesthesia for thyroplasty in the average 70 kg patients is as follows: initially, Versed, 1–2 mg intravenously, is used in the holding area. Fentanyl citrate, 50 µg/ml, is used in the holding area or on the way to the operating room. In the operating room, fentanyl, 25 µg (2), is used at the beginning of the operation. Incremental doses of propofol are then used until the desired level of sedation is reached.

One nasal cavity is sprayed with a mixture of 3% Xylocaine and 2% phenylephrine hydrochloride or packed with a pledget saturated with 4% cocaine hydrochloride solution. The pack remains in place until the introduction of the fiberoptic laryngoscope. The line of the incision and the underlying musculature are injected with 2% Xylocaine and 1:100,000 epinephrine hydrochloride.

Two to 5 min prior to insertion of the implant, 50–100 mg of lidocaine hydrochloride is administered intravenously to prevent laryngospasm and coughing.

Surgical Technique

The horizontal incision begins approximately 2 cm from the midline on the contralateral side of the neck, midway between the thyroid notch and in the inferior margin of the thyroid cartilage. It extends to the ipsilateral side of the neck, just to the anterior border of the sternocleidomastoid muscle. Subplatysmal skin flaps are raised superiorly and inferiorly. The sternohyoid muscles are separated in the midline so as to identify the thyroid notch, the thyroid lamina anteriorly, and the cricothyroid membrane.

The strap muscles are undermined and retracted laterally. If exposure is difficult, they may be transected at a level midway between the thyroid notch and the cricothyroid membrane. Exposure is accomplished with two Wietlander-type self-retaining retractors.

The thyrohyoid muscle is transected so as to expose the thyroid lamina. The inferior thyroid tubercle is found and exposed about midway along the inferior border of the thyroid lamina. Afterwards, the inferior border of the thyroid lamina is exposed anterior and posterior to the tubercle.

findings were comparable to those reported in previous studies of phonatory outcomes after thyroplasty by other authors [4–10].

Conclusion

The Montgomery Thyroplasty Implant System and operative technique provides a reliable means of attaining excellent voice results in the majority of patients treated. The system requires no intraoperative carving and is standardized so as to reduce operative time while not sacrificing results.

The ability to close the posterior glottis without an arytenoid adduction is also a significant advantage over other techniques. This places the technique into the hands of the community otolaryngologist as well as the fellowship-trained laryngologist. Ultimately this increases accessibility for patients with vocal cord paralysis to clinicians who can provide optimal care for their affliction, impacting positively upon their quality of life.

References

1. Montgomery WW, Blaugrund SM, Varvares MA (1993) Thyroplasty: a new approach. Ann Otol Rhinol Laryngol 102:571–579
2. Montgomery WW, Montgomery SK (1997) Montgomery Thyroplasty Implant System. Ann Otol Rhinol Laryngol (Suppl) 106:170
3. Muse AM, Montgomery WW, Hillman RE, Varvares MA, Bunting G, Dyle P, Eng J (2000) Montgomery thyroplasty implant for vocal fold immobility: phonatory outcomes. Ann Otol Rhinol Laryngol 109:393–400
4. Adams SG, Irish JC, Durkin LC, Wong DL, Brown DH (1996) Evaluation of vocal function in unilateral vocal fold paralysis following thyroplastic surgery. J Otolaryngol 25:165–170
5. Bryant NJ, Gracco C, Sasaki CR, Vining E (1996) MRI evaluation of vocal fold paralysis before and after type I thyroplasty. Laryngoscope 106:1386–1392
6. D'Antonio LL, Wigley TL, Zimmerman GJ (1995) Quantitative measures of laryngeal function following Teflon injection or thyroplasty type I. Laryngoscope 105:256–262
7. Gorham MM, Avidano MA, Crary MA, Cotter CS, Cassisi NJ (1998) Laryngeal recovery following type I thyroplasty. Arch Otolaryngol Head Neck Surg 124:739–742
8. Gray SD, Barkmeier J, Jones D, Titze I, Druker D (1992) Vocal evaluation of thyroplastic surgery in the treatment of unilateral vocal fold paralysis. Laryngoscope 102:415–421
9. LaBlance GR, Maves MD (1992) Acoustic characteristics of post-thyroplasty patients. Otolaryngol Head Neck Surg 107:558–565
10. Lu F, Casiano RR, Lundy DS, Xue J (1996) Longitudinal evaluation of vocal function after thyroplasty type I in the treatment of unilateral vocal paralysis. Laryngoscope 106:573–577

Insertion of Implant

The thyroplasty implant is grasped with forceps. The posterior tip of the medial triangular portion of the implant is inserted first through the window. The tiered base of the implant is engaged into the posterior rim of the window in the thyroid lamina. The implant-inserter instrument (Fig. 9.2.2) is applied against the implant anteriorly, and the prosthesis is snapped into place.

If the implant requires change at the time of surgery, or change or removal at a later date as a secondary procedure, the anterior end of the external portion of the implant is grasped with forceps or a hemostat and removed.

Closure

The muscle and subcutaneous tissues are approximated with 3–0 chromic catgut, and the skin incision is repaired with 6–0 mild chromic catgut. Steri-Strips are then applied. Butterfly-closed suction draining is used.

Postoperative Care

Patients are admitted for observation due to the possibility of laryngeal edema or intralaryngeal bleeding that could interfere with the laryngeal airway. Pain medication is given as required. Antibiotics are given preoperatively and are continued for 1 week following surgery. Intravenous Decadron (8–12 mg) is also given at the beginning of the operation and continued for two additional doses at 8-h intervals. The suction drainage tubing is removed the morning following surgery and the patient is discharged. If indicated, the exact position of the prosthesis can be easily determined with computed tomography, as the implant is radio opaque. Patients are evaluated postoperatively by videofibrolaryngoscopy or videostroboscopy and voice analysis as described above.

Complications

The Montgomery Thyroplasty Implant System was designed to overcome such potential difficulties as incorrect implant position or size, or implant displacement [1, 2]; thus, complications related to this system are infrequent. In 176 consecutive cases of unilateral vocal cord paralysis treated with the system, there were no major complications [2]. There were no reactions to the silicone implant. No implants were noted to have displaced medially or laterally, or to have rotated out of position. Two cases of laryngeal edema occurred requiring an extra day in the hospital for intravenous steroid therapy. No patients required tracheotomy related to the procedure. Four of 176 cases required an increase in size of the implant in order to improve vocal function. Several patients have had implantation performed following radiotherapy to the head and neck, and there has been no difficulty noted in those patients related to placement of the implant into an irradiated field.

Results

In a recent study by Muse et al. [3] to evaluate phonatory outcomes, 43 patients with a diagnosis of unilateral vocal fold immobility underwent thyroplasty type I with the Montgomery Thyroplasty Implant System. Preoperative and postoperative evaluations were completed by means of videostroboscopic, acoustic, and aerodynamic measures. Clinicians' perceptions of vocal quality and patients' satisfaction with the surgery and vocal quality were also determined.

Improvements after surgery were observed for glottal closure, vocal fold amplitude, mucosal wave activity, average intensity, maximum intensity range, maximum phonation time, glottal air flow, average sound pressure, and subglottal pressure.

An overall average of 80% of patients were judged to exhibit an improvement in post-implant voice quality by clinical experts. Also, patients indicated high satisfaction with surgery (95%) and with vocal quality (80%). These

Method for Cutting Window

A small, tangential electric saw has been specifically designed for the thyroplasty type-I operation and other laryngeal framework surgery (Stryker Corp.). This saw can be used regardless of whether or not the cartilage has undergone ossification. Cutting the window should be accomplished with great care so as not to injure the underlying soft tissue. Once the window is free, it is grasped with the sharp hook (Fig. 9.2.2) and is carefully elevated form the underlying perichondrium with the chisel elevator designed for this purpose (Fig. 9.2.2). The cartilage is then removed. Following removal of the cartilage from the window, the inner perichondrium is elevated form the underlying cartilage in all directions with the duckbill elevator (Fig. 9.2.2), especially posteriorly towards the arytenoid. If there is no perforation of the inner perichondrium by this point, a longitudinal incision is made in this layer in the mid-portion of the window.

This is necessary in order to completely seat the large, obtuse inner portion of the implant. Extrusion is prevented by the tiered plates of the outer portion of the implant, which lock the implant into the thyroid window.

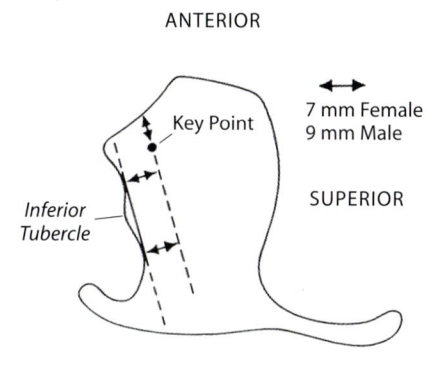

Fig. 9.2.3. Window measurement. The appropriate-size window caliper is used to measure from inferior border of thyroid cartilage, anterior and posterior to inferior thyroid tubercle, to superior border of thyroplasty window. A line is extended anteriorly through these points. The key point is then measured with the same caliper from anterior midline of thyroid cartilage, marking the anterior–superior angle of thyroplasty window. (From [2])

Implant Measurement

Implant measuring devices included in the Montgomery Thyroplasty Implant System are inserted through the window in the thyroid lamina. There are five sizes each for male and female larynges, corresponding to the appropriately sized implant. The vocal folds can be observed with a fiberoptic laryngoscope during this process. The end point is complete closure of the glottic chink during phonation, from anterior to posterior commissure. The ideal measurement is recorded so that the correct-size implant can be selected.

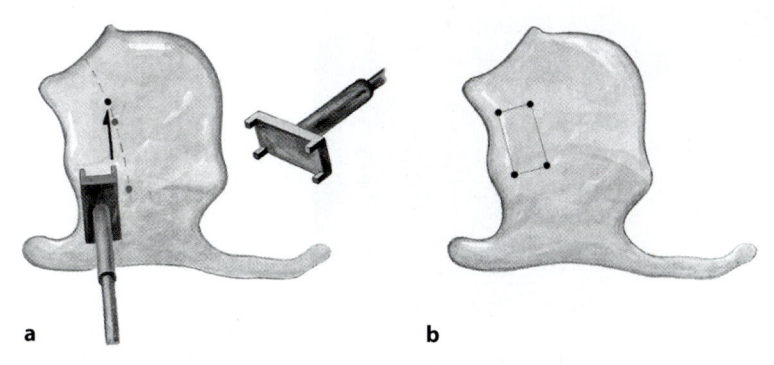

Fig. 9.2.4. Window outline. **a** The anterior–superior point of the window outline instrument is placed on the key point. The posterior–superior point of the instrument is placed along the line indicating superior border of window. **b** Cautery is applied, making four marks that locate the four corners of thyroplasty window. The four corners are connected with a surgical marking pen. (From [2])

Window Measurement

Instruments have been designed to accurately locate and outline the window in the thyroid lamina (Fig. 9.2.2). The window calipers, 7 mm wide in women and 9 mm wide in men, are used to locate the superior border and anterosuperior angle (key point) of the window (Fig. 9.2.3). One arm of the caliper touches the inferior border of the thyroid lamina, anterior to the inferior thyroid tubercle, and the other, a point directly superior. As the inferior arm is lifted free, electrocautery is applied to the measuring device to mark the superior point. A cautery mark is made in similar fashion beginning on the inferior border posterior to the inferior thyroid tubercle. The anterior and posterior cautery marks are then connected with a marking pen. This line is extended to the anterior midline of the thyroid lamina. The line corresponds with the superior margin of the window. One arm of the same caliper is placed at the anterior midline at the same level, and a cautery mark is made where the second arm comes to rest along this line. This cautery mark is the point of the anterosuperior angle (key point) of the thyroid lamina window (Fig. 9.2.3).

Window Outline

The window outline instrument (Fig. 9.2.2) is a modified cautery tip. The instrument is inserted into a Bovie handle and placed so that the anterosuperior angle and superior border correspond to the key-point mark and line on the thyroid lamina (Fig. 9.2.4). Current is applied and four marks appear on the cartilage surface, thus marking the border of the thyroid window. The four points are then connected to complete the rectangular window outline (Fig. 9.2.4). It is emphasized that the superior and inferior borders of the window must be parallel to the inferior boarder of the thyroid lamina for correct positioning. The window measures 5×10 mm for the female larynx and 7×12 mm for the male larynx.

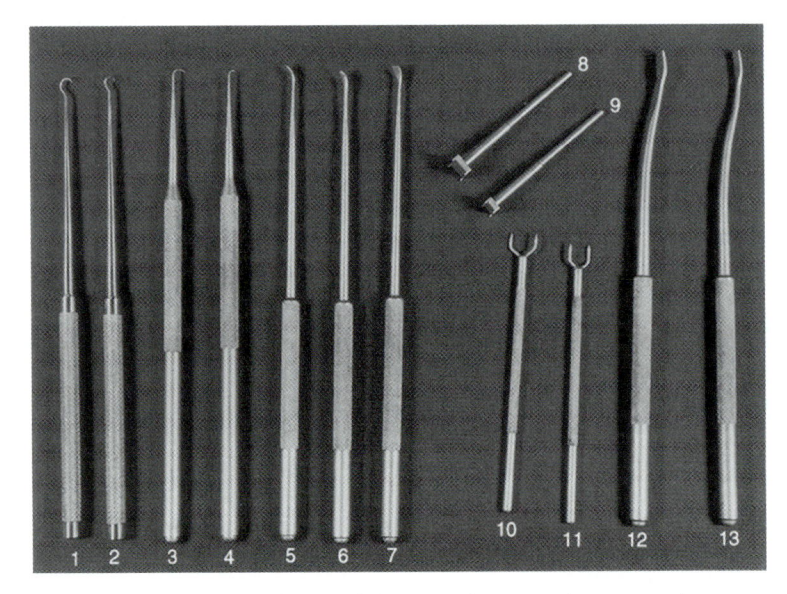

Fig. 9.2.2. Instruments for medialization laryngoplasty. *1,2* curved hooks for traction on thyroid cartilage; *3,4* sharp hooks to elevate cartilage from thyroplasty window; *5,6* duckbill elevator to elevate inner perichondrium from thyroid cartilage; *7* chisel elevator used to separate inner perichondrium from cartilage; *8,9* window outline instrument, male and female; *10,11* window calipers, male (9 mm) and female (7 mm); *12,13* implant inserters. (From [2])

Chapter 9

Medialization Thyroplasty Using the VoCoM Vocal Cord Medialization System

9.3

Tanya K. Meyer, Andrew Blitzer

Introduction

The VoCoM thyroplasty method [1] is a self-contained system of implants and instruments to allow accurate vocal fold medialization. The VoCoM system can provide membranous vocal fold medialization in addition to moderate medialization of the vocal process of the arytenoid. The implants come in five sizes, and are secured with one of four shims allowing placement of the implant in several different positions. Specifically, the implant can be secured in a horizontal or vertical orientation, with variability of anterior/posterior and superior/inferior positioning within the thyroplasty window (Fig. 9.3.1).

There are several advantages inherent in the design of this system which streamline the actual surgical procedure. This is critical to the success of the thyroplasty technique as tissue edema, which develops from excessive operative time or manipulation, can make it difficult for the surgeon to judge the appropriate vocal endpoint. A specially designed surgical instrument set facilitates window placement, determination of implant size and optimal location, and insertion of the implant. The graduated pre-fabricated implants and shims obviate the need to hand carve implants on the back table during the procedure, saving valuable operative time. The implant is made of hydroxylapatite with proven biocompatibility that generates a thin fibrous encapsulation. In some individuals, there may be osteogenesis in the region of the fenestra creating lamellar bone bridging between the implant and the thyroid lamina [2]. For individuals with paresis and residual motion, this provides implant stability and minimizes the risk of migration or extrusion. Although the osteogenesis is localized and does not preclude implant removal, this system

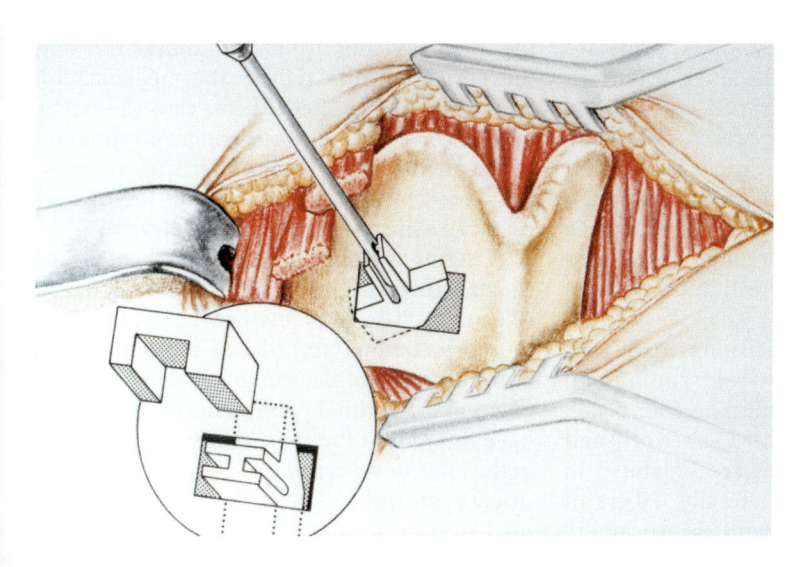

Fig. 9.3.1. The VoCoM implant and shim system for vocal cord medialization

should not be used in individuals in whom removal is anticipated.

The main disadvantage of the system is that the firm nature of the implant does not allow further carving, and additional modification of the shape must be done with a diamond drill. Additionally, osteointegration in the area of the thyroid lamina may make the procedure less easily reversible than other implants such as silastic.

Surgical Technique

This procedure is usually performed under local anesthesia to allow vocal feedback when determining implant size and position; therefore, sedation should be given to minimize anxiety while still allowing the patient to follow commands. Pre-operative antibiotics and decadron are given just prior to the incision. Glycopyrrolate or an equivalent anticholinergic can be used to inhibit secretions. Some surgeons prefer to perform the case with the flexible laryngoscope in place during part or all of the procedure to visualize the adequacy of medialization; others rely solely on auditory feedback. At our institution we use the laryngoscope only during the manipulation of the sizing devices.

The patient is placed in a supine position with a shoulder roll to enhance neck extension as tolerated. All efforts are made to enhance patient comfort and minimize movement during the procedure (pillow under knees, arms are tucked comfortably, etc.). The anterior portion of the neck is prepped and draped with a folded towel over the mandibular area to leave the nose and mouth exposed. An adhesive dressing can be suspended to provide a barrier between the exposed face and the surgical field. The area of the incision and corresponding surgical field is injected with 1% lidocaine with 1:100,000 epinephrine solution.

A 4- to 5-cm horizontal incision is made over the lateral aspect of the thyroid lamina and extended 1 cm across the midline (Fig. 9.3.2). Subplatysmal flaps are elevated superiorly and inferiorly, the strap muscles are separated in the midline and retracted laterally. Fibers of the thyrohyoid are divided with electrocautery to delineate the inferior boarder of the thyroid cartilage, and the thyroid lamina is exposed by retraction of the strap muscles laterally and rotating the larynx to the contralateral side using a single hook placed at the thyroid notch.

To prevent coughing during implant manipulation, topical anesthetic can be injected into the subglottic airway or 50–100 mg of lidocaine can be given intravenously just prior to entry through the thyroid lamina. Interestingly, no local anesthetic is needed in the paraglottic tissues during implant manipulation.

The position of the cartilage window is determined. The superior aspect of the window should be placed at the level of the true vocal fold. This position lies at halfway between the fundus of the thyroid notch and the anterior inferior edge of the thyroid cartilage. A line from this point extending posteriorly parallel to the inferior boarder of the thyroid cartilage will approximate the level of the TVF. For females, the anterior aspect of the window is positioned 5–8 mm lateral to the midline, and for males 8–10 mm. The window is then carefully outlined using the template, and the outer perichondrium and cartilage are removed taking care to accurately maintain the dimensions of the window. This is important to ensure a snug fit of the prosthesis. The cartilage can be removed using a scalpel, a Kerrison punch, or a small otologic drill. If possible, the integrity of the inner perichondrium is preserved.

Some experts place the implant external to the inner perichondrium, and others feel that the perichondrium tethers the medialization and strip it away. Regardless, care should be taken to ensure hemostasis and avoid violation of the airway. The paraglottic tissues are carefully freed from the inner table of the thyroid cartilage using the perichondrial elevator.

A series of trial implants are then placed ranging from 3 to 7 mm of displacement (Fig. 9.3.3). The implants can be rotated into four orientations and placed throughout the four quadrants of the window to determine the position for optimal phonation (Fig. 9.3.4). We have found that the most common position is in the inferior posterior quadrant in the vertical orientation with the bevel facing inferiorly. To medialize the vocal process of the arytenoid, the

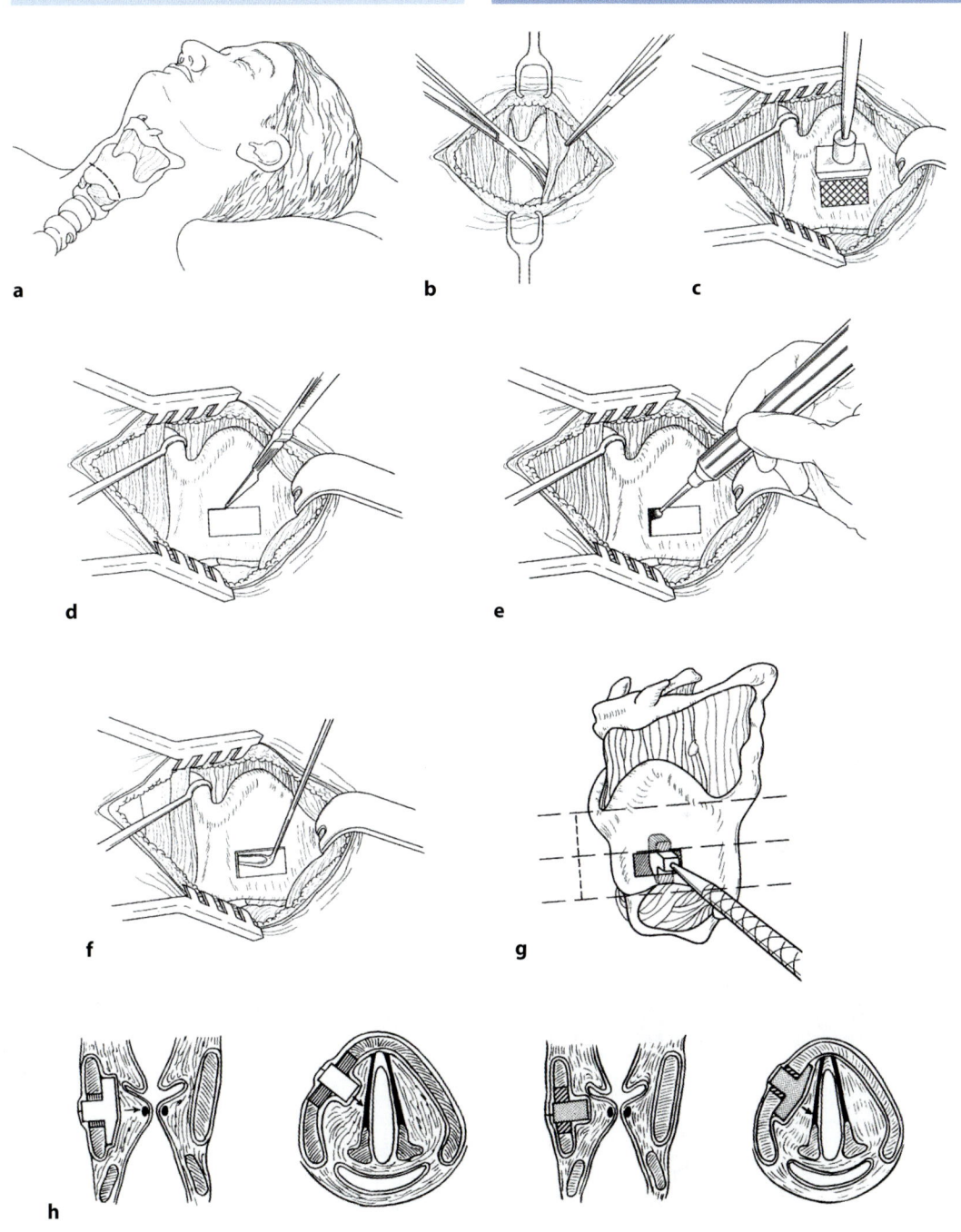

Fig. 9.3.2. Thyroplasty technique. **a** Skin incision. **b** After elevation of subplatysmal flaps, the strap muscles are divided and retracted laterally. **c** The larynx is rotated using a single hook and the fenestra template tool is used to mark the location of the window. **d,e** The window can be fashioned using a scalpel, Kerrison punch, or an otologic drill. **f** The paraglottic tissues are freed from the inner table of the thyroid cartilage. **g** A series of trial inserts are placed to determine optimum implant size and position, after which the final implant is placed and secured with the appropriate shim. The position of the vocal fold relative to external landmarks is shown. **h** The implants can be placed vertically or horizontally to achieve optimum phonation. (From [3])

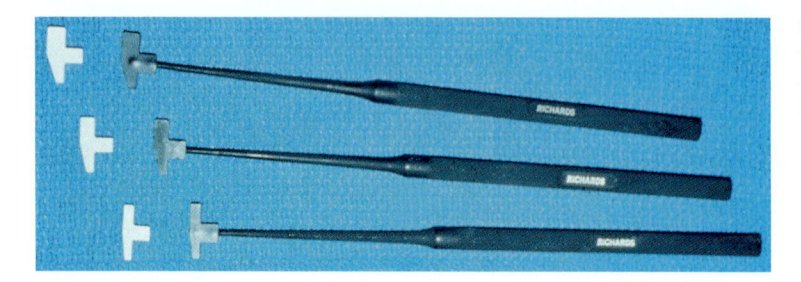

Fig. 9.3.3. Trial implant tools alongside the corresponding final implants

implant can be rotated to the horizontal position and placed posteriorly. The patent is asked to vocalize to confirm optimal placement. We advocate using the largest implant that gives good voicing without airway compromise, to prevent deterioration in voice quality as postoperative edema resolves. The trial implant is then removed.

If inadequate voicing is obtained, and if a persistent posterior glottic gap is evident on laryngoscopy, an arytenoid adduction procedure can be considered at this point, prior to placement of the final implant. Medialization thyroplasty does not affect the level of the vocal fold in the vertical plane. If there is significant discrepancy, it may be necessary to add an arytenoid repositioning procedure to the medialization.

Once the window is created, it is important to proceed with implant placement with alacrity to minimize distortion of the voice from glottic edema. The appropriate implant and shim are chosen. Just before placement of the final prosthesis, the field is flooded with saline and the patient asked to perform a Valsalva maneuver. Appearance of air bubbles suggests violation of the airway in which case the procedure should be terminated.

Assuming the integrity of the airway has been maintained, the implant is loaded onto the handle of the implant inserter and placed in the proper position. The correct shim is then placed using a smooth dressing forceps, thus securing the implant in the desired position within the fenestra (Fig. 9.3.5).

The wound is irrigated with antibiotic solution. A drain is placed deep to the strap muscles. The strap muscles and platysma are closed with an absorbable suture and skin closed as desired.

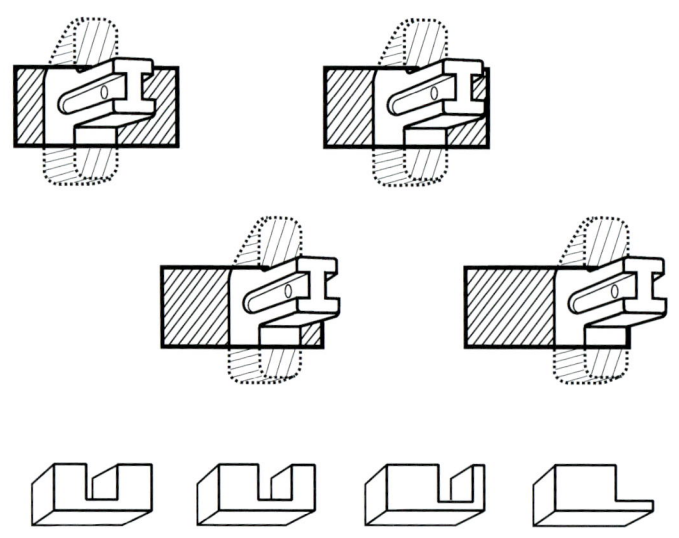

Fig. 9.3.4. Depending on the shim used, the implant can be variably positioned along the anterior/posterior and superior/inferior axis of the fenestra.

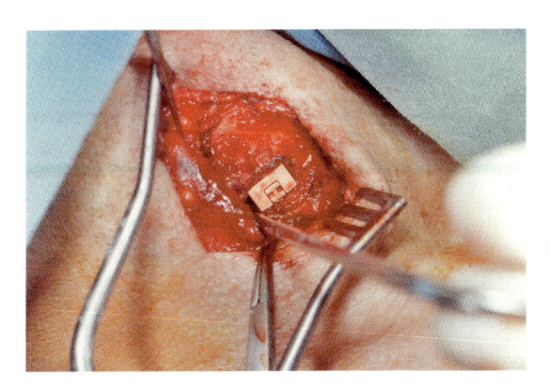

Fig. 9.3.5. An implant in situ just prior to closure

Post-operatively, the patient is monitored overnight in the hospital for possible hematoma formation and airway obstruction. The drain is removed on post-operative day 1. The patient is given a regular diet but encouraged to minimize aggressive vocal behavior such as coughing, throat clearing, or yelling, although absolute voice rest is not required. Patients are told that the voice may deteriorate on post-operative day 1, and the true voice will not emerge for 3–5 days. Prophylactic antibiotics are continued for 5 days.

Revision

The surgical approach for revision is the same as for the primary surgery. After exposure of the implant, any osteogenesis is disrupted using a Freer elevator or a diamond drill. Closure and post-operative care are the same as in the original surgery.

Complications

The most serious complication is post-operative airway compromise. In light of this, all patients are monitored in the hospital overnight. The performance of concomitant arytenoid adduction increases this risk and also the risk of hematoma formation. Other complications include perforation of the endolaryngeal mucosa, implant migration, infection, chondritis, and implant extrusion.

Results

A study from Johns Hopkins University evaluated 35 patients implanted for vocal fold paralysis and reported subjective improvement in 89% [3]. In our series of 25 patients we had a 92% improvement with no complications. There were two complications including one implant extrusion and one case of airway obstruction. These results compare favorably with the results of other implant techniques in the literature.

Conclusion

The VoCoM implant system is a simple, efficient, and flexible method to achieve accurate vocal fold medialization. It is compatible with concomitant arytenoid adduction, although it may provide modest medialization of the vocal process. The implant material is biocompatible with nearly a decade of clinical use. The procedure is technically reversible, although it should be used in patients who are candidates for permanent implantation.

References

1. http://www.gyrus-ent.com.
2. Flint PW, Corio RL, Cummings CW (1997) Comparison of soft tissue response in rabbits following laryngeal implantation with hydroxylapatite, silicone rubber, and Teflon. Ann Otol Rhinol Laryngol 106:399–407
3. Cummings CW, Purcell LL, Flint PW (1993) Hydroxylapatite laryngeal implants for medialization. Preliminary report. Ann Otol Rhinol Laryngol 102:843–851

Chapter 9

Titanium Medialization Implant

9.4

Berit Schneider

Titanium as a Biomaterial

Titanium (Ti, anatomic number 22) was a laboratory rarity until William Kroll (1889–1973) developed a process for commercial production of titanium alloys by combining titanium tetrachloride with calcium to produce ductile titanium (the "Kroll Process"). Titanium is the fourth most abundant structural metal on Earth. Today, it is widely used in medical devices, dental applications, and surgical implants due to its superior biological performance. About as strong as steel, titanium is 50% lighter. Its high strength-to-weight and stiffness-to-weight ratios, outstanding corrosion resistance, and other highly desirable attributes have been made this material attractive as biomaterial. It is physiologically hypoallergenic and immune to corrosion, especially microbiologically influenced corrosion. In biological tissue titanium is inert: the oxide layer that is in contact with the tissue is hardly soluble and in particular no ions are released that could react with other molecules [8].

Titanium has an extremely low toxicity and is well tolerated by both bone and soft tissue. Animal experiments have revealed that the material may be implanted for an extensive length of time; fibrous encapsulation of the implants is minimal to nonexistent. Histopathological examinations have revealed no cellular changes adjacent to titanium implants.

The mechanical properties of titanium compare favorably with those of surgical-quality stainless steel. The low modulus results in a material that is less rigid and deforms elastically under applied loads.

Titanium is virtually nonmagnetic, making it ideal for applications where electromagnetic interference must be minimized. Titanium, as a nonferromagnetic material, does not interfere with MRI or CT [2]; thus, postoperative imaging examinations with respect to necessary tumor follow-up are possible.

Titanium Vocal Medialization Implant

The titanium vocal medialization implant (TVFMI; Fig. 9.4.1) has been introduced recently by Friedrich [3] in cooperation with Kurz Medical, Inc. (Germany) for external medialization of a unilaterally paralyzed vocal fold. Three sizes are commercially available (Kurz Medical, Inc.). The large implant normally used in men measures 6×15 mm; the next smaller one, normally used in women, 6×13 mm. For external medialization in very small larynges, a third size of 4.5×11 mm is available. Except for a bending pliers and a marking stamp, as shown in Fig. 9.4.2, no special instruments are necessary to perform the thyroplasty.

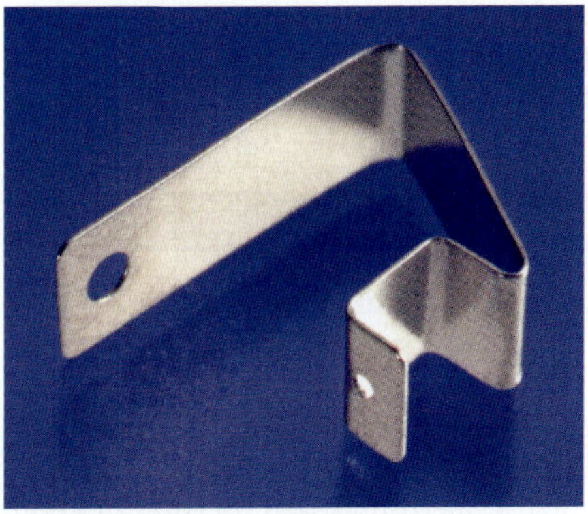

Fig. 9.4.1. Titanium vocal fold medialization implant (TVFMI)

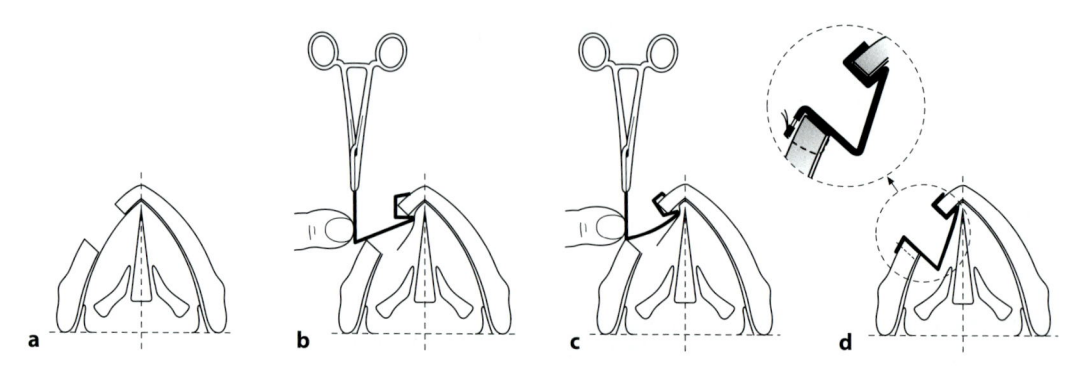

Fig. 9.4.2 a–d. Principle of external vocal fold medialization using the TVFMI

Preoperative Medication

Preoperative sedation (e.g., midazolam hydrochloride), single-dose intravenous cortisone (about 250 mg prednisolone hemisuccinate natrium), and a prophylactic single-dose broad-spectrum antibiotic are recommended 30 min preoperatively.

Anesthesia

Local anesthesia supplemented by intravenous sedation is recommended for this procedure. This allows an optimum positioning of the implant under audiophonatory control. In addition, the use of a respiratory tube would interfere with the vocal fold medialization.

The patient should be monitored intraoperatively by the anesthesiologist. A continuous intraoperative propofol infusion is recommended.

Surgical Technique

The technique used for medialization of the vocal folds has been previously reported by Friedrich [3].

After infiltration with lidocaine hydrochloride 1% (plus epinephrine hydrogen tartrate 1:200,000), a horizontal skin incision of about 3 cm is made at the level of the mid-thyroid ala of the appropriate side. The thyroid cartilage is exposed with the perichondrium preserved from the midline laterally. The overlying strap muscles are cut using the electrocautery. A reference line is drawn parallel to the inferior thyroid margin, beginning from the anterior midline at the midpoint between the superior and inferior thyroid notches. This line corresponds to the free edges of the vocal folds endolaryngeally. With a preformed silicone template the cartilage window should be marked caudal to the reference line and near the oblique line of the thyroid ala.

For the 13 mm implant the window size is 6×11 mm, for the 15 mm one 6×13 mm, and for the small size 4.5×9 mm. The cartilage and osteoid material are drilled out with a steel drill until the inner perichondrium becomes visible. For irrigation, local anesthesia solution as described above is recommended. The edges and corners of the window can be smoothed using a small diamond burr. The inner perichondrium is incised along the window's rim with a Colorado needle or a low-energy electrocautery. It is very important not to enter the paraglottic space or to cut the endolaryngeal vessels during dissection of the perichondrium.

After careful mobilization of the endolaryngeal tissue the TVFMI can be placed in the subperichondrial pocket (Fig. 9.4.3). The anterior (ventral) flange is inserted first. The implant has to be positioned under slight tension through the cartilage into the larynx, because the implant is 2 mm larger than the window. Under audiophonatory control, the optimum medial-

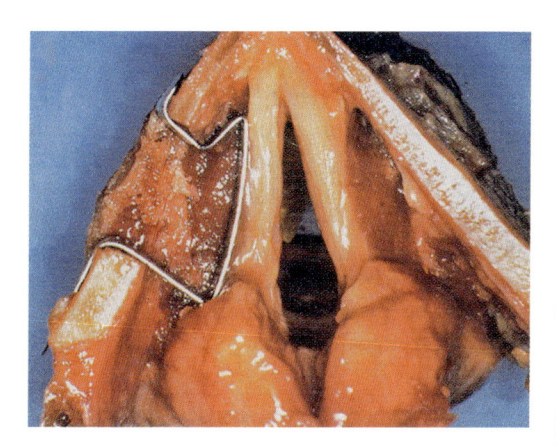

Fig. 9.4.3. The TVFMI placed in a cadaver larynx

ization depth of the dorsal flange is determined and the position is marked. The dorsal flange is bent at the marked point with the bending pliers. The TVFMI is re-seated precisely and fixed with monofil nonabsorbable sutures (one to fix the ventral flange and two to fix the dorsal one).

After reanastomosis of the strap muscles, a drain is placed, which can be removed after approximately 2 days.

Objective Outcome Measures

Five years of clinical experience with the TVFMI have yielded excellent and stable functional results and satisfying improvements of phonation and swallowing without any fixation or migration problem of the implant [4]. Primary goals of this technique are to improve phonation, vocal efficacy and force of cough, and to decrease subjective dysphagia and aspiration without a negative influence on the glottal resistance. The type, completeness, and duration of glottal closure are important for the vocal outcome, airway control, and the airway protection during swallowing. After thyroplasty, patients regularly demonstrate improved glottal closure. Maximum medialization is possible with the TVFMI, especially in subjects with a large posterior gap and vocal fold bowing, by adjusting the length of the posterior flange.

The anamnestic, perceptual, videostroboscopic, acoustic, videocinematographic, and aerodynamic data investigated underline the clinical benefit after external medialization thyroplasty with the TVFMI [4, 5, 7]. As for the swallowing function, a convincing improvement of the degree of aspiration and subjective dysphagia in most patients can be observed. Comprehensive aerodynamic measurements have not revealed any increase in extrathoracic obstruction after thyroplasty surgery [6].

Advantages

The customized design ensures safe implant placement and reduces the operation time significantly. This is, on the one hand, convenient for both the patient and the surgeon, and on the other hand, important for achieving optimal results because of reduced intralaryngeal swelling and hematoma. While other implant techniques presume very experienced and specialized surgical skills, the TVFMI is simple to handle even for less experienced surgeons and allows precise and atraumatic vocal fold medialization. It eliminates free-hand shaping of a suitable implant, and permits the use of a commercially available template to outline the thyroplasty window, which simplifies the surgery and shortens the operating time.

Under phonatory control, an exact positioning of the implant is possible intraoperatively and optimum medialization with the TVFMI can be achieved.

Implant materials have occasionally been reported to migrate or shift. Migration of the TVFMI can be largely eliminated by fixation with nonabsorbable thread.

In patients with a very lateral position of the paralyzed vocal fold, a combination of medialization thyroplasty with approximation of the cricoid and thyroid cartilages, or with endoscopic fat augmentation, is possible.

Complications

Our experiences showed no major intraoperative complications. In only less than 1% of patients, a repositioning of the implant was necessary after flexible endoscopic laryngoscopy because of respiratory deficits reported by the patient resulting from "over"-correction of the vocal fold position.

Postoperatively, major complications after medialization thyroplasty (e.g., tracheostomy) did not occur in any patients treated. About 25% of the patients developed mild local hematoma for some days without any negative permanent effect on the vocal outcome.

In very rare cases (two women in our own patient group) the implant had to be removed because of tissue atrophy and granulation tissue neoformation in the anterior third of the vocal fold. It is very important to consider the thickness of the thyroid cartilage and to adapt if necessary the length of the anterior flange of the implant to the cartilage. The anterior flange should fit exactly to the cartilage and should not be placed too loosely.

Other Titanium Implant Devices

To complement the TVFMI, another implant device has been introduced. In 1993 Desrosiers et al. reported preliminary experiences using a standard double-titanium–vanadium miniplate and screws (LUHR Minifixation System) in two fresh cadaver larynges. With this system, a cartilage window can be moved horizontally, and pressure can be transmitted directly to the underlying vocal fold.

Eight years later, Dean and coworkers [1] reported the use of an adjustable laryngeal implant which has three distinct parts: the titanium plate; a micrometric screw; and an adjustable titanium block. The plate allows fixation of the implant to the thyroid cartilage. It is contiguous with an adjustable titanium block which can be medialized by means of a micrometric screw. The implant is available in different sizes: the block in 4- and 6-mm thicknesses, and the degree of angulation in the adjustable part in 0, 1, 2, and 3 mm. Although the authors gathered satisfactory postoperative results with regard to voice and swallowing improvements, a relatively high number of complications (five airway problems, one death, two malpositions of the implant, and six inadequate medializations in 53 patients) are noteworthy. We are not able to report personal experience with the adjustable laryngeal implant.

References

1. Dean CM, Ahmarani C, Bettez M, Heuer RJ (2001) The adjustable laryngeal implant. J Voice 15:141–150
2. Desrosiers M, Ahmarani C, Bettez M (1993) Precice vocal cord medialization using an adjustable laryngeal implant: a preliminary study. Otolaryngol Head Neck Surg 109:1014–1019
3. Friedrich G (1999) Titanium vocal fold medializing implant: introducing a novel implant system for external vocal fold medialization. Ann Otol Rhinol Laryngol 108:79–86
4. Schneider B, Denk DM, Bigenzahn W (2003a) Functional results after external vocal fold medialization thyroplasty with the Titanium vocal fold medialization implant. Laryngoscope 113:628–634
5. Schneider B, Bigenzahn W, End A, Denk DM, Klepetko W (2003b) External vocal fold medialization in patients with recurrent nerve paralysis following cardiothoracic surgery. Eur J Cardiothorac Surg 23:477–483
6. Schneider B, Kneussl M, Denk DM, Bigenzahn W (2003c) Aerodynamic measurements in medialization thyroplasty. Acta Otolaryngol 123:883–888
7. Schneider B, Denk DM, Bigenzahn W (2003d) Acoustic assessment of voice quality prior to and after medialization thyroplasty using the Titanium vocal fold medialization implant (TVFMI). Otolaryngol Head Neck Surg 128:815–822
8. Suzuki R, Frangos JA (2000) Inhibition of inflammatory species by titanium surfaces. Clin Orthop 372:280–289

Chapter 9

Medialization Laryngoplasty with Gore-Tex (Expanded Polytetrafluoroethylene)

9.5

Timothy M. McCulloch, Henry T. Hoffman

Introduction

Although the ideal implant material for medialization laryngoplasty has not been defined, there has been increased enthusiasm for the utilization of expanded polytetrafluoroethylene or Gore-Tex as the implant of choice in the treatment of unilateral vocal cord paralysis. This material has many advantages not found in solid implant types; however, there is more to Gore-Tex medialization laryngoplasty than simply an alternative implant material. The technique of implantation is altered to ensure success and limit serious complications such as implant extrusion. In this chapter we emphasize the following:

1. The biological rationale for utilizing Gore-Tex as an intralaryngeal implant.
2. The modifications in approach to the laryngeal framework surgery to maximize the benefit of the Gore-Tex implantation.
3. The utilization of Gore-Tex in combination with arytenoid reduction to facilitate posterior glottic closure.
4. A step-by-step procedural methodology
5. Possible areas where extra caution should be utilized in order to prevent poor voice results or postoperative complications.

Gore-Tex (W.L. Gore and Associates, Flagstaff, Ariz.) has been utilized as a biocompatible implant material since the early 1970s [1]. Medical-grade Gore-Tex is a semiporous implant material which allows for limited vascular ingrowth without significant inflammatory response (Fig. 9.5.1) [2, 3]. The report on the first series of cases of Gore-Tex medialization laryngoplasty was presented at the Second International Symposium on Laryngeal and Tracheal Reconstruction at Monte Carlo, Monaco, in May 1996, and the technique was first discussed in a review article by Hoffman and McCulloch in the same year [4]. A patient case series was subsequently published in the "Annals of Otolaryngology-Head and Neck Surgery" in May 1998, which formally describes the initial findings in 16 patients treated for vocal cord paralysis with Gore-Tex as the medialization material [5]. Initially, a modification of an already available Gore-Tex product, a cardiac patch cut into a spiral ribbon, was described; however, since 1999 the W.L. Gore company has produced an FDA-approved thyroplasty "device" in a pre-

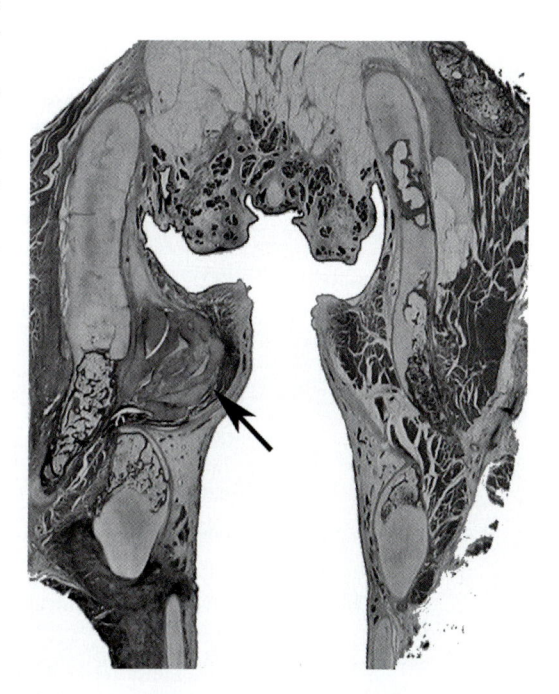

Fig. 9.5.1. Gore-Tex-implanted human larynx, 5 months post-implantation. Human larynx coronal section mid-vocal-cord level. Arrow indicates Gore-Tex implant

on the surgical approach were also described in that article and, as expected, improved glottic closure resulted from the combined approach. Other authors [7–10] have also reported their technique and results utilizing Gore-Tex as a medialization material (Table 9.5.1), identifying similar outcomes as initially described by Hoffman and McCulloch [4].

Technique of Gore-Tex Thyroplasty

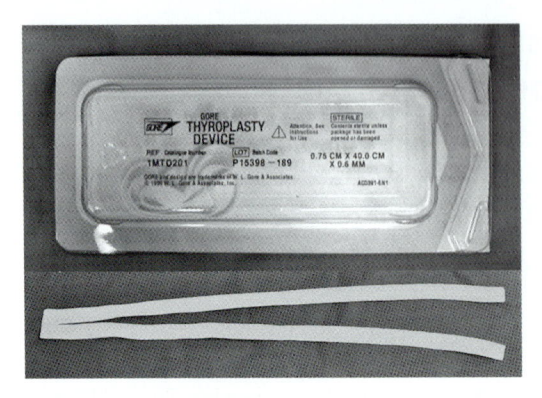

Fig. 9.5.2. Sterile Gore-Tex thyroplasty device as supplied by W.L. Gore and Associates (Scottsdale, Ariz.)

formed ribbon shape, 0.6 mm in thickness and with a pore size desirable for tissue in-growth yet which preserves ease of removal if required (Fig. 9.5.2). We compared the results of Gore-Tex medialization alone with Gore-Tex medialization and arytenoid adduction combined in a group of 72 patients in 2000 [6]. Further details

In obtaining the patient consent, we mention the need for local anesthesia to numb the neck and topical anesthesia for fiberoptic scope placement. We describe a small skin incision and exposure of the larynx and the possible use of a small drill if the larynx is significantly calcified. We review potential complications: bleeding; infection; reaction to the anesthesia; a less-than-perfect voice postoperatively; possible dyspnea; and the potential need for intubation or tracheotomy. We also discuss the fact

Table 9.5.1. Gore-Tex medialization laryngoplasty case series results. *AA* arytenoid adduction

Reference	Number	Descriptive results	Maximum phonation time
[5]	16	Ten patients with pre- and post-op voice data: mean improvement in voice "grade"[b] from 2.3 to 1.1 and „breathiness"[b] from 2.0 to 0.4	Not reported
[6]	72 (25 Gore-Tex and 19 plus AA)	Mean changes	Mean changes
		Gore-Tex alone: grade 2.2 to 1.5; breathiness 1.9 to 0.9	Gore-Tex Alone: 8.3 to 9.9 s Plus AA: 6.9 to 16.7 s
		Plus AA grade 2.1 to 0.8; breathiness 1.9 to 0.3	Not reported
[7]	13	Ten patients with pre- and post-op data: mean improvement in voice "grade"[b] from 2.8 to 0.8; jitter form 14.5 to 0.88	
[8][a]	26	69% with post-op "good voice," 27% with satisfactory voice	Mean changes 8.1 to 13.1 s
[9]	142	Overall very positive results; details not reported	Not reported
[10]	24	Mean improvement post-op in: jitter (2.9); shimmer (8.6); and noise:harmonic ratio (0.2)	Mean postoperative results: 7 s

[a]Utilized a small fenestration technique. All patients in this report had Gore-Tex alone without arytenoid adduction
[b]GRBAS scale of Hirano [16]

that the voice will change during the first several weeks after surgery and there may be a need for future procedures to fine-tune the result.

No significant special instrumentation is required. We request a minor otolaryngology instrument tray, with a few different small elevators, tracheotomy and skin hooks, and two Richards adjustable double fork retractors. Sometimes a simple custom bend on a small flat elevator can improve its usefulness around the edges of the laryngeal cartilage. Also needed are the otologic electric drill, a tray of small bone rongeurs, a bipolar forceps, and a flexible fiberoptic laryngoscope. The FDA-approved Gore-Tex laryngeal implants are now available sterilely packaged in a variety of widths and lengths.

Patient Preparation Steps

The patient preparation steps are as follows:
1. Although general anesthesia may be used in selected cases (e.g., anticipated poor patient compliance), local anesthesia is preferred to permit voice assessment intraoperatively and to avoid laryngeal distortion due to the presence of endotracheal tube. Supplemental oxygen by nasal prongs is reasonable in any sedated patient. Preoperative mediations should include Glycopyrrolate 0.1 mg intramuscular on call to operating room, and Decadron (dexamethasone) 10 mg and antibiotic of choice delivered intravenously as soon as the IV is started.
2. The skin is marked at a level between the midportion of the thyroid cartilage and the cricothyroid space using a neck skin crease when possible. Bupivacaine, 0.25%, with 1:100,000 epinephrine is injected at this site.
3. Topical nasal decongestion and anesthesia is achieved with Oxymetazoline HCL nasal spray, 0.05% and Tetracaine hydrochloride, 2%.
4. The patient should be reasonably comfortable. The head of bed is elevated 30° and the neck is extended with a small shoulder roll, and pillows are placed under feet and knees.
5. Standard neck preparation is carried out from clavicles to chin. The neck is draped and a half sheet is used to separate neck and face with access to face for oxygenation, anesthesia monitoring, voice assessment, and transnasal scope placement.

Operative Steps

The operative steps are as follows:
1. Incision is made over the midportion of thyroid cartilage on the side of paralysis.
2. The strap muscles are separated in the midline. Cutting the muscle bellies over the thyroid cartilage simplifies deeper dissection.
3. Supplement injection to deeper tissue with 1% lidocaine with 1:100,000 epinephrine is administered as needed as the dissection continues.
4. A tracheotomy hook is inserted through the laryngeal prominence, permitting medial traction on the larynx with improved exposure.
5. The ipsilateral thyroid cartilage is exposed inferiorly to the cricothyroid membrane and posteriorly to its lateral edge. Limiting dissection to the oblique line is adequate for placement of the prosthesis, but restricts exposure and orientation, and is inadequate for arytenoid adduction.
6. Slips of the cricothyroid muscle inserting on the lateral border of the muscular process (inferior tubercle) of thyroid cartilage are detached (Fig. 9.5.3).
7. One percent lidocaine with 1:100,000 epinephrine is injected into the cricothyroid membrane immediately below the lower border of thyroid cartilage.
8. The window location is defined. The window measures approximately 5–8 mm. Its lower border rests 3–5 mm above cricothyroid membrane, and its anterior border of window at least 10 mm posterior to midline. Usually the best location is just superior to the inferior thyroid tubercle, which is approximately at the midportion of the vocal fold. A small drill is used to make the window if thyroid cartilage is calcified.

9. Small elevators are used to elevate the inner perichondrium from the undersurface of thyroid cartilage through the window. The perichondrium is also detached from inferior edge of thyroid cartilage, making this space continuous with the window. We attempt to maintain intact anterior inner perichondrium; however opening the perichondrium posteriorly, inferiorly, and superiorly may be needed to ensure adequate medialization.
10. From the inferior approach, a small, bent elevator is placed under lower border of thyroid cartilage and into the window to depress the contents of the paraglottic space medially while assessing phonation. From this testing it is possible to estimate the primary point for medialization and the volume of Gore-Tex that may be required.
11. The Gore-Tex strip is placed under the thyroid cartilage from the inferior approach, adding and positioning material until the optimal voice is achieved. It is important to keep in mind that many patients have developed compensatory voicing habits which may persist despite medialization. Having a speech pathologist in the OR may be useful to address these during the voice testing. Also, a slight over-correction until the voice sounds mildly "pressed" may provide a more durable long-term result (Fig. 9.5.4).
12. The strip of Gore-Tex is secured primarily by wedging it between the contents of the paraglottic space (perichondrium and LCA/TA muscle group) and the overlying thyroid cartilage. The addition of a 4-0 Prolene suture placed around lower strut of cartilage and through the Gore-Tex may add security in the early stages of healing.
13. Any excess Gore-Tex is divided, and the wound is closed in a layered fashion over a small passive drain.

Gore-Tex medialization laryngoplasty can be easily combined with arytenoid adduction to ensure closure of a posterior glottic gap. In order to accomplish this, additional steps are added prior to Gore-Tex placement:

1. The laryngeal attachments of the inferior constrictor muscle are removed, exposing the lateral border of the thyroid cartilage lamina. The larynx is rotated with a double hook and the pyriform sinus mucosa is carefully separated away from the posterior larynx, allowing visualization and palpation of the arytenoid muscular process. The removal of a small amount of thyroid lamina along the posterior–lateral border can aid in this procure [11]. Care must be taken not to injure the pyriform during this step of the

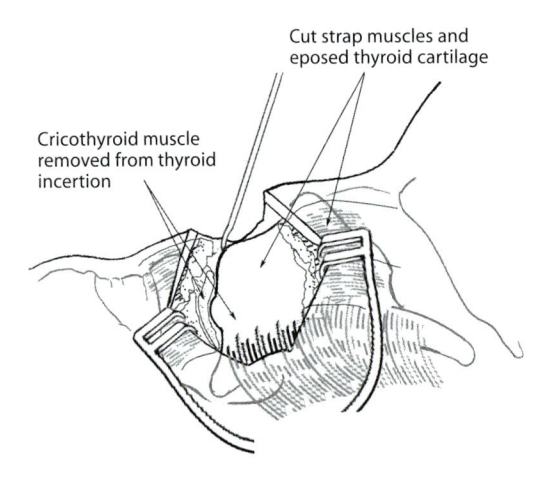

Fig. 9.5.3. Standard external approach with land marks identified

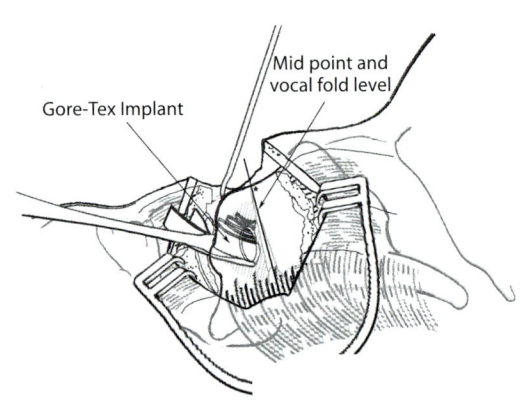

Fig. 9.5.4. Gore-Tex implantation inferior to thyroid lamina (arrows)

procedure, as any mucosal opening would preclude the placement of Gore-Tex.
2. Once the muscular process is identified, two 4-0 Prolene sutures are placed through its tendinous attachments and tied. The previously dissected lateral paraglottic space should easily be connected to the area adjacent to the muscular process. The sutures are then passed from posterior to anterior and brought out under the thyroid cartilage in the cricothyroid space. A small hole is drilled approximately 5 mm posterior to the location of the anterior commissure through which one of the suture pairs is passed via an 18-G hollow needle.
3. The final step is tying the suture pairs together over the anterior thyroid cartilage lamina strut; however, this step is completed only after the implant is inset and secure. It is essential that the suture lie medial to the Gore-Tex as this provides the proper vector of pull on the arytenoids, which produces rotation of the vocal process in to the phonatory position. It is also essential that these sutures not be over-tightened leading to posterior glottic over-closure and airway compromise (Fig. 9.5.4).

One of the primary advantages of Gore-Tex medialization laryngoplasty is its overall simplicity. It allows the surgeon to incrementally medialize the vocal fold until an appropriate on-table voice is obtained. The surgeon may quickly remove material if over-correction is identified and/or shortness of breath occurs. The surgeon does not need to refashion an implant or modify an implant with each correction, but simply add or remove Gore-Tex. Also, utilizing an inferior approach to implant placement essentially ensures that the implant

Table 9.5.2. Possible complications and management suggestion

Complication	Management suggestion
Intra-operative airway swelling: edema or hematoma	Pre-operative steroids
	Intubation with small endotracheal tube, controls bleeding, check coagulation status; post-op steroids; controlled extubation after resolution
	Assess implant: insure that implant size or location is not the cause of airway obstruction
Post-operative airway swelling	Same as above: tracheotomy only if conservative airway management fails
Complaints of shortness of breath or exertional dyspnea	Glottic evaluation for over-correction and/or contralateral weakness
	Bilateral weakness will require addition work-up with airway management based on clinical findings. Over-correction can diminish with time if airway is otherwise safe. Revision procedure will be required if improvement not seen during the first few months
Persistent breathy voice	Assess glottis for under-correction
	Revision procedures may required: – Augmentation Gore-Tex laryngoplasty – Injection laryngoplasty – Arytenoid adduction
Gore-Tex extrusion	Intraoperative, endolaryngeal Gore-Tex removal with secondary procedure after healing, or Transcutaneous removal with strap muscle augmentation

will be appropriately positioned in the paraglottic space, allowing medialization of only the true vocal fold region of the larynx. Other authors have reported utilization of a standard thyroplasty window for Gore-Tex insertion with adequate and reasonable voice results [7–9]. These articles emphasize the need to properly place the window below the level of the true vocal fold and reiterate the simplicity of this approach, as a specific size or shape to the window is not required. In fact, a smaller fenestra is often better than a larger one, retaining the additional thyroid lamina to assist in the retention of the Gore-Tex and the subsequent medialization of the vocal fold. In our personal experience an inferior approach from the cricothyroid space can be utilized without the creation of any window at all. This provides maximal cartilaginous barrier to ensure stable medialization. Sutures are placed through the Gore-Tex and passed through the cartilaginous portion of the midthyroid lamina for further stability. The disadvantage of this technique is the inability to manipulate the Gore-Tex within the paraglottic space to the same degree that a small fenestra allows. Also, an inferiorly ossified laryngeal cartilage precludes suture passage through the lamina without creation of at least a small drill hole.

The decision to combine Gore-Tex thyroplasty with arytenoid adduction is made individually by each surgeon and is based on the preoperative position of the paralyzed vocal fold. Patients with a large posterior glottic gap are more likely to benefit from an arytenoid adduction suture than those with a closed posterior glottis and primarily midvocal fold bowing. The literature supports arytenoid adduction in combination with implant medialization for maximum vocal benefit regardless of the implant material [6, 10, 12]; however, posterior glottic procedures are associated with higher risk of postoperative airway complications [13].

Complications

Overmedialization of a paralyzed vocal fold beyond the midline can lead to persistent patient dyspnea and shortness of breath on physical exertion [6]. Postoperative edema may require prolonged hospital observation and steroid use or reintubation [9]. Postoperative hematoma has also been described and can require re-operation, intubation, or short-term tracheotomy [9]. Undermedialization can lead to complaints of persistent vocal fatigue and breathiness and may require future augmentation procedures (Table 9.5.2) [9, 14].

Although rare, extrusion is a possibility, as with any implant material. Gore-Tex extrusion has been reported at three primary locations: in the subglottic region; at the region of the ventricular floor; and posteriorly through the pyriform mucosa [7, 14, 15]. In all cases it is most likely that mucosa was violated during or prior to implant placement, or inappropriately thinned or devascularized, leading to subsequent breakdown and Gore-Tex exposure intraluminally. Once any implant material becomes thus exposed, it requires removal in all cases. Removal of Gore-Tex is relatively simple and can be accomplished either transmucosally with endoscopic techniques or through external incisions, allowing for the opportunity to complete a simultaneous secondary augmentation with native materials such as adjacent strap muscle or fat. A staged re-medialization is also a prudent option.

Steps that should be taken to decrease the potential of extrusion of Gore-Tex include maintaining caution in elevating soft tissues prior to implantation to ensure that mucosal surfaces are not violated. The areas at primary

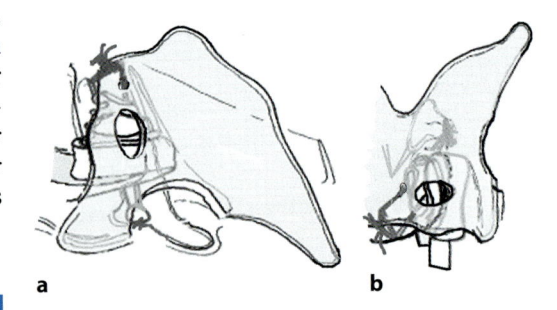

Fig. 9.5.5. Position of arytenoid adduction suture relative to implant within the paraglottic space. a Lateral view. b Anterior view

risk are anteriorly in the region just adjacent to the anterior commissure, superiorly at the mucosal floor of the ventricle, and posteriorly at the pyriform sinus region during arytenoid adduction. Also, if the material is placed too far anterior–inferior, the subglottic tracheal mucosa may also be violated. In most cases, if the Gore-Tex is appropriately placed in the midbody of the vocal fold and adjacent to the vocal process, it remains deep to both the vocalis muscle and lateral cricoarytenoid muscle, which provide an additional barrier to extrusion.

Conclusion

In conclusion, Gore-Tex medialization laryngoplasty remains a simple surgical technique for the restoration of voice and airway function after unilateral vocal cord paralysis. It allows great flexibility for individual surgeons to modify their technique to suit their comfort level and patient population. It is easily combined with arytenoid adduction in patients requiring closure of a posterior glottic gap. It is reversible and revisable, and the complications are quite limited. When they do occur they are commonly managed with simple procedures that allow future restoration of vocal cord position and quality of voice.

References

1. Soyer T, Lempinen M, Cooper P, Norton L, Eiseman B (1972) A new venous prosthesis. Surgery 72:864–872
2. Neel HB (1983) Implants of ePTFE. Arch Otolaryngol 109:427–433
3. Schoenrock L, Chernoff WG (1995) Subcutaneous implantation of ePTFE for facial reconstruction. Otolaryngol Clin North Am 28:325–340
4. Hoffman HT, McCulloch TM (1996) Anatomic considerations in the surgical treatment of unilateral laryngeal paralysis. Head Neck 18:174–187
5. McCulloch TM, Hoffman HT (1998) Medialization laryngoplasty with expanded polytetrafluoroethylene. Ann Otol Rhinol Laryngol 107:427–432
6. McCulloch TM, Hoffman HT, Andrews BT, Karnell MP (2000) Arytenoid adduction combined with Gore-Tex medialization thyroplasty. Laryngoscope 110:1306–1311
7. Giovanni A, Vallicioni JM, Gras R, Zanaret M (1999) Clinical experience with Gore-Tex for vocal fold medialization. Laryngoscope 109:284–288
8. Stasney CR, Beaver ME, Rodriguez M (2001) Minifenestration type I thyroplasty using an expanded polytetrafluoroethylene implant. J Voice 15:151–157
9. Zeitels SM, Mauri M, Dailey SH (2003) Medialization laryngoplasty with Gore-Tex for voice restoration secondary to glottic incompetence: indications and observations. Ann Otol Rhinol Laryngol 112:180–184
10. Nouwen J, Hans S, De Mones E, Brasnu D, Crevierbuchman L, Laccourreye O (2004) Thyroplasty type I without arytenoid adduction in patients with unilateral laryngeal nerve paralysis: the Montgomery implant versus the Gore-Tex implant. Acta Otolaryngol 124:732–738
11. Maragos NE (1998) The posterior thyroplasty window: anatomical considerations. Laryngoscope 108:1697–1703
12. Miller FR, Bryant GL, Netterville JL (1999) Arytenoid adduction in vocal fold paralysis. Oper Tech Otolaryngol Head Neck Surg 10:36–41
13. Ronsen CA (1998) Complications of phonosurgery: results of a national survey. Laryngoscope 108:1697–1703
14. Cohen JT, Bates DD, Postma GN (2004) Revision Gore-Tex medialization laryngoplasty. Head Neck Surg 131:236–240
15. Laccourreye O, Hans S (2003) Endolaryngeal extrusion of expanded polytetrafluoroethylene implant after medialization thyroplasty. Ann Otol Rhinol Laryngol 112:962–963
16. Hirano M (1981) Clinical examination of voice. Springer, Berlin Heidelberg New York

Chapter 10

Arytenoid Repositioning Surgery

Gayle E. Woodson

Introduction

Surgical correction of arytenoid position is an effective means of managing patients with posterior glottic incompetence due to laryngeal paralysis [1–3]. Many surgeons avoid arytenoid procedures because they perceive this approach to be difficult and fraught with complications [4]. Additionally, most patients with laryngeal paralysis respond to either injection augmentation or open thyroplasty; however, persisting posterior gap is a common reason for failure of medialization procedures. A review of 20 cases of failed medialization laryngoplasty found that 12 patients had persisting posterior gaps, which were subsequently corrected by arytenoid adduction [5]. Other clinical reports, as well as experimental studies in animals, indicate that arytenoid adduction is much more effective than type-I thyroplasty in closing the posterior glottis [6, 7]. Successful management of patients with flaccid laryngeal paralysis requires attention to the posterior gap; therefore, it is important that all surgeons who care for patients with laryngeal paralysis be familiar with the indications for arytenoid repositioning. With knowledge of local anatomy and understanding of key technical principles, the procedure can be mastered, with a complication rate comparable to that of medialization thyroplasty [8]. A study of type-I thyroplasty in 237 patients compared outcomes with and without arytenoid adduction. Average operative time and hospital stay were both longer with arytenoid adduction (73 vs 45 minutes and 1.8 vs 1.1 days), but there was no significant difference in incidence or severity of complications [9]. In fact, neither of the two patients who required emergency tracheotomy for airway obstruction had undergone arytenoid adduction.

Indications

The symptoms of laryngeal paralysis vary greatly, ranging from no symptoms to glottal incompetence, with aphonia and aspiration. When the arytenoid cartilage of the paralyzed vocal fold is in an internally rotated position, the vocal process is near the midline, so that during phonatory closure the membranous vocal folds are essentially parallel and separated by a gap of less than 3 mm. Many such patients are able to compensate by increasing adduction of the normal vocal fold. Those patients who do not develop effective compensation can usually achieve a good voice after either vocal fold augmentation or medialization thyroplasty; however, when the vocal process of the arytenoid is not near the midline, the membranous folds diverge posteriorly, so that there is a wide glottic gap during phonation and sometimes aspiration during swallowing. Such a gap is too wide for closure to be achieved by injection augmentation or thyroplasty. The vertical position of the paralyzed vocal fold may also affect function. For example, the vocal process may be displaced superiorly and laterally, due to external rotation of the cricoarytenoid joint. In other patients, the arytenoid "sags" forward, so that the vocal process is at or below the phonatory plane. In either case, the vocal folds do not make contact, even when they seem to be adjacent when viewed from above. Surgical correction of arytenoid position can be an effective tool for correcting the position of the vocal process in both the horizontal and vertical planes.

Vocal Fold Motion

When viewed from above, by mirror examination or endoscopy, the vocal folds appear to open and close in an axial plane, pivoting at the anterior commissure, like opposing windshield wipers; however, vocal fold motion is considerably more complex. The chief major moving parts of the larynx are the arytenoid cartilages, which articulate with the cricoid cartilage in shallow, ball, and socket-type joints and rotate around variable axes. The membranous vocal folds are rigidly fixed anteriorly to the thyroid cartilage and posteriorly to the vocal processed of the arytenoid cartilages. Opening and closing of the glottis is achieved by motion of the arytenoids, so that the vocal processes move medially and laterally. The membranous vocal folds are passively dragged to and from, varying the angle between the vocal folds. The only muscles that abduct the vocal fold are the posterior cricoarytenoid muscles (PCA), which originate on the posterior cricoid and insert on the muscular process of the arytenoid. During PCA contraction, the arytenoids rotate externally, around a nearly vertical axis, so that the vocal process moves up and out (Fig. 10.1) [10]. All other muscles that insert on the arytenoid exert a closing force, but with differing vectors of pull. For example, contraction of the lateral cricoarytenoid muscle rotates the arytenoid internally so that the vocal processes move inwardly and caudally. The "criss-crossing" fibers of the unpaired interarytenoid muscle internally rotate the arytenoid in a coronal plane, pulling the apices medially. Because each muscle has a different vector of force, the cricoarytenoid joint has a wide range of motion. The vocal process moves superolaterally with active abduction and inferomedially with active adduction; however, a paralyzed vocal fold need not lie within the trajectory of normal motion. Many authors have reported superior displacement of the paralyzed vocal fold [11, 12]. But in some patients with flaccid paralysis, the vocal process is displaced caudally as the arytenoid tips forward, due to lack of support from the PCA muscle [13]. Cadaver specimens from patients with laryngeal paralysis have demonstrated caudal displacement of the paralyzed vocal fold and shift of the conus elasticus to a horizontal plane [14, 15]. During phonation, the mobile vocal fold can compensate to some degree for vertical misalignment. But a vertical gap that cannot be easily appreciated during routine laryngeal exam can substantially impair phonation.

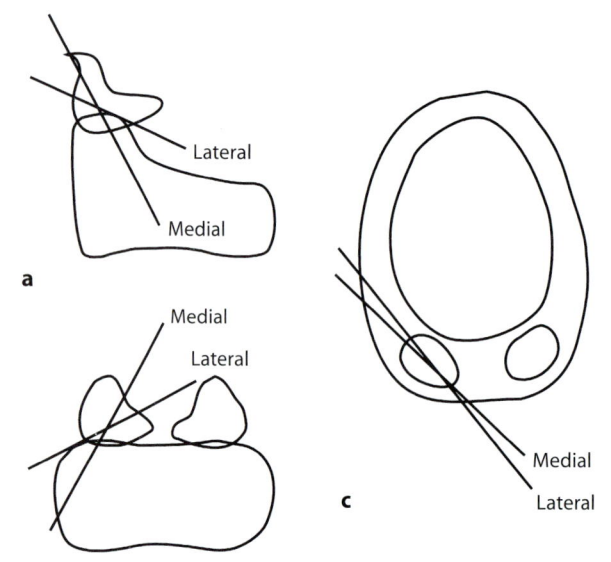

Fig. 10.1. Action of posterior cricoarytenoid muscle: medial and lateral compartments. a Sagittal view. b Axial view. c Coronal view

What Is a Posterior Gap?

The term "posterior gap" is somewhat misleading. A true posterior gap normally occurs in phonation. The vocal processes are apposed, but there is usually a small gap between the arytenoid bodies [16, 17]. Frequently, this space is not visible during transoral examination, as it is obscured by overhanging posterior glottic tissue, and may actually be filled in by soft tissue. The posterior glottis can be best observed in patients with a tracheotomy, by retrograde flexible endoscopy via the stoma. This posterior gap is usually aerodynamically insignificant, as induction of glottic vibration requires parallel apposition of the membranous folds [18].

In patients with posterior glottic incompetence, the maximal glottic opening is actually between the vocal processes. In the abducted glottis, the posterior glottic walls actually converge posterior to the vocal process. When a vocal fold is paralyzed in this abducted position, the posterior body of its arytenoid blocks the normal one from achieving vocal process contact; thus, the vibratory portion of the vocal folds are not parallel, but diverge posteriorly. Another factor that contributes to glottic incompetence in flaccid paralysis is that the paralyzed vocal process is not stable but can be driven laterally by the force of the mobile vocal fold during adduction. Finally, as mentioned above, the vocal process may be vertically displaced, above or below the plane of phonation.

History of Arytenoid Surgery

The first surgical approaches to the arytenoid were to remove or lateralize it in patients with airway obstruction due to bilateral laryngeal paralysis [18]. In 1948, Morrison described surgical displacement of the arytenoid to medialize a unilaterally paralyzed vocal fold. He called his operation the "reverse King" procedure [19]. Via a lateral approach to the larynx, the cricoarytenoid joint was opened, and the capsule was completely divided to mobilize the arytenoid. The arytenoid was then moved medially and fixed to the cricoid cartilage with a suture. In 1977 Ballenger stated that the Morrison procedure had "been supplanted by intrachordal injections" [20]. Indeed, Teflon injection, as described by Arnold in 1962, was the prevailing treatment for unilateral laryngeal paralysis for many years [21]. Over time, it became apparent that Teflon injection had a significant incidence of delayed complications, specifically, granuloma formation. Additionally, injection laryngoplasty was ineffective in patients with a large glottal gap and did not close the posterior glottis. In 1975 Isshiki et al. reported the used of thyroplasty type-I as an alternative to injection [22]. Their procedure was similar in concept to the thyroid cartilage flap that had been described by Payr in 1915 [23]. Within a few years, type-I thyroplasty had become widely accepted as the procedure of choice for unilateral laryngeal paralysis; however, it was noted that type-I thyroplasty, like injection laryngoplasty, was not effective in closing the posterior glottis.

In 1978 Isshiki reported arytenoid adduction as a means of treating patients with large glottal gaps [1]. They noted that the normal motion of the arytenoid was rotational, rather than translational, and that rotating the arytenoid through its natural range of motion was much more effective in closing the glottis than attempting to move the entire arytenoid medially along the cricoid (Fig. 10.2). This procedure

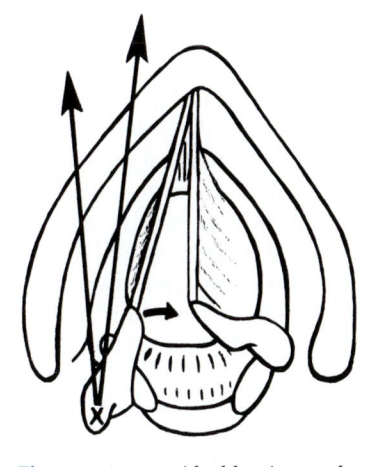

Fig. 10.2. Arytenoid adduction, as described by Isshiki et al. [1]. *Large arrows* indicate vectors of suture pull; *small arrow* indicates resultant motion of vocal process

dure gained acceptance more slowly than type-I thyroplasty, due to concerns about technical difficulty and complications. In addition, the procedure, as originally described, included dividing the cricothyroid joint and opening the cricoarytenoid joint. In a series of 12 arytenoid adduction procedures, Slavit and Maragos found over-rotation of the arytenoid and shortening of the vocal fold in 1 patient, presumably due to destabilization of the arytenoid by opening the joints [24]. Netterville et al. also noted unfavorable voice results that seemed to result from over-rotation or anterior displacement of the larynx [25]. Woodson subsequently reported modification of the technique to preserve the cricothyroid and cricoarytenoid joints, which prevented anterior arytenoid dislocation and resulted in more consistent vocal process position, and to dissect lateral to the strap muscles, to improve exposure and reduce risk to the carotid [2]. In addition to improved vocal quality, mean phonation time was substantially increased in these patients. Subsequently, larger series have demonstrated the efficacy of arytenoid adduction [8, 26].

Zeitels et al. [3] has developed a different approach to arytenoid surgery, the "adduction arytenoidopexy," which is similar in concept to the "reverse King procedure" developed by Morrison [19]. In adduction arytenopexy, the lateral wall of the cricoarytenoid joint is opened widely. A single suture is then placed through posterior cricoid and through the body or the muscular process of the arytenoid. The suture is positioned so that it draws arytenoid posteriorly, superiorly, and medially. The goal is to mimic combined motion of lateral cricoarytenoid, thyroarytenoid, and interarytenoid muscles. Published results in a series of 12 patients supports the efficacy of the procedure [3]. Zeitels et al. developed his approach to overcome perceived shortcomings of arytenoid adduction. Firstly, they states that the normal vocal fold contour is straight during adduction, and arytenoid adduction "hyperrotates" the arytenoid, so that the vocal process is too medial, resulting in a persisting chink persists behind the vocal processes. Adduction arytenopexy was designed to translate the entire arytenoid medially, rather than rotate it. The goal of his procedure is to medialize and lengthen the paralyzed vocal fold, and to achieve a straight vocal fold edge; however, there is considerable evidence that during normal phonation the vocal fold is not straight and there is usually a problem behind the vocal processes [16, 17].

Adduction arytenopexy is technically more difficult and less standardized than arytenoid adduction. The suture should pass through either the body or vocal process of the arytenoid. There are no guidelines for determining exact suture placement, as the description of the procedure states, "The completion of the stabilizing suture can be done in several ways and is individualized to each patient and to surgeon preference." Furthermore, the vector of pull is essentially localized in the posterior glottis, in the coronal plane with narrowly spaced points of fixation, and lateral stability is sacrificed by the opening of the joint. The sutures exert a medial force on the body of the arytenoid but do not prevent slight rotation with lateral displacement of the vocal process during phonatory closure. At present, arytenoid adduction is more widely used than adduction arytenopexy.

Mechanics of Arytenoid Surgery

Medialization procedures, which focus on displacing the anterior vocal fold, do have some influence on the position of the vocal process, since the two structures are connected; however, the torque achieved by medial displacement of the muscular portion of the vocal fold is inadequate to effect significant internal rotation of the arytenoid cartilage. The vector of force in medialization is linear, toward the midline, while arytenoid motion is actually rotational. The rationale for arytenoid repositioning surgery is to restore the phonatory position of the paralyzed vocal process and to stabilize the arytenoid cartilage in internal rotation, preventing passive displacement during glottal closure. The objective is effective glottal closure, with a minimum of compensatory hyperfunction. Repositioning of the arytenoid does not restore bulk to the atrophic muscles of the paralyzed vocal fold, and so concomitant medialization procedure may be required.

The mechanics of the arytenoid adduction procedure have been studied in cadaver larynges. Three-dimensional coordinates of laryngeal cartilages were determined by CT at rest and after arytenoid adduction, and then rotation and translation was computed in three planes, using rigid body mechanics [27]. The arytenoid rotates about a nearly vertical axis with the vocal process moving downward and medially. The paralyzed vocal fold generally appears shorter than the mobile side [28]. In patients, as viewed from above, arytenoid adduction appears to lengthen the paralyzed vocal fold; however, research in cadaver larynges indicates that the arytenoid adduction procedure does not actually lengthen the vocal fold, but moves the vocal process caudally [29]. It is this vertical component of motion that is endoscopically perceived as a length change. An abducted vocal fold appears shorter when viewed from above, because the vocal process has moved rostrally; the vocal fold slopes upward, out of the plane of the image. In arytenoid adduction the vocal process is displaced caudally, toward the level of the anterior commissure, so that the vocal fold is parallel to the image plane, and apparently longer. With bilateral arytenoid adduction in cadaver larynges, vocal processes are pulled together, and resistance to air flow is increased [27].

Other studies in cadaver larynges explored the influence of varying the site of attachment of the anterior sutures, and have also assessed induced phonation. Results indicate that fine adjustment of the arytenoid in three planes can be achieved by varying the anterior site of attachment of the adduction suture. Such adjustments are more evident in phonatory function than in visually detectable variation in position [30, 31].

Zeitels et al. [3] has compared the results of arytenoid adduction and adduction arytenopexy in cadaver larynges, by performing the two procedures on opposing sides of several specimens. The vertical positions of the two vocal folds were compared by placing a ruler between the vocal processes. The length of each vocal fold was measured with calipers and the angle of the arytenoid measured from a cranial perspective. Finally, the displacement of the arytenoid along the cricoid was measured with calipers. The findings indicated no vocal fold length change with arytenoid adduction, consistent with prior studies, but a 2-mm increase after adduction arytenopexy. Vertical position measurement indicated that the vocal process was 2 mm higher on the side of the adduction arytenopexy [3]. The downward displacement of the vocal process is appropriate when the paralyzed vocal fold lies above the plane of glottic closure. But in some patients with flaccid laryngeal paralysis, the arytenoid "sags" anteriorly. In such cases the arytenoid adduction cannot correct, and may exacerbate, the vertical gap between the vocal processes during closure. A second suture can be attached to the vocal process and secured posteriorly, to provide posterior suspension, essentially replacing the force of normal resting tone in the PCA muscle [32].

Technique of Arytenoid Adduction

Arytenoid adduction is usually performed under local anesthesia. This allows the vocal results to be assessed intraoperatively, and avoids the problem of an endotracheal tube that blocks adduction of the glottis; however, it can be performed under general anesthesia by placing sufficient tension on the adducting suture to achieve maximal anterior motion of the muscular process. This generally results in appropriate adduction of the vocal fold when the patient is awake and extubated. A general anesthetic is most useful in anxious or immature patients or in those where surgical dissection is hindered by scarring, obesity, or presence of a tracheotomy.

A horizontal incision is made in the neck over the lower thyroid ala, similar to the incision used for thyroplasty, but extending somewhat further posteriorly. In most cases a thyroplasty window should be created at this point. Such a window is a very good route for passing the adduction suture. It also prepares the field for a thyroplasty, either planned, or to correct a persistent anterior gap after arytenoid adduction.

The most effective exposure of the posterior thyroid lamina is achieved by dissecting lateral to the cervical strap muscles. This allows the entire laryngotracheal complex to be rotated as a unit, providing broad access to the posterior larynx. This approach also decreases the risk to the carotid sheath, since the larynx is displaced away from that structure (Fig. 10.3). The omohyoid muscle can be grasped to aid in rotating the larynx during dissection, but stable rotation during arytenoid surgery is provided by sturdy hook on the superior cornu or the hyoid bone. If necessary, the thyrohyoid ligament can be divided to allow more rotation and greater exposure.

To access the cricoarytenoid joint, it is necessary to go through the inferior pharyngeal constrictor muscle and then displace the mucosa of the pyriform sinus. One can accomplish this by sharply dividing the inferior constrictor muscle along the posterior edge of the thyroid lamina. The nerve to the cricothyroid can usually be located and preserved, although the functional consequences of sacrificing this nerve would be minimal. Another means of managing the constrictors is to incise the perichondrium anterior to their attachment, and reflecting that flap posteriorly [33]. The pyriform sinus is then dissected off the PCA muscle and displaced superiorly and anteriorly, until the muscular process of the PCA is located. It can usually be easily identified by following the fibers of the PCA muscle until they converge at the muscular process (Fig. 10.4). If exposure is unsatisfactory, it can be improved by removing a portion of the posterior edge of the thyroid cartilage. An alternate surgical approach is the posterior thyroplasty window, as described by Maragos [34].

Patients with paralysis due to a vagus nerve injury frequently have dysphagia with aspiration, due to unilateral pharyngeal constrictor paralysis in the face of continued activity in the bilaterally innervated cricopharyngeus muscle. In such cases, a cricopharyngeal myotomy can dramatically improve swallowing function, and is easily added to this procedure, by an inferior extension of the incision of the through the inferior constrictor muscle, onto the cricoid cartilage [2].

As originally described, the next steps in the procedure would be to disarticulate the cricothyroid joint and then open the cricoarytenoid joint; however, most authors now recommend preserving natural biomechanics by leaving these structures intact. The muscular process is exposed by further refection of the pyriform sinus. It is important not to violate that mucosa by tearing during dissection or puncturing it with a suture needle, as a leak could contaminate the field and possibly result in a fistula; thus, identification and preservation of the margins of the pyriform sinus can be the most challenging part of the procedure. An awake

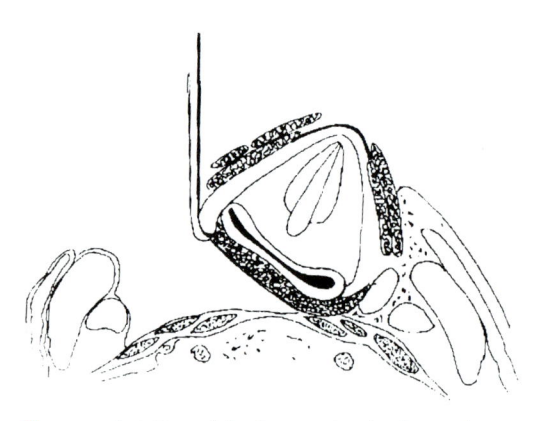

Fig. 10.3. Rotation of the laryngotracheal complex to expose the posterior larynx

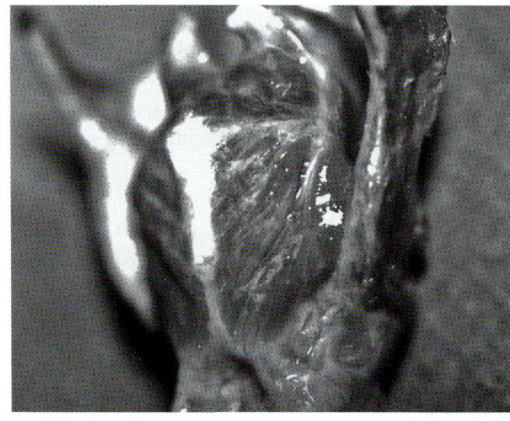

Fig. 10.4. Location of muscular process at convergence of posterior cricoarytenoid muscle fibers

and cooperative patient can be instructed to produce positive intraoral pressure (Say "puppy"), which distends and clearly delineates the pyriform.

The adducting suture should be placed horizontally through the muscular process, assuring that a good "bite" of cartilage is obtained. The suture should be tied securely, leaving two long ends.

A key step in the procedure is to clear a tunnel as a path for the suture to follow to the anterior larynx. If the suture passes through any connective tissue or muscle en route, that tissue could act as a pulley that alters the vector of force and prevents adequate adduction. If the suture is through muscle or tendon, the resulting torque will be inadequate. It is important that this dissection be through the paraglottic space, medial to perichondrium and external to muscle, to decrease the chance of hemorrhage.

Once the tunnel is created, a small hemostat can be used to pass one end of the arytenoid suture through the tunnel and out through the thyroplasty window. Ultimately, both suture segments will be passed forward and secured to the lower thyroid cartilage. But initially only one segment is passed forward, so that alternating tension on the two sutures can be used to test the efficacy of rotation. The anterior tension should be sufficient to move and maintain the vocal process as far anteriorly as possible. This generally requires very little force. Increasing tension after the arytenoid has reached maximal internal rotation is counterproductive, and can distort the vocal fold, or even result in avulsion of the suture. The larynx should be observed from above by endoscopy to confirm adequate vocal process adduction. If satisfactory position is not achieved, the suture insertion should be re-evaluated and may need to be revised. If the adduction is satisfactory, then the other end of the suture is passed forward through the tunnel. Adequate position is reassured, and then secured with a surgeon's knot, and several throws. This author has found that the most satisfactory means of securing the suture anteriorly is to bring one end through the thyroplasty window and the other through the cricothyroid space, below the posterior inferior corner of the window. This permits subsequent medialization of the anterior vocal fold with an implant (Fig. 10.5); however, research by Inagi and colleagues in cadaver larynges suggests that optimal medialization is achieved by anchoring the suture as far inferiorly and anteriorly as possible in the thyroid cartilage [31].

A posterior suspension suture should be considered if the arytenoid is tipped anteriorly, with caudal displacement of the vocal process [32]. The location of this suture on the arytenoid should be superior to that of the primary suture. Careful examination and palpation of the arytenoid will reveal a ridge that runs from the muscular process to the apex of the arytenoid. The lateral cricoarytenoid muscle attaches to the anterior surface of this ridge, while the interarytenoid muscle attaches posteriorly. The suspension suture should be attached to this ridge, about 1 cm away from the primary suture. Inferior traction should be applied to rock the arytenoid posteriorly, while observing the larynx endoscopically to assure improved laryngeal posture, without lateral displacement of the vocal process. This suture is then secured inferiorly by passing one end around or through the inferior cornu of the thyroid cartilage.

A drain is prudent, as well as overnight observation, since bleeding into the paraglottic space can cause airway obstruction. This author has encountered one patient in 15 years

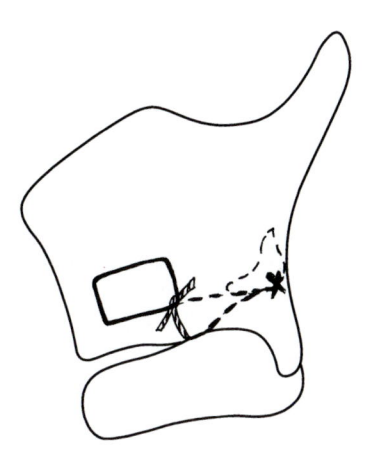

Fig. 10.5. Location of arytenoid adduction suture in posterior inferior corner of medialization thyroplasty window, to permit concomitant medialization implant

who required emergency tracheotomy because of an obstructing hematoma. Another potential source obstruction is herniation of pyriform mucosa, as reported by Weinman and Maragos [35]. They noted this complication after arytenoid adduction via a posterior thyroplasty window, and have found that tacking down the pyriform mucosa is effective in preventing airway obstruction.

Conclusion

Surgical adjustment of the arytenoid cartilage is a valuable tool in the surgical armamentarium for the treatment of laryngeal paralysis. While this approach is technically more difficult and requires more operative time than a type-I thyroplasty, it is much more effective in patients with a large glottic gap and posterior glottic incompetence.

References

1. Isshiki N, Tanabe M, Masaki S (1978) Arytenoid adduction for unilateral vocal cord paralysis. Arch Otolaryngol Head Neck Surg 14:555–558
2. Woodson GE (1997) Cricopharyngeal myotomy and arytenoid adduction in the management of combined laryngeal and pharyngeal aralysis. Otolaryngol Head Neck Surg 117:339–343
3. Zeitels SM, Hochman I, Hillman RE (1998) Adduction arytenoidopexy: a new procedure for paralytic dysphonia with implications for implant medialization. Ann Otol Rhinol Laryngol (Suppl) 107:173
4. Koufman JA, Isaacson G (1991) Laryngoplastic phonosurgery. Otolaryngol Clin North Am:1151–1173
5. Woo P, Pearl A, Hsiung M, So P (2001) Failed medialization laryngoplasty: management by revision surgery. Otolaryngol Head Neck Surg 124:615–621
6. Noordzij JP, Perrault DF, Woo P (1998) Biomechanics of combined arytenoid adduction and medialization laryngoplasty in an ex vivo canine model. Otolaryngol Head Neck Surg 119:634–642
7. Green DC, Berke GS, Ward PH (1991) Vocal fold medialization by surgical augmentation versus arytenoid adduction in the in vivo canine model. Ann Otol Rhinol Laryngol 100:280–287
8. Kraus DH, Orlikoff RF, Rizk SS et al. (1999) Arytenoid adduction as an adjunct to type I thyroplasty for unilateral vocal cord paralysis. Head Neck 21:52–59
9. Abraham MT, Gonen M, Kraus DH (2001) Complications of type I thyroplasty and arytenoid adduction. Laryngoscope 111:1322–1329
   Arnold GE (1962) Vocal rehabilitation of paralytic dysphonia IX: technique of intrachordal injection. Arch Otolaryngol 76:358
10. Bryant NJ, Woodson GE, Kaufman K, Rosen C, Hengesteg A, Chen N, Yeung D (1996) Human posterior cricoarytenoid muscle compartments. Anatomy and mechanics. Arch Otolaryngol Head Neck Surg 122:1331–1336
11. Leden H von, Moore P (1961) The mechanics of the cricoarytenoid joint. Arch Otolaryngol 73:541–550
12. Isshiki N, Ishikawa T (1986) Diagnostic value of tomography in unilateral vocal cord paralysis. Laryngoscope 86:1573–1578
13. Blitzer A, Jahn AF, Keidar A (1996) Semon's law revisited: an electromyographic analysis of laryngeal synkinesis. Ann Otol Rhinol Laryngol 105:764
14. Bridger GP (1977) Unilateral laryngeal palsy: a histopathological study. J Laryngol Otol 91:303–307
15. Kirchner JA (1966) Atrophy of laryngeal muscles in vagal paralysis. Laryngoscope 76:1753–1765
16. Hirano M, Yoshida T, Kurita S, Kioykawa K, Sata K, Tateishi O (1987) Anatomy and behavior of the vocal process. In: Baer T, Sasaki C, Harris K (eds) Laryngeal function in phonation and respiration. College-Hill, Boston, pp 3–13
17. Murry T, Xu JJ, Woodson G (1998) Glottal configuration associated with fundamental frequency and vocal register. J Voice 12:44–50
18. King BT (1939) A new and function-restoring operation for bilateral abductor cord paralysis: preliminary report. J Am Med Assoc 112:814–823
19. Morrison LF (1948) The "reverse King operation." A surgical procedure for restoration of phonation in cases of aphonia due to unilateral vocal cord paralysis. Ann Otol Rhinol Laryngol 57:943–946
20. Ballenger JJ (1977) Neurologic disease of the larynx. In: Ballenger JJ (ed) Disease of the nose, throat, and ear. Lea and Febiger, Philadelphia, p 467
21. Arnold GE (1962) Vocal rehabilitation of paralytic dysphonia, vol VII. Technique of intrachordal injection. Arch Otolaryngol 76:358
22 Isshiki N, Okamura H, Ishikawa T (1975) Thyroplasty type I (lateral compression) for dysphonia due to vocal cord paralysis or atrophy. Acta Otolaryngol 80:465–473
23. Payr E (1915) Plastik am Schildknorpel zur Behebung der Folgen einseitiger Stimmbanclahmung. Dtsch Med Wochenschr 43:1265–1270
24. Slavit D, Maragos N (1992) Physiologic assessment of arytenoid adduction. Ann Otol Rhinol Laryngol 101:321–327

25. Netterville JL, Stone RE, Lukens ES et al. (1993) Silastic medialization and arytenoid adduction. The Vanderbilt experience. A review of 116 phonosurgical procedures. Ann Otol Rhinol Laryngol 102:413–424
26. Slavit DH, Maragos NE (1994) Arytenoid adduction and type I thyroplasty in the treatment of aphonia. J Voice 8:84–91
27. Neuman TR, Hengesteg A, Lepage RP, Kaufman KR, Woodson GE (1994) Three-dimensional motion of the arytenoid adduction procedure in cadaver larynges. Ann Otol Rhinol Laryngol 103:265–270
28. Brewer DW, Woo P, Casper JK et al. (1991) Unilateral recurrent laryngeal nerve paralysis: a re-examination. J Voice 5:178–185
29. Woodson GE, Rosen CA, Yeung D (1997) Changes in length and spatial orientation of the vocal fold with arytenoid adduction in cadaver larynges. Ann Otol Rhinol Laryngol 106:552–555
30. Inagi K, Connor NP, Suzuki T, Bless DM, Kamijo T (2003) Visual observations of glottal configuration and vocal outcomes in arytenoid adduction. Am J Otolaryngol 24:290–296
31. Inagi K, Connor NP, Suzuki T, Ford CN, Bless DM, Nakajima M (2002) Glottal configuration, acoustic, and aerodynamic changes induced by variation in suture direction in arytenoid adduction procedures. Ann Otol Rhinol Laryngol 111:861–870
32. Woodson GE, Picerno R, Yeung D, Hengesteg A (2000) Arytenoid adduction: controlling vertical position. Ann Otol Rhinol Laryngol 109:360–364
33. Netterville JL, Billante CR (2003) The immobile vocal cord. In: Ossoff RH, Shapshay SM, Woodson GE Netterville J (eds) The larynx. Lippincott, Williams and Wilkens, Philadelphia, pp 269–305
34. Maragos NE (1999) The posterior thyroplasty window: anatomical considerations. Laryngoscope 109:1228–1231
35. Weinman EC, Maragos NE (2000) Airway compromise in thyroplasty surgery. Laryngoscope 110:1082–1085

Part III

Special Topics

Chapter 11
Laryngeal Reinnervation *189*
Randal C. Paniello

Chapter 12
**Electrical Stimulation
for Vocal Fold Paralysis** *203*
Michael Broniatowski

Chapter 13
Bilateral Medialization Laryngoplasty *219*
Gregory N. Postma, Peter C. Belafsky

Chapter 14
Vocal Fold Paralysis in Children *225*
Marshall E. Smith

Chapter 15
Bilateral Vocal Fold Immobility *237*
George Goding

# Chapter 11

Laryngeal Reinnervation

Randal C. Paniello

Introduction

Laryngologists have dreamed of restoring functional innervation to the paralyzed larynx ever since they have been able to make the diagnosis of paralysis. The ideal method of laryngeal reinnervation would result in vocal folds that voluntarily adduct during phonation, that abduct during inspiration, and that reflexively adduct during deglutition (i.e., that have a normal glottic closure reflex). No current reinnervation technique satisfies this ideal.

Laryngeal reinnervation has been used most often in cases of unilateral paralysis involving the recurrent laryngeal nerve (RLN), and this is the primary focus of this chapter. Other types of laryngeal reinnervation are discussed in the latter sections.

Rationale for Reinnervation in UVFP

Patients with unilateral vocal fold paralysis (UVFP) often ask, "If the nerve is damaged, can't it be fixed?" With reinnervation techniques, the injured RLN is usually not repaired but replaced with an alternative nerve. The goal of such reinnervation is to provide neural input to the vocal fold adductor muscles [primarily the thyroarytenoid (TA) and lateral cricoarytenoid (LCA) muscles], resulting in enough muscle tone to prevent atrophy and bowing of the paralyzed fold. Electromyographic (EMG) studies show that most patients with UVFP have some degree of active innervation, even if there is no videostroboscopic evidence of movement of the involved arytenoid. This may represent residual innervation from a partial injury, or spontaneous reinnervation; these two possibilities cannot be distinguished. During a reinnervation procedure, any existing innervation is sacrificed when the RLN is divided (in order to connect it to the new nerve); therefore, reinnervation procedures are performed in the hope and expectation that the ultimate number of live axonal connections following the procedure will exceed the number that existed prior to the procedure. The number of intact neuromuscular units required for arytenoid movement is unknown, as EMG is not generally quantitative, but it is probably something greater than 50%. Careful consideration should be given as to whether a reinnervation procedure is likely to result in more functional motor units than the patient has already. On the other hand, it has also been hypothesized that patients with UVFP who have some neural activity may be better candidates for reinnervation than those with electrical silence, as the existing partial innervation may serve a "babysitter" function and prevent or reduce atrophy of the laryngeal muscles.

The RLN has virtually no topographic orientation along its length until it reaches the cricoarytenoid joint, at which point it becomes organized into an adductor division and an abductor division [1, 2]. Since most RLN injuries occur proximal to this point, any spontaneous reinnervation that occurs will follow a random pattern, i.e., the regenerating adductor fibers may grow into either adductor or abductor muscles. The abductor fibers similarly may randomly reinnervate either type of muscle. Since there are normally about three times as many adductor fibers as abductor fibers, a regenerating adductor fiber has approximately a 75% chance of connecting to an adductor muscle, while an abductor fiber has only a 25% chance of reaching the posterior cricoarytenoid (PCA) muscle. But either type of reinnervation is most likely a random process, and would be expected to follow a normal distribution (a "bell curve").

The condition in which adductor fibers grow into abductor axonal tubules to reinnervate the PCA muscle, or in which abductor fibers reinnervate an adductor muscle, is called laryngeal synkinesis. Rarely, severe synkinesis involving abductor fibers innervating the adductor muscles may cause the vocal fold to adduct during inspiration, causing variable degrees of stridor, "laryngeal asthma," or frank airway obstruction. More commonly, some adductor fibers innervate the PCA. During phonation, contraction of the PCA can antagonize the adductors, resulting in a more lateral vocal fold position, and causing dysphonia. Laryngeal synkinesis can usually be diagnosed by electromyography [3]. Dividing the RLN for reinnervation effectively eliminates synkinesis. As a result, some patients actually report immediate voice improvement from a reinnervation procedure. Such improvement can also be achieved by selective chemodenervation with botulinum toxin [3].

Any new nerve that is anastomosed to the common trunk of the RLN will send fibers into both the adductor and abductor muscles. This is a desirable result. Maintenance of some tone in the PCA serves to support the arytenoid vertically on the cricoarytenoid joint. Complete denervation of the PCA would lead to unopposed anteromedial pull on the arytenoid by the TA muscle, causing the vocal process to shift inferiorly with resultant dysphonia. Because of the 3:1 ratio of adductor to abductor fibers, the chronic tone created in the reinnervated muscles favors adduction, and the vocal fold may gradually drift into a more medial position (depending on the total number of restored motor units). This explains the frequent reports from reinnervation patients that voice quality continues to improve for several months following the initial onset of benefit; thus, the absolute number of restored axonal connections is probably just as important to the final voice product as the degree of synkinesis.

Crumley [4, 5] lists the following potential advantages of reinnervation for UVFP (over "static" medialization techniques):

1. It is possible to restore normal or near-normal voice without synthetic materials placed inside the laryngeal framework.
2. It does not alter the stiffness of the vocal folds.
3. It restores bulk to the thyroarytenoid muscle.
4. It improves vocal fold positioning due to muscular contraction of the lateral cricoarytenoid, interarytenoid, and posterior cricoarytenoid muscles.
5. It is reversible (by nerve section).
6. It does not preclude static methods if it should fail.
7. It eliminates dysphonia due to synkinesis if present (by sectioning the RLN).

Potential disadvantages include:
1. The need for an intact donor nerve.
2. The distal stump of the RLN must be identifiable.
3. Cost (as compared with medialization).
4. A several-month delay before reinnervation becomes effective.

Titze has also stated that adductor reinnervation may be superior to medialization because it restores tone to the thyroarytenoid muscle. He notes that while medialization procedures may restore geometric symmetry to the phonating glottis, they do not restore viscoelastic symmetry, which reinnervation may achieve [6, 7].

Choice of Donor Nerve

The ideal donor nerve would have the following properties: (a) minimal donor site morbidity; (b) a large number of axons; and (c) adequate length to perform neurorrhaphy without the need for a nerve graft. There is no nerve that has all of these properties, but the ansa cervicalis, the hypoglossal nerve, and the RLN itself come close. Some axons are lost across any neurorrhaphy due to scarring, perhaps as many as 50%, so nerve grafts, with at least two neurorrhaphy sites, should be avoided. Adequate length must be provided so that the normal vertical excursion of the larynx during deglutition will not pull the anastomosis apart as soon as the patient wakes up; usually 1 cm of extra length meets this requirement. Another possible ideal attribute to consider is appropriate natural temporal activity. However, the merits of this feature are not necessarily as obvious as they seem. While it makes sense to consider a donor nerve that mimics the neural activation pattern of the original RLN, it is also conceivable that too much neural input during phonation could cause hyperadduction, uncoordinated vocal fold motion, inconsistent adduction, or some other anomaly that could be deleterious to the voice product. This potential problem has not yet been reported in clinical series.

The ansa cervicalis has been used most frequently for RLN reinnervation [8]. It has little or no donor site morbidity and is usually long enough to perform primary anastomosis. The strap muscles that it innervates are naturally active during vertical laryngeal posturing, especially with swallowing, and they also serve as accessory respiratory muscles; thus, the ansa's normal activity is not exactly synchronous with phonatory adduction. The ansa cervicalis is a fairly small nerve, providing only a modest number of axons. When possible, it is usually preferable to use the ansa branches that innervate more than one strap muscle (commonly, sternohyoid plus omohyoid) [9]. Crumley [4, 5] refers to the ansa cervicalis as a "quiet little nerve" that provides enough axons to provide suitable muscle tone to the adductor muscles, without the risk of inappropriate temporal interference patterns.

The hypoglossal nerve was recently studied by Paniello et al. as an alternative to the ansa cervicalis [10, 11]. Significant experience using the hypoglossal nerve for facial reanimation had shown that the donor site morbidity was acceptable, although it was clearly greater than that of the ansa cervicalis. The hypoglossal nerve has substantially more axons than the ansa, and in fact is has many more axons than the RLN as well. In a series of neck dissections, it was found that the maximum reach of the hypoglossal nerve required that there be about 3.5–4.0 cm of intact RLN stump in order to perform a primary anastomosis [12]. The other unique feature of the hypoglossal nerve was that its natural activity correlates well with that of the RLN: it is most active during deglutition, when tight glottal closure is desired, and also very active during phonation, especially during connected speech. These features together created the potential for active arytenoid adduction, which was an enticing prospect, although it was not known initially whether this would turn out to be problematic (as discussed above).

The original RLN is occasionally available for reanastomosis. If a clean transection injury is recognized during a thyroidectomy, for example, a primary reanastomosis can be performed. There is a significant risk of synkinesis when this is done, but there is also a good chance of a reasonable result. In terms of donor nerve criteria, the proximal RLN stump, if available, would have no donor site morbidity, a fair number of axons (more than the ansa but less than the hypoglossal), and presumably adequate length if primary anastomosis is considered. But there is little extra length of the RLN available. If an injured segment is identified, only a few millimeters can be resected and still allow primary anastomosis.

Choice of Anesthesia / Contingency Plans

Most patients undergo reinnervation surgery under general anesthesia. It is desirable for the patient to lie still during the microneural anastomosis. It is also possible to perform reinnervation procedures with the patient under local anesthesia with deep sedation (monitored anesthesia care, or MAC). The latter approach should be avoided in patients with back problems or other issues that might make it difficult for them to lie comfortably without moving for about 2 h.

In patients who have undergone previous neck surgery, the availability of the ansa cervicalis is often unknown prior to neck exploration. Similarly, in patients with previous surgery near the RLN, such as thyroid surgery, the availability of an adequate length of RLN stump is unknown. A contingency plan for such cases is advisable. If the ipsilateral ansa cervicalis is found to have been previously divided, and the RLN stump is long enough, the opposite ansa cervicalis may be used. This nerve could cross the neck anterior to the larynx, at about the level of the cricothyroid membrane, or it could be passed posterior to the larynx through a tunnel dissected in the party wall. If the latter option is selected, care must be taken to avoid injuring the contralateral RLN during the dissection.

Another contingency plan is to start the neck exploration with the patient under MAC anesthesia, so that if the RLN or the donor nerve is unavailable, the patient could instead undergo a thyroplasty procedure. Once the adequacy of both nerves has been established, induction to general anesthesia and intubation can be performed. However, at this point most of the procedure has been completed, so the author usually just finishes the case with the patient under MAC. Thyroplasty may also be performed under general anesthesia, although the potential for voice feedback from the patient is lost. Another possibility would be to abort the case if reinnervation cannot be performed. The wound is closed and alternative plans are performed on another date.

A third back-up plan would be to switch to the hypoglossal nerve as the donor nerve. If this option is considered, it must be discussed with the patient pre-operatively, especially with respect to the donor site morbidity (which can be pre-tested, as discussed below). This possibility may also affect the choice of neck incision.

Overall, the author has found a need to utilize some form of contingency plan in about 10% of cases.

Technique of Ansa Cervicalis to RLN Anastomosis

The neck is extended using a shoulder roll, then prepped and draped in a sterile manner. A horizontal incision is made in a skin crease at about the level of the lower edge of the cricoid cartilage. Immediately after dividing the platysma muscle, care must be taken to avoid injury to the ansa cervicalis; sometimes it is very superficial and can be injured at this early stage of the procedure. The fascia along the anterior edge of the sternocleidomastoid muscle is carefully incised, watching for the ansa cervicalis that will be crossing horizontally beneath it. The ansa can usually be found traversing the jugular vein; it can also be located by careful examination of the posterior aspect of the omohyoid or sternohyoid muscles. Once identified, the nerve is dissected proximally to the lateral edge of the jugular vein, and distally into the omohyoid, sternohyoid, and sternothyroid muscles. A loose suture or vessel loop is placed around the proximal nerve for easy subsequent identification.

The recurrent laryngeal nerve is identified next. A single hook is placed around the posterior aspect of the thyroid cartilage, just superior to the cricothyroid joint. Anterior traction on this hook causes the larynx to rotate, allowing dissection posterior to the cricothyroid joint, where the RLN is found entering the larynx. The nerve is then dissected several centimeters inferiorly. Alternatively, the RLN may be identified inferior to the thyroid gland and dissected superiorly along the tracheoesophageal groove. With either approach, the RLN should be dissected to be as long as possible.

Before either nerve is divided, it is useful to confirm that there is enough length to allow a tension-free anastomosis. If the procedure cannot be performed for technical reasons, it would be better to leave both nerves intact. The RLN may contain some intact fibers that provide tone to the intralaryngeal muscles, and the intact ansa cervicalis may provide some small advantage for swallowing. A ruler may be used to measure the length of both nerves, or a vessel loop may be laid on top of each nerve to determine whether their ends, when cut, will reach one another.

It is desirable to incorporate as many axons as possible from the ansa cervicalis. It is possible to create an anastomosis between the RLN and both the omohyoid and sternohyoid branches of the ansa cervicalis (a two-to-one anastomosis). This approach may be useful if the RLN diameter is significantly larger than the ansa branches. If the RLN is long enough, it can be anastomosed to the ansa cervicalis proximal to the branching point, so that the proximal axons of two or more branches will be included in a single anastomosis.

When it has been determined that there is adequate length for successful anastomosis, both nerves are divided. The patient under sedation may be converted to a general anesthetic if desired, although most of the procedure is completed at this point.

In order to approximate the nerve ends, a tunnel is created through the sternohyoid and sternothyroid muscles and the nerve is passed through this tunnel. Alternatively, the strap muscles may be divided without added morbidity (since they were just denervated). End-to-end neurorrhaphy is performed using standard microneural technique. Typically, about four or five sutures of 8–0 nylon are placed circumferentially. An operating microscope or loupe magnification is used.

If there is an adequately sized (about 3–4 mm) vein readily available, it may be helpful to harvest a 1- to 2-cm segment of this vein early in the case and keep it in saline in a specimen cup. Prior to performing the anastomosis, the RLN is passed through the lumen of the vein, which is slid back a few millimeters from the end. After the anastomosis is completed, the vein is slid over the anastomosis, forming a cuff around it. This cuff serves to keep neurotrophic factors secreted by the freshly cut nerve endings from diffusing away from the site, and also may help to direct regenerating axons into the RLN.

Placement of a drain is optional. Final hemostasis is achieved and the wound is closed.

Technique of Hypoglossal Nerve to RLN Anastomosis

This procedure is similar to the ansa cervicalis to RLN anastomosis, except that more length of the RLN is required for it to reach the hypoglossal nerve. It is imperative that confirmation of adequate length of both nerves is obtained prior to sacrificing the hypoglossal nerve. If the hypoglossal nerve and RLN cannot be coapted with a single anastomosis (i.e., if a nerve graft is needed to get adequate length), there is probably no advantage of this approach over the ansa-RLN and the tongue innervation should not be sacrificed [11].

The incision may be placed in a horizontal skin crease, but it needs to be a little higher and more lateral than the ansa-RLN incision in order to allow complete dissection of the hypoglossal nerve in the submandibular triangle. Alternatively, two smaller horizontal incisions may be made, one high in the neck as if approaching the submandibular gland, and one lower in the neck as for thyroidectomy. A third choice is to use an oblique incision along the anterior border of the sternocleidomastoid muscle, as is sometimes used for carotid endarterectomy. If the patient has any pre-existing neck scars, such as from previous neck surgery, these are incorporated in the planned approach.

After subplatysmal flaps are elevated, the RLN is identified and dissected throughout its length, from the cricothyroid joint superiorly to the thoracic inlet inferiorly. It is necessary to dissect the RLN inferiorly as far as possible in order to maximize the available length. Usually this means dissecting it behind the clavicle or manubrium. If it is found that the RLN is significantly damaged along this course, a hypoglossal reinnervation should probably not be attempted. When the dissection has been maximized, the RLN is divided as low as possible.

The hypoglossal nerve is identified high in the neck as it crosses the carotid artery, and is then dissected distally until it penetrates the mylohyoid muscle. The nerve can be traced further be spreading some mylohyoid fibers to gain a few millimeters of additional length. At this point, a vessel loop is laid atop the hypoglossal nerve, from the most distally dissected point (where it will be divided) to the anterior edge of the carotid artery; the latter is taken as the pivot point. Holding the vessel loop stationary at the pivot point, the distal end is rotated toward the larynx, and the RLN is rotated superiorly to meet it. At this point the critical assessment of adequacy of nerve lengths is made. The two nerves should overlap by at least 10 mm, so that later there is no tension on the anastomosis when the larynx moves vertically during swallowing. If adequate length is confirmed, the hypoglossal nerve is divided as distally as possible.

The hypoglossal nerve may appear at first to be significantly larger than the RLN, but under the microscope it is seen that much of its larger diameter is made up of non-neural supporting tissue. Some of this extra adventitia should be trimmed at the distal end. A vein graft cuff is desirable to help direct the hypoglossal axons into the RLN, as described above. Standard microneural anastomosis is performed with 8-o nylon sutures. Hemostasis is obtained, a drain is optionally placed, and the wound is closed.

Postoperative Care

Routine care for neck incisions is all that is necessary. It may be preferable to use a soft diet for the first week, so that muscle action during swallowing is not excessive. Voice rest is unnecessary. For either type of reinnervation, division of the RLN will result in loss of any intact axons that were present. If there were many such axons, the patient may feel their voice is worse postoperatively. This possibility should be explained to the patient preoperatively ("your voice may get a little worse before it gets better"). Also, care should be taken that the patient does not have a significant increase in aspiration; if symptomatic, they should be instructed to swallow with the head turned toward the paralyzed side. The acute changes in voice and swallowing usually improve within a week or two. Patients usually report improvement in their voice starting about 4 months post-operative, but further improvement often continues for up to a year.

Results of Animal Studies

Several animal studies of laryngeal reinnervation using the ansa cervicalis have been reported. Small animal series by Zheng et al. [13], Marie et al. [14], and van Lith-Bijl et al. [15, 16] showed some restoration of spontaneous adduction, although reflex adduction was not observed. More typically, ansa cervicalis reinnervation does not result in movement of the arytenoids, although adduction can usually be induced with electric stimulation of the nerve. This finding was reported by Green et al. [17], by Brondbo et al. [18], and by Paniello et al. [11]. Several studies also reported "physiologic motion" after reinnervating the adductor muscles with the ansa cervicalis and the PCA muscle with another nerve, such as the phrenic or its roots [14, 15, 19]. In each of these cases, restoration of adduction was greater than that of abduction.

A series of canine studies using the hypoglossal nerve for laryngeal reinnervation was reported by Paniello et al. [10, 11]. Six months following hypoglossal-to-RLN neurorrhaphy, the reinnervated vocal folds showed full adduction to midline during deglutition, then a brisk return to the resting position. The relaxation abductory motion is presumed secondary to the natural elastic forces of the laryngeal ligaments. Induced phonation was achieved by stimulating the hypoglossal nerve while passing air through the vocal folds from below. Retrograde labeling confirmed that the hypoglossal nucleus was indeed the source of the innervating axons. It was found that a split hypoglossal nerve resulted in similar vocal fold motion, with less atrophy of the donor hemitongue; however, the human hypoglossal nerve is not organized into fascicles like that of the canine, and a split hypoglossal nerve in a human would not be expected to give these same results. Dogs treated using a full hypoglossal nerve with a 2-cm interposition nerve graft, and comparison dogs that underwent an ansa cervicalis reinnervation, showed tone but no active motion. It was concluded that if there is not adequate length to perform a primary hypoglossal-RLN anastomosis, so that a nerve graft is needed, then there is probably no advantage of the hypoglossal reinnervation approach over the ansa cervicalis, and the tongue donor morbidity should be avoided [11].

The problem of synkinesis is under current study in our laboratory, using a canine model. A method for quantifying synkinesis has been studied using a functional measure, which we termed the "laryngeal adductory pressure (LAP)" [20]; however, this approach is not sensitive enough to demonstrate small differences in synkinesis. Currently, we are using the ratio of myosin isoform expression, which has been well characterized in the canine and other species [21], based on the work of Buller et al. who showed that cross-innervation induces a change in the histochemical properties of the reinnervated muscle [22]. Interventions intended to promote appropriate adductor reinnervation, and to inhibit synkinesis, are under study.

Clinical Results

Crumley has been using the ansa-RLN reinnervation technique for over 20 years, periodically reporting his consistently positive results [4, 5, 8, 23]. His experience has shown that this approach for treating UVFP compares favorably to thyroplasty and injection techniques, on the basis of several variables: surgical time; ease of performance; time interval to improvement; reversibility; changes in vocal structure; complications; cost; as well as phonatory results [4].

Ansa-RLN

Other authors have reported very favorable clinical experiences with ansa-RLN transfer. Olson et al. performed perceptual analyses on 12 patients following this operation, with excellent results [24]. Several of their patients underwent reinnervation several years after the onset of their paralysis. El-Khashlan et al. [25] and Zheng et al. [26] also reported excellent voice results in small series. May and Beery reported significant improvement in voice in 19 of 20 patients reinnervated using the ansa-nerve muscle pedicle technique [27].

Some interesting findings were reported by Maronian et al. [28] Nine patients who underwent ansa-RLN reinnervation had «near-normal» voice results as judged by three speech pathologists. Electromyography was performed on each patient at both an early (5 months) and late (12–16 months) time interval. The early EMGs of the thyroarytenoid muscle confirmed active motor unit recruitment during head lift (a strap muscle / ansa cervicalis activity, with the patient supine), but none during active phonation. The late EMGs did show recruitment during phonation (as well as head lift).

It is unknown whether this activity represents central reorganization, spontaneous supplemental reinnervation by some other motor neurons (presumably related to the RLN), or some other phenomenon.

Several recent cadaveric studies of the anatomy of the ansa cervicalis nerve and RLN have been published [29, 30]. Chhetri et al. [31], Damrose et al. [32], and Sun et al. [33] all found that division of the human RLN into adductor and abductor divisions usually occurs just before the nerve enters the larynx at the cricothyroid joint. Maranillo et al. studied the variable innervation of the PCA muscle and found it suitable for selective reinnervation [34].

Ansa-RLN and Medialization

Another surgical option that has been proposed is to combine reinnervation with medialization thyroplasty. Some surgeons have found that the initial benefit of a thyroplasty tends to diminish with time, often over a course of 6–12 months [35]. Few longer-term follow-up studies have been published to verify or refute this. The cause of this fading benefit is unknown, but hypotheses include: (a) atrophy of the denervated TA muscle, leading to a more lateral position of the phonatory free margin of the vocal fold; (b) slow, gradual resolution of perioperative edema from the medialization procedure; (c) weakening or other loss of compensation from the non-paralyzed vocal fold; and (d) subtle shift of the thyroplasty implant to a more "relaxed" position, with lateralization of the vocal fold. All of these mechanisms are plausible and may play a role, but the atrophy idea is cited most often. The idea of combining reinnervation with thyroplasty is to prevent such atrophy, as well as to reduce the chances that the other listed mechanisms will have significant impact.

Tucker compared a series of 52 patients who underwent either combined medialization and reinnervation or medialization alone in a non-randomized study [35, 36]. The voice samples, as evaluated by a panel of blinded listeners, showed significantly better voice results in the patients who underwent the combined procedure; however, Chhetri et al. did a similar study in a group of 19 patients, and found no difference in results between their two study groups [37]. The question of whether to perform the combined procedures has not been adequately answered yet and merits further study.

Hypoglossal Nerve

Before the hypoglossal nerve could be used clinically, two significant questions required study: (a) whether the human hypoglossal nerve would be long enough to reach the RLN without the need for a nerve graft, and (b) whether the combined morbidity of the paralyzed ipsilateral hypoglossal nerve and RLN would be acceptable. For the first question, data was collected from a series of 89 patients who underwent open neck procedures for a variety of reasons (mostly neck dissections for malignancy) [12]. The available length of the hypoglossal nerve, and the consequent required length of the RLN, were measured and recorded. It was found that a minimum of 3 cm of RLN stump was required for the nerves to comfortably reach one another in most cases, if the hypoglossal nerve length was maximized as described above (but 4-5 cm would be preferable). For the second question, the combined morbidity was studied by temporarily paralyzing the hypoglossal nerve in 25 patients with UVFP. Recordings were made of the patients' voices while reading sets of words with specific phonemes, chosen to include the consonant sounds most likely affected by the loss of the hypoglossal nerve. These recordings were analyzed by a speech pathologist. More importantly, an assessment of aspiration was made. It was found that only a few patients had any articulation changes, and these were judged as being fairly minor. There were no significant aspiration problems. It is noteworthy that these assessments were made during the acute phase of hypoglossal paralysis. With time, natural compensation would be expected to diminish any impact. It was concluded that the combined morbidity of hypoglossal and RLN paralysis would be acceptable.

A series of patients who had undergone hypoglossal lidocaine injections went on to have hypoglossal-to-RLN anastomosis performed [12]. The first case was a young woman who had previously had two neck explorations for anterior cervical spine fusion procedures. At the time of her reinnervation procedure, the RLN stump was identified, but the ansa cervicalis had been divided and could not be used. This possibility had been anticipated and she was prepared for hypoglossal nerve transfer, which was performed without difficulty. Postoperatively, she noted a sudden, dramatic return to a completely normal voice at 18 weeks. There was no significant donor site morbidity and she was completely satisfied with her result. The 18-week recovery time was noted by several additional patients in this series, and most patients noted continued improvement for up to a year after surgery. Subjectively, it was the author's impression that these patients as a group had the best results of any group of patients with UVFP that he had treated; however, although the patients expressed few complaints about the donor morbidity to the tongue (other than occasionally biting it for the first few weeks), the question remains as to whether the voice benefit is worth this additional morbidity. Because the ansa cervicalis approach has also been very successful, it seems likely that the hypoglossal nerve will, for now, remain as a secondary option for cases in which the ansa cervicalis is not available, as it was for the index case [12].

Original RLN

The most common scenario in which the original RLN is used for reinnervation is when it is inadvertently injured during thyroid surgery, and the injury is recognized intraoperatively. If the site of injury is small, there may be enough laxity in the two stumps to allow primary re-anastomosis. When the nerve damage is found at a secondary procedure, the stumps will usually have retracted, and bringing them together is less likely to succeed. Horsley is usually credited with reporting the first successful reinnervation of this type, performed during a neck exploration following a gunshot wound [38].

Although the reported voice result was good, no mention was made of return of active adduction. If a segment of the RLN must be sacrificed due to involvement by malignancy, such as in some thyroid carcinoma cases, the remaining ends will not reach and primary repair will not be possible. As mentioned previously, a nerve graft should be avoided due to the loss of axons across each anastomotic site.

There have been a number of case reports of primary or secondary repair of the RLN over the years. If such repair can be performed, most surgeons will do so whenever possible. Chou et al. reported significant improvement in 8 patients in which a transected RLN was repaired primarily, compared with 4 similar patients who did not undergo repair but who later required a thyroplasty procedure [39]. There seems to be little down side from this approach, since there may be a satisfactory result, and no other options are precluded if it fails; however, either secondary reinnervation or thyroplasty would require a return trip to the operating room. Crumley recommends avoiding this possibility by performing immediate reinnervation with the ansa cervicalis, with reliable good results [40].

Reinnervation or Medialization?

When reinnervation or medialization options are presented to patients with UVFP, there is unfortunately no data presently available to recommend one option over the other. It is true that the initial results of thyroplasty are achieved within days to weeks, whereas those of reinnervation are not realized for several months. This latter issue can be ameliorated by performing an injection laryngoplasty with a collagen product at the same time that reinnervation is performed. Some patients who are very ill may have other reasons to avoid the delayed benefit of reinnervation. Some patients will choose reinnervation because they feel it is the most logical approach to treating their problem – "replace a bad nerve with a good nerve" – or because they have an aversion to any sort of implant. But most patients are interested in undergoing whichever procedure will give them the better voice result. Yet, all we can tell them currently is that both operations can reasonably be expected to make them better, but that we do not know which procedure is likely to be better for them.

To address this question, the author is currently the principal investigator of a multicenter, prospective, randomized clinical trial comparing these two approaches head to head. Data will include acoustic, aerodynamic, videostroboscopic, and EMG data to be collected preoperatively and at 6 and 12 months postoperatively. The voice samples will be evaluated by volunteer listeners. We are hoping that this study will enable us to make recommendations as to which future patients will be better served by which operation.

Cricothyroid Reinnervation

The cricothyroid (CT) muscle is innervated by the external (motor) branch of the superior laryngeal nerve (SLN). It is generally considered a vocal fold tensor and weak adductor, although its activation pattern, by EMG, suggests it is a respiratory muscle. The CT muscle is clearly used in pitch elevation. The SLN may be injured during dissection of the superior pole of the thyroid gland, and this injury is probably much more common than is generally recognized because the findings in SLN paralysis are often quite subtle. In addition to reduced frequency range, the patient may have diplophonia from asymmetric vocal fold tension. Reinnervation of the CT muscle is a logical therapeutic alternative that has received little attention.

Hogikyan et al. have investigated the use of a muscle–nerve–muscle (M–N–M) technique for laryngeal reinnervation in a feline model [41]. In this procedure one end of a free nerve graft is implanted into an intact donor muscle, and the opposite end is implanted into the target paralyzed muscle. In this series of cats, there was EMG evidence of successful neurotization in the implanted TA of most of the animals, using the CT as the donor muscle. This group also reported on the results of three patients who underwent M–N–M reinnervation of the CT muscle, using the contralateral CT as the donor [42]. These patients had suffered high vagal lesions and were simultaneously undergoing ansa-RLN reinnervation. All three patients regained normal voice quality, and also demonstrated successful CT and TA reinnervation by EMG. This interesting approach merits further study.

Abductor Reinnervation

In patients with bilateral vocal fold paralysis, the resting position of the vocal folds is often at or near the midline, making their phonation reasonably good but their airway severely compromised, often requiring a tracheotomy. In this group of patients, the notion of dynamic abductor reinnervation is quite attractive as it would offer the potential for decannulation. Vocal fold lateralization procedures, cordectomy, and arytenoidectomy procedures may also achieve decannulation, but at the expense of voice quality and/or increased aspiration risk.

The ideal donor nerve for abductor reinnervation would (a) have phasic activity with inspiration, (b) contain a large number of axons, (c) be anatomically proximate enough to allow neurorrhaphy with a single anastomosis, and (d) have minimal donor site morbidity. No nerve meets all of these criteria. The phrenic nerve would be ideal except for the potential donor site morbidity of a paralyzed hemidiaphragm, which may be problematic in some patients. The superior laryngeal nerve has activity in both adduction and abduction, although it is nearby and of good size. The ansa cervicalis innervates the "strap" muscles, which function as accessory respiratory muscles, but this activity is weak. Some of the intercostal nerves have the desired phasic activity, but are not anatomically proximate enough to allow primary neurorrhaphy.

Abductor reinnervation surgery is technically difficult. In order to direct all of the reinnervating axons into the PCA muscle, the adductor division of the RLN must be dissected and ligated. Often, this branching occurs within the laryngeal framework.

The branch to the PCA is also fairly small, making microneurorrhaphy challenging. In some cases the nerve–muscle–pedicle (NMP) technique, or possible direct suturing of a nerve into the PCA muscle, is used.

Phrenic Nerve

Some creative approaches to abductor reinnervation with the phrenic nerve have been reported in animal models, working around some of these technical difficulties. In a series of cats, Mahieu et al. performed phrenic-RLN anastomosis, and also implanted the adductor division of the RLN into the ipsilateral PCA [43]. They observed "near-normal" abduction in eight of nine animals. Doyle et al. used a direct phrenic-to-PCA implantation technique, and found phasic respiratory abduction in 9 of 12 cats [44]. Baldissera et al. performed phrenic-RLN anastomosis, and implanted the adductor division into the contralateral PCA muscle [45]. Bilateral abduction was observed in five of six cats, and histochemical analysis showed strong, appropriate reinnervation. In a canine study, Rice performed phrenic-RLN anastomosis and ligated the adductor division, obtaining normal abduction in six of eight dogs [46].

A split phrenic donor nerve would theoretically preserve some fibers to the diaphragm. Crumley was the first to report this approach, using a canine model, but abductor function was only seen in 5 of 12 dogs [47, 48]. Marie et al. performed a reinnervation experiment of the sternohyoid muscle using only one to two cervical roots in a series of 36 rabbits [49]. Appropriate abduction was obtained, and movement of the diaphragm was maintained.

Reports of clinical experience with phrenic reinnervation have been limited, as has the success of this approach. Crumley observed a slight increase in glottal gap, but no abduction, using phrenic-RLN reinnervation in a series of five patients [50]. Zheng et al. reported good abduction in five of six patients who underwent phrenic-RLN anastomosis, whereas the contralateral side, following ansa-PCA NMP reinnervation, had no motion [51].

The present author has recently addressed the question of donor site morbidity by performing a trial of hemidiaphragm paralysis using a lidocaine block of the left phrenic nerve of a 57-year-old woman. A successful block was confirmed by fluoroscopy, then pulmonary function tests (PFTs) were performed. The reduction in forced vital capacity (FVC) of about 25% matched literature reports of studies of phrenic paralysis from other causes. This change was well tolerated by the patient. This patient subsequently underwent phrenic-RLN neurorrhaphy with ligation of the adductor division (similar to Rice's procedure above). The PFT results a few days post-operative were virtually identical to the lidocaine-paralyzed numbers, indicating that the lidocaine block was a good predictor of the potential morbidity. The vocal fold has moved to a more lateral position, and the patient is tolerating increasing periods with the tracheotomy plugged, preparing for possible decannulation (publication pending).

Ansa Cervicalis

It is a medical curiosity that the same nerve can be used effectively for both adductor and abductor reinnervation of the larynx. The ansa cervicalis has been used for abductor reinnervation in a number of animal experiments, with mixed results. In a series of dogs, the ansa was anastomosed directly to the abductor branch of the RLN by Attali et al. [52]. The EMG confirmed successful reinnervation in 80%. However, in a cat study, Fata et al. observed abduction only with electrical stimulation (not spontaneously), using the NMP technique [53]. A similar experiment in dogs by Crumley revealed no motion at all, even with electrical stimulation of the ansa branch [48].

Tucker has reported a series of over 200 patients in which the PCA was reinnervated using the ansa-NMP technique. He reports a 74% success rate with 2 years follow-up [54]. However, most surgeons with smaller series have had less positive results, similar to Zheng et al. [51].

In a canine study, Brondbo et al. compared PCA reinnervation with the RLN, the ansa, and the phrenic nerve [55]. The phrenic nerve group had phasic respiratory motion. The other two groups only showed motion during electrical stimulation of the nerves.

Combined Adductor and Abductor Reinnervation

Efforts to restore appropriate activity to both adductor and abductor muscles have been reported by several authors, usually by using separate nerves for each division. If the natural activity of each reinnervating nerve does not match that of the normal larynx, there is the risk of overlapping activity, with both nerves activated simultaneously and effectively antagonizing one another. For example, reinnervating both functions with branches of the ansa cervicalis, although feasible based on the discussion above, would clearly be unlikely to result in any functional activity.

Bidirectional Motion: Animal Models

Crumley used the phrenic nerve to reinnervate the PCA and the ansa to reinnervate the adductors in a series of dogs [19]. He reported good adduction, but no abduction. Another group, van Lith-Bijl et al., used this same combination in a series of cats, and found spontaneous bidirectional motion, but no reflex adduction [15, 16]. Marie achieved bidirectional motion in a canine series using the ansa and one to two cervical roots, maintaining some innervation to the diaphragm [56].

Reinnervation for Laryngeal Transplantation

Transplantation of the larynx, if it becomes an accepted option, will only be successful if functional bidirectional motion can be achieved. As a technical demonstration, Peterson et al. carefully harvested NMPs from each intrinsic laryngeal muscle in a series of four beagle pairs [57]. Laryngeal transplantation was performed and the NMPs were implanted into the appropriate recipient muscles. Good adduction and slightly weak abduction was observed bilaterally.

A single human laryngeal transplantation case has been reported by Strome et al., in which a severely traumatized larynx was replaced [58]. Both SLNs (motor and sensory branches) and the right RLN were anastomosed to the matching nerves in the transplanted larynx. Within a few months, the patient had a reasonable voice, tactile sensation of the supraglottis, and good enough glottic closure that he could swallow a normal diet. His voice improved further with time, but his vocal folds remained near midline and he could not be decannulated. The EMG confirmed volitional motor activity in both PCA muscles and in both TA muscles. The apparent spontaneous reinnervation of the left TA muscle occurred by an unknown mechanism.

Conclusion

Laryngeal reinnervation is a logical approach to treating laryngeal paralysis. There continues to be some exciting work in this field, and our ability to treat patients with unilateral or bilateral vocal fold paralysis continues to improve. The clinical studies underway may eventually provide guidance as to optimum utilization of these techniques in the management of our patients.

References

1. Gacek RR, Malmgren LT, Lyon MJ (1977) Localization of adductor and abductor motor nerve fibers to the larynx. Ann Otol Rhinol Laryngol 86:771–776
2. Malmgren LT, Gacek RR (1981) Acetylcholinesterase staining of fiber components in feline and human recurrent laryngeal nerve. Topography of laryngeal motor fiber regions. Acta Otolaryngol 91337–352
3. Maronian NC, Robinson L, Waugh P, Hillel AD (2004) A new electromyographic definition of laryngeal synkinesis. Ann Otol Rhinol Laryngol 113:877–886
4. Crumley RL (1991) Update: ansa cervicalis to recurrent laryngeal nerve anastomosis for unilateral laryngeal paralysis. Laryngoscope 101:384–388
5. Crumley RL (1990) Teflon versus thyroplasty versus nerve transfer: a comparison. Ann Otol Rhinol Laryngol 99:759–763
6. Titze IR (1994) Principles of voice production. Prentice-Hall, Englewood Cliffs, New Jersey
7. Titze IR (1979) Comments on the myoelastic–aerodynamic theory of phonation. J Speech Hear Res 23:495–510
8. Crumley RL, Izdebski K (1986) Voice quality following laryngeal reinnervation by ansa hypoglossi transfer. Laryngoscope 96:611–616
9. Goding GS Jr (1991) Nerve–muscle pedicle reinnervation of the paralyzed vocal cord. Otolaryngol Clin North Am 24:1239–1252
10. Paniello RC, Lee P, Dahm JD (1999) Hypoglossal nerve transfer for laryngeal reinnervation: a preliminary study. Ann Otol Rhinol Laryngol 108:239–244
11. Paniello RC, West SE, Lee P (2001) Laryngeal reinnervation with the hypoglossal nerve. I. Physiology, histochemistry, electromyography, and retrograde labeling in a canine model. Ann Otol Rhinol Laryngol 110:532–542
12. Paniello RC (2000) Laryngeal reinnervation with the hypoglossal nerve: II. Clinical evaluation and early patient experience. Laryngoscope 110:739–748
13. Zheng H, Li Z, Zhou S, Cuan Y, Wen W, Lan J (1996) Experimental study on reinnervation of vocal cord adductors with the ansa cervicalis. Laryngoscope 106:1516–1521
14. Marie JP, Dehesdin D, Ducastelle T, Senant J (1989) Selective reinnervation of the abductor and adductor muscles of the canine larynx after recurrent nerve paralysis. Ann Otol Rhinol Laryngol 98:530–536
15. van Lith-Bijl JT, Stolk RJ, Tonnaer JA, Groenhout C, Konings PN, Mahieu HF (1997) Selective laryngeal reinnervation with separate phrenic and ansa cervicalis nerve transfers. Arch Otolaryngol Head Neck Surg 123:406–411
16. van Lith-Bijl JT, Mahieu HF (1998) Reinnervation aspects of laryngeal transplantation. Eur Arch Otorhinolaryngol 255:515–520
17. Green DC, Berke GS, Graves MC (1991) A functional evaluation of ansa cervicalis nerve transfer for unilateral vocal cord paralysis: future directions for laryngeal reinnervation. Otolaryngol Head Neck Surg 104:453–466
18. Brondbo K, Jacobsen E, Gjellan M, Refsum H (1992) Recurrent nerve/ansa cervicalis nerve anastomosis: a treatment alternative in unilateral recurrent nerve paralysis. Acta Otolaryngol 112:353–357
19. Crumley RL (1984) Selective reinnervation of vocal cord adductors in unilateral vocal cord paralysis. Ann Otol Rhinol Laryngol 93:351–356
20. Paniello RC, West SE (2000) Laryngeal adductory pressure as a measure of post-reinnervation synkinesis. Ann Otol Rhinol Laryngol 109:447–451

21. Wu YZ, Crumley RL, Armstrong WB, Caiozzo VJ (2000) New perspectives about human laryngeal muscle: single-fiber analyses and interspecies comparisons. Arch Otolaryngol Head Neck Surg 126:857–864
22. Buller AJ, Kean CJC, Ranatunga KW (1987) Transformations of contraction speed in muscle following cross reinnervation: dependence on muscle size. J Muscle Res Cell Motil 8:504–516
23. Crumley RL, Izdebski K, McMicken B (1988) Nerve transfer versus Teflon injection for vocal cord paralysis: a comparison. Laryngoscope 98:1200–1204
24. Olson DE, Goding GS, Michael DD (1998) Acoustic and perceptual evaluation of laryngeal reinnervation by ansa cervicalis transfer. Laryngoscope 108:1767–1772
25. El-Kashlan HK, Carroll WR, Hogikyan ND, Chepeha DB, Kileny PR, Esclamado RM (2001) Selective cricothyroid muscle reinnervation by muscle-nerve-muscle neurotization. Arch Otolaryngol Head Neck Surg 127:1211–1215
26. Zheng H, Li Z, Zhou S, Cuan Y, Wen W (1996) Update: laryngeal reinnervation for unilateral vocal cord paralysis with the ansa cervicalis. Laryngoscope 106:1522–1527
27. May M, Beery Q (1986) Muscle-nerve pedicle laryngeal nerve reinnervation. Laryngoscope 96:1196–1200
28. Maronian N, Waugh P, Robinson L, Hillel A (2003) Electromyographic findings in recurrent laryngeal nerve reinnervation. Ann Otol Rhinol Laryngol 112:314–323
29. Nguyen M, Junien-Lavillauroy C, Faure C (1989) Anatomical intra-laryngeal anterior branch study of the recurrent (inferior) laryngeal nerve. Surg Radiol Anat 11:123–127
30. Nguyen M, Junien-Lavillauroy C (1990) Anatomy of the larynx, study of the anterior branch of the recurrent laryngeal nerve. Rev Laryngol Otol Rhinol (Bord) 111:153–155
31. Chhetri DK, Berke GS (1997) Ansa cervicalis nerve: review of the topographic anatomy and morphology. Laryngoscope 107:1366–1372
32. Damrose EJ, Huang RY, Ye M, Berke GS, Sercarz JA (2003) Surgical anatomy of the recurrent laryngeal nerve: implications for laryngeal reinnervation. Ann Otol Rhinol Laryngol 112:434–438
33. Sun SQ, Zhao J, Lu H, He GQ, Ran JH, Peng XH (2001) An anatomical study of the recurrent laryngeal nerve: its branching patterns and relationship to the inferior thyroid artery. Surg Radiol Anat 23:363–369
34. Maranillo E, Leon X, Ibanez M, Orus C, Quer M, Sanudo JR (2003) Variability of the nerve supply patterns of the human posterior cricoarytenoid muscle. Laryngoscope 113:602–606
35. Tucker HM (1997) Combined surgical medialization and nerve–muscle pedicle reinnervation for unilateral vocal fold paralysis: improved functional results and prevention of long-term deterioration of voice. J Voice 11:474–478
36. Tucker HM (1999) Long-term preservation of voice improvement following surgical medialization and reinnervation for unilateral vocal fold paralysis. J Voice 13:251–256
37. Chhetri DK, Gerratt BR, Kreiman J, Berke GS (1999) Combined arytenoid adduction and laryngeal reinnervation in the treatment of vocal fold paralysis. Laryngoscope 109:1928–1936
38. Horsley J (1909) Suture of the recurrent laryngeal nerve with report of a case. Trans South Surg Gynecol Assoc 22:161
39. Chou FF, Su CY, Jeng SF, Hsu KL, Lu KY (2003) Neurorrhaphy of the recurrent laryngeal nerve. J Am Coll Surg 197:52–57
40. Crumley RL (1990) Repair of the recurrent laryngeal nerve. Otolaryngol Clin North Am 23:553–563
41. Hogikyan ND, Johns MM, Kileny PR, Urbanchek M, Carroll WR, Kuzon WM Jr (2001) Motion-specific laryngeal reinnervation using muscle–nerve–muscle neurotization. Ann Otol Rhinol Laryngol 110:801–810
42. El-Kashlan HK, Carroll WR, Hogikyan ND, Chepeha DB, Kileny PR, Esclamado RM (2001) Selective cricothyroid muscle reinnervation by muscle-nerve-muscle neurotization. Arch Otolaryngol Head Neck Surg 127:1211–1215
43. Mahieu HF, van Lith-Bijl JT, Groenhout C, Tonnaer JA, de Wilde P (1993) Selective laryngeal abductor reinnervation in cats using a phrenic nerve transfer and ORG 2766. Arch Otolaryngol Head Neck Surg 119:772–776
44. Doyle PJ, Chepeha DB, Westerberg BD, Schwarz DW (1993) Phrenic nerve reinnervation of the cat's larynx: a new technique with proven success. Ann Otol Rhinol Laryngol 102:837–842
45. Baldissera F, Tredici G, Marini G, Fiori MG, Cantarella G, Ottaviani F, Zanoni R (1992) Innervation of the paralyzed laryngeal muscles by phrenic motoneurons. A quantitative study by light and electron microscopy. Laryngoscope 102:907–916
46. Rice DH (1982) Laryngeal reinnervation. Laryngoscope 92:1049–1059
47. Crumley RL, Horn K, Clendenning D (1980) Laryngeal reinnervation using the split-phrenic nerve-graft procedure. Otolaryngol Head Neck Surg 88:159–164
48. Crumley RL (1982) Experiments in laryngeal reinnervation. Laryngoscope 92 (Suppl 30):1–27
49. Marie JP, Lerosey Y, Dehesdin D, Jin O, Tadie M, Andrieu-Guitrancourt J (1999) Experimental reinnervation of a strap muscle with a few roots

of the phrenic nerve in rabbits. Ann Otol Rhinol Laryngol 108:1004–1011
50. Crumley RL (1983) Phrenic nerve graft for bilateral vocal cord paralysis. Laryngoscope 93:425–428
51. Zheng H, Zhou S, Li Z, Chen S, Zhang S, Huang Y, Wen W, Shen X, Wu H, Zhou R, Cui Y, Geng L (2002) Reinnervation of the posterior cricoarytenoid muscle by the phrenic nerve for bilateral vocal cord paralysis in humans. Zhonghua Er Bi Yan Hou Ke Za Zhi 37:210–214 [in Chinese]
52. Attali JP, Gioux M, Henry C, Urtassun A, Vital C, Traissac L (1988) Vocal cord abduction rehabilitation by nervous selective anastomosis. Laryngoscope 98:398–401
53. Fata JJ, Malmgren LT, Gacek RR, Dum R, Woo P (1987) Histochemical study of posterior cricoarytenoid muscle reinnervation by a nerve–muscle pedicle in the cat. Ann Otol Rhinol Laryngol 96:479–487
54. Tucker HM (1989) Long-term results of nerve–muscle pedicle reinnervation for laryngeal paralysis. Ann Otol Rhinol Laryngol 98:674–676
55. Brondbo K, Hall C, Teig E, Dahl HA (1986) Functional results after experimental reinnervation of the posterior cricoarytenoid muscle in dogs. J Otolaryngol 15:259–264
56. Marie JP (2000) Functional reinnervation of the canine larynx. Presented at the Meeting of the Neurolaryngology Subcommittee, American Academy of Otolaryngology – Head and Neck Surgery, Washington D.C., 25 September
57. Peterson KL, Andrews R, Manek A, Ye M, Sercarz JA (1998) Objective measures of laryngeal function after reinnervation of the anterior and posterior recurrent laryngeal nerve branches. Laryngoscope 108:889–898
58. Strome M, Stein J, Esclamado R, Hicks D, Lorenz RR, Braun W, Yetman R, Eliachar I, Mayes J (2001) Laryngeal transplantation and 40-month follow-up. N Engl J Med 344:1676–1679

Chapter 12

Electrical Stimulation for Vocal Fold Paralysis

Michael Broniatowski

Introduction

The restoration of workable dynamics to the paralyzed larynx is long overdue. Whatever its etiology, the problem is usually clinically expressed through a variable mix of deficits affecting swallowing, breathing, and phonation. Traditional approaches to rehabilitation fail to return appropriate tone and coordination to the organ because they lack a dynamic profile. Inertia inherent to paralysis further leads to muscular atrophy from disuse.

While the effects of electric current on contractile tissue are well documented, activation of neuromuscular groups endowed with specific functions has only been recently considered. This dynamic approach to rehabilitation is called functional electrical stimulation (FES) or pacing. It enlists varieties of neuroprostheses designed to bypass the disabled central nervous system (CNS) power centers normally responsible for smooth integration of laryngeal dynamics. The electronics are modeled on nature with a central core to which are attached afferent (sensory) and efferent (motor) limbs constituting an artificial reflex arc. Afferent information may be gathered from sensors interrogating allied functions spared by the pathological process. Efferent commands may reach the muscle(s) either directly or via perineural electrodes, considering the physiological unity and plasticity of the nerve-muscle complex.

Functional electrical stimulation has been beneficial in improving neuromuscular deficits such as diaphragm paralysis and the control of gait and voiding in paraplegics. While options for artificial rehabilitation of failed vocal fold dynamics have been more recently considered, the pivotal role of the larynx in swallowing, respiration, and phonation should make applications to the organ quite attractive. Pacing has so far focused on glottic closure for aspiration, and opening after inspiratory compromise. While animal experimentation remains critical for further progress, human applications have not yet reached the full potential implied in the laboratory. Further developments will likely depend on increased public awareness of the clinical advantages offered by laryngeal pacing as a more convenient and cheaper alternative to currently available palliative approaches.

Background and Justification

The Problem

Paralysis is defined as a loss of power of voluntary movement in a muscle through injury or disease of it or its nerve supply [1]. Another aspect of this problem is the damage to accessory pathways from the cortex that normally inhibit brain stem control, accompanied by increased muscular tension and hyperactive reflexes [2]. Regardless of their etiologies, laryngeal paralyses clinically reflect the inability for one or both vocal folds to appropriately either adduct or abduct from fixed positions. In a number of cases, the organ's normal axial excursion is also compromised. While the causes and symptoms of laryngeal paralyses are more fully described elsewhere in this text, this particular chapter concentrates on exposing incremental levels of sophistication in electrodynamic rehabilitation seen through this author's experience in laboratory and clinical settings.

Typical lower motor neuron paralyses of one vocal fold usually produces dysphonia and some degree of aspiration until compensation or recovery eventually seals the glottic chink.

Sometimes, glottic closure is slow to materialize or just unworkable. Bilateral paralyses usually carry higher morbidities. While incapacity for the vocal folds to abduct induces airway compromise, adduction failure will, conversely, allow secretions originating upstream to be aspirated into the unprotected trachea. The CNS insults originating above the lower motor neuron usually allow the preservation of some degree and coordination of vocal fold motion, due to crossed neural distribution. This may be expressed as series of ill-timed and conflicting contracting sequences of either weakened, or conversely hyperactive laryngeal muscles (spasm). Since undue tone increase indicates a failure of CNS control over typical inhibitory signals, spasm may also qualify as a form of paralysis.

Critique of Traditional Management of Laryngeal Paralyses

It would certainly make sense to restore laryngeal dynamics by returning normal reinnervation to the paralyzed organ. Unfortunately, anastomosing the severed ends of the current laryngeal nerve (RLN) or suturing peripheral motor nerve stumps to suitable laryngeal counterparts often results in axonal mismatching and muscular synkinesis, even when the conduits can be clearly identified [3, 4]. Alternatives remain limited to merely palliative rearrangements of the incompetent organ's anatomy. Basically, the closed glottic chink may be bypassed by an alternate airway (e.g., tracheostomy) or thrown open (e.g., arytenoidectomy) to restore airway permeability. Conversely, the chronically open laryngeal lumen may be occluded (e.g., by vocal fold suturing) or diverted from incoming secretions (e.g., by cranial suspension) to curtail aspiration of material originating upstream (as accomplished more radically by total laryngectomy). Static laryngeal rearrangements are unable to restore dynamic sequences essential to safe and fine-tuned inspiration, swallowing, and voice, because they ignore the mutually exclusive nature of vocal fold adduction and abduction [5]. An alternative to this conceptually flawed design considers electrodynamic stimulation of the larynx, which is viewed as an otherwise healthy neuromuscular system merely disconnected from its CNS power centers upstream.

Physiological Bases for Laryngeal Stimulation

Striated laryngeal musculature normally responds to CNS commands along direct (e.g., α motor neurons) and self-regulatory (e.g., γ loop) pathways analogous to those driving nerve-muscle systems elsewhere (e.g., the agonist/antagonist system of flexion/extension of the limbs) [6]. These fundamental attributes of nerve-muscle interactions are dependent on proprioception which supports natural synergistic and opposing muscular coupling and smooth integration of the laryngeal power works [7].

Stimulation may be delivered to paralyzed muscles either via anatomically intact nerves, "foreign" motor implants (nerve pedicles, NPs, with or without a peripheral fragment of donor muscle) or directly through implanted needle electrodes. The NPs are particularly convenient as conduits when the paralysis follows severance of the neuroanatomical link with the CNS within the lower motor neuron. Nerve-muscle stimulation (a) has the further advantage of targeting the reimplanted muscle exclusively, (b) requires only low levels of current to ensure robust long-term contraction (once reinnervation has taken place), (c) can be anatomically extended for longer reach, and (d) may prolong muscle viability (i.e., prevent atrophy) by "babysitting." Using the nerves is further attractive because (a) they allow stimulation at a distance from the targeted larynx, (b) potentially facilitates interactions between multiple implants, (c) allows charges accurately reproducing action potentials [8], and (d) elicits naturally influenced muscular contraction after depolarization through the release of neurohumors (e.g., acetylcholine) at the motor end plate [9]; however, NPs remain, at least in our current state of knowledge, still unable to fully return neuromuscular power present before paralysis [10], despite their abilities to promote satisfactory long-term contractile capabilities to the reinnervated muscles [11].

Since denervated myofibers, particularly when atrophied, lack an appropriate number of occupied motor end plates, it is no surprise that effective direct stimulation will require stronger (from 10 to 100 times) charges than when applied via NPs and normal nerve-muscles (Table 12.1) [11]. Stronger charges have the potential inconvenience to spill beyond the muscle(s) they activate, engaging functions not intended to be reanimated. They may, conversely, not be sufficiently effective to elicit appropriate responses due to high resistance from electrode corrosion or fibrosis [12].

Challenges in Approaches to Laryngeal Stimulation

RLN stimulation appears attractive in paralyses originating above the level of the lower motor neuron since this link to the CNS is readily available. Unfortunately, standard RLN stimulation does not necessarily allow focused ILM activation. The problem is due to scattered distributions within the nerve of the muscles' subtending axons, as opposed to organized bundles which would favor more accurate targeting. Also, electrical activation of nerve-muscle complexes as traditionally applied authorizes muscles endowed with larger motor units to contract before their smaller counterparts. This attribute is in line with higher excitabilities of larger axons and their subtended motor units when compared with thinner neurofibers [13]. In nature, however, and according to Henneman's size principle, the smaller, less excitable axons subtending the less populated motor units are recruited earlier [14].

Intricacies in the recruiting process may not be an issue in systems running tasks of a more straight forward nature, such as the strap muscle bound ansa hypoglossi and cervicalis

Table 12.1. Published pacing parameters for normal nerve-muscles and reinnervated and paralyzed striated muscles. *CT* cricothyroideus, *PCA* posterior cricoarytenoideus, *TA* thyroarytenoideus, *TD* thoracodorsal nerve, *RLN* recurrent laryngeal nerve

Reference	Year	Muscle	Frequency (Hz)	Intensity (mA)	Potential (V)	Pulse (ms)
[64]	1964	N (phrenic)	60–90			0.05–5
[42]	1977	P (CT)	10	7		30
[65]	1984	P (PCA)	30	50		1
[66]	1984	P (PCA)	20–40		2–3	20
[67]	1985	P (PCA)	30		5	12.5
[39]	1985	R (strap)	60	1	0.5	2.5
[23]	1985	P (PCA)	50		1,8	2
[12]	1986	R (strap)	60		0.5	2.5
[30]	1988	R (PCA)a	40		2.2	4.5
[44]	1989	R (facial)	40	0,5		0.1–10
[38]	1990	N (TA)	40–45	1–2		0.02
[68]	1990	P (TA)	50	3.5–5		5
[69]	1991	P (PCA)	10–200			2.4
[70]	1991	P (PCA)	30	1–50		1
[34]	1991	P (PCA)	30	0.2–0.7		0.18
[31]	1994	P (PCA)	50	1–4		0.002
[71]	1994	P (PCA)	30	4–15		0.01–1000
[72]	1996	P (PCA)	30	1.5–7		2
[73]	1997	R (strap)	50	0.1–0.8		0.2
[22]	2001	R (strap)	42	1		0.05–0.132
[41]	2003	R (strap)	30–40		2–7	1–2

Charges necessary to achieve contraction via nerves are 10–100 times lower than when the muscle is directly stimulated. aLaryngeal reimplantation: *N* normal; *P* paralyzed; *R* reinnervated. (From [11], with a few additions)

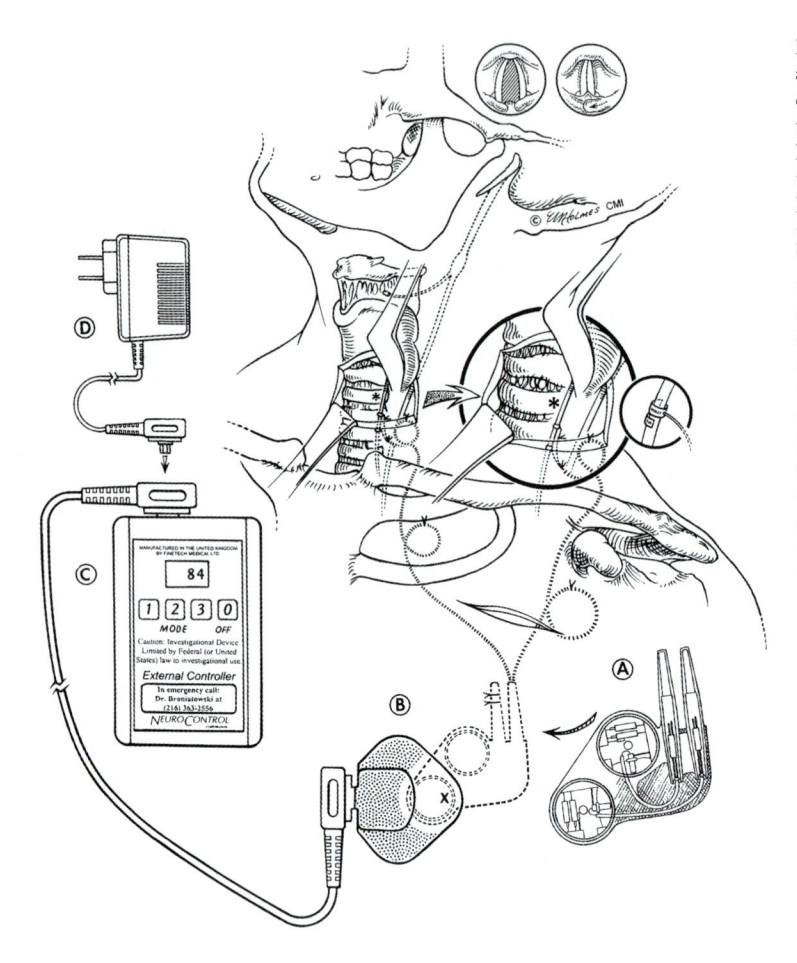

Fig. 12.1. Block diagram of a fully implantable circuit designed for glottic closure to control aspiration in the human. This first-generation system has no afferent limb and activation is under patients' voluntary control. The perineural electrode on the RLN (inset) is linked to a receiver stimulator (**A**) on the chest wall. The external stimulator transmits pulses via an external transmitter (**B**) to the implanted stimulator underneath the skin. Stimulating parameters (intensity, frequency, pulse duration) programmed through the external controller (**C**) through buttons (1, 2, 3, and 0) appearing on the screen. With stimulation ON, vocal fold adduction ensues to effect glottic closure (below) This design has also received FDA approval for NP stimulation for vocal fold abduction. (From [22])

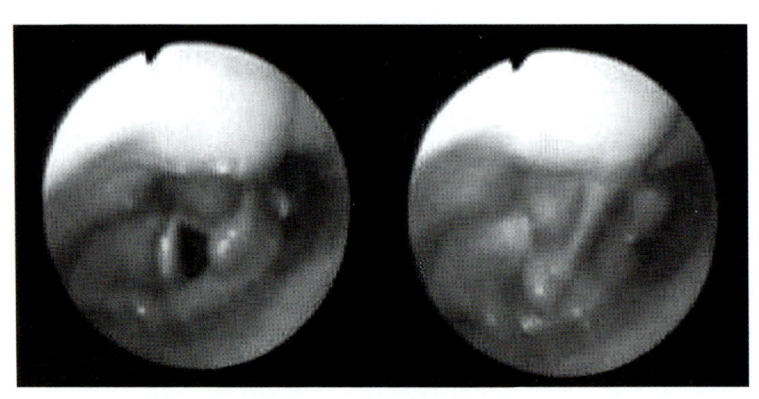

which control airway excursion, the superior laryngeal nerve (SLN) serving the cricothyroideus (CT) which elongates the vocal folds, and, as one would expect, NPs deliberately aimed at any of the individual ILMs.

Laryngeal Stimulating Strategies

Neuroprosthetic devices act as purpose-oriented electrodynamic substitutes for CNS territories rendered unable to drive specified nerve-muscle groups. The circuits may receive afferent information from activities normally associated with the missing function, but unaffected by the paralytic process (e.g., inspiratory signals as information for glottic opening). In this manner, the combination of a central electronic core fitted with afferent and efferent limbs constitutes an artificial reflex arc.

Patterns of stimulation traditionally delivered to biological tissue consist of pulse trains of variable frequencies (Hz), amplitudes (mA), and durations (ms), which may be variably adjusted depending on the expected outcome downstream. Injected waveforms can take monophasic, or preferably biphasic, shapes, better able to avoid long-term nerve injury from electrochemical tissue damage. Variations in amplitude and pulse durations of currents administered are expected to manipulate contractile forces by varying the amounts of injected charges.

Clinical RLN stimulation (e.g., for vocal fold monitoring during thyroidectomy) typically produces adduction [15] because activities of the PCA as the lone abductor are overwhelmed by those of the dominating adductors. Perineural electrodes assuming a bipolar configuration (i.e., a positively charged anode and a negatively charged cathode) are equally effective when adductor contractile patterns are expected for pacing purposes. In clinical situations of inappropriately elevated muscular tone, suppression along an inverted mirror image may be considered over an appropriate baseline. Blocking strategies use choices of circuits and electrode designs assuming either special asymmetric [16] or tripolar [17] configurations. Because their ability is limited to arrest incoming action potentials "across the board," individual ILMs may not be curbed by this approach.

Specific ILM targeting is challenging due to the muscles' small sizes, diverging vectorial anatomies, crowding within a relatively inaccessible space, and especially their non-homogeneous myofiber-type distributions. Like other muscles, the ILMs comprise a variable mix of slow (oxidative, type I) and fast (glycolytic, type II) fibers designating them to respond variably to stimulation irrespectively of their specific motor unit arrangements [18]. Regardless, focused activation may be achieved either via implanted electrodes, NPs, and selective blockage of opposing ILMs.

Issues of Long-Term Stimulation and Biocompatibility of Implanted Circuits

Even in this early stage in development, it is probably accurate to state that technology has outgrown the pool of potential FES applications in laryngology. Fully implantable miniaturized neuroprostheses designed with various nerve-muscle systems in mind may currently be appropriately modified to fit most basic needs of laryngeal pacing as defined above. The electronics have reached a point of high tolerance due to excellent insulation techniques of non-reactive materials within biocompatible shells. Perineural electrodes have an equally good record considering the few side effects reported with long-term vagus nerve stimulation for epilepsy. Problems, when present, remain limited to rupture at connecting sites with either the sensor or the electrode, perineural electrolytic damage, and fibrosis necessitating a boost in charges injecting the nerves [21]. Electrolysis can be avoided by using appropriate alloys and waveforms. Perineural fibrosis occurs normally as nerve-electrode encapsulation; however, excess collagen production is usually associated with motion. The placement of electrodes at a distance from the moving larynx fortunately obviates this problem.

Current Human Applications

Due to the vital roles they play in breathing and lung protection, respiratory and sphincteric functions of the larynx qualify to be first in line for rehabilitation after paralysis. Paced vocal fold closure for the control of aspiration has been first to materialize clinically [22] due to a large number of potential candidates and a relatively straightforward approach to securing a glottic seal. By contrast, paced vocal fold opening has been slower to develop despite earlier interest in the laboratory [23]. The problem is due to a limited number of available patients, the necessity to selectively target the posterior cricoarytenoid muscle (PCA) which is the lone adductor of the larynx, and a debate about the most effective approach.

Dynamic Laryngotracheal Closure for Aspiration

Dynamic control of aspiration probably constitutes the most desirable application of FES to the larynx considering the number of potential candidates. About three-quarters of a million new patients suffer cerebral hemisphere or brain stem stroke-related dysphagia each year in the United States alone [24, 25], and approximately half of these will experience aspiration, defined as the passage of food or secretions into the trachea beyond the vocal folds. Stroke patients have a 20-fold increase in pneumonia as compared with non-aspirators [26]. These problems can also be observed in conditions attacking the CNS either above or below the brain stem such as tumors, amyotrophic lateral sclerosis, multiple sclerosis, Parkinson's disease, Guillain-Barré syndrome, and so forth [27].

When rehabilitative maneuvers and special diet ordered by the speech-language pathologist fail to control aspiration, the inability to secure safe esophageal passage necessitates the placement of a PEG tube to supply appropriate caloric intake, as well as a tracheostomy. While this procedure is chiefly indicated to improve pulmonary toilet under the circumstances, it unfortunately also promotes aspiration on its own account by tethering the normally axially mobile aerodigestive tract to the surrounding soft tissues. Unfortunately, and despite all precautions, too many aspirating patients develop pneumonia and die [24-26]. Surgeries designed to control the problem have not been satisfactory because their palliative nature fails to return a mobile profile to the organ's mutually exclusive functions. Also, their irreversible nature makes them unappealing to most candidates.

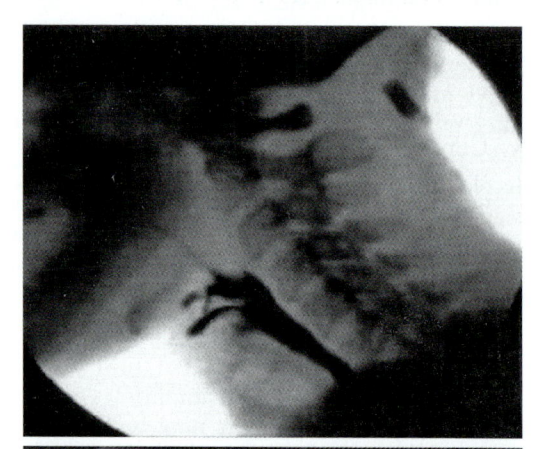

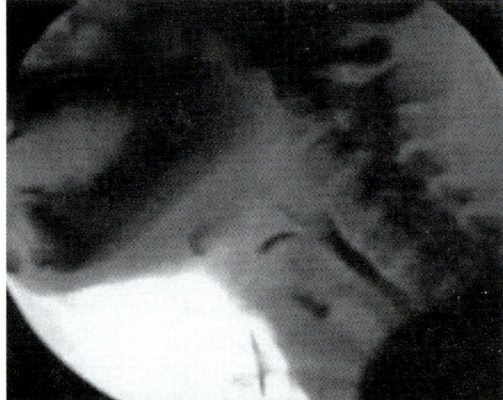

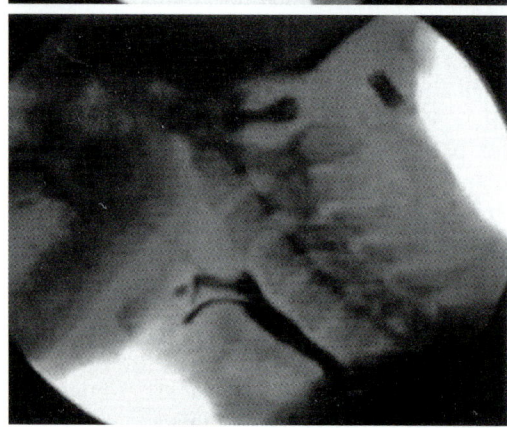

Fig. 12.2. On these fluoroscopic images (modified barium swallow) using honey-thick liquids, tracheal aspiration occurs in the absence of stimulation (middle) but is checked when applied (upper and lower views) (From [22])

Pilot experimentation in the canine has shown that RLN stimulation was able to produce frank vocal fold adduction when cued from afferent information originating from pharyngeal pressure [28–31]; however, human application had to await the availability of suitable implantable electronics. The first and only system currently available to run electrodynamic laryngotracheal separation is based on a hybrid unit appropriately modified from the extensively implanted Vocare bladder stimulator otherwise used to restore voiding in paraplegics [32]. The device is further fitted with electrodes analogous to those safely implanted in thousands of epileptic patients for the control of seizures [21, 33]. Since no afferent limb has as yet been integrated into the circuit, triggering is left to the patients. While this disposition appears satisfactory for the control of food intake, the integration of automated responses based on afferent sensors would probably (a) pick up all stimuli suitable to trigger timely glottic closure, (b) require no particular attention from the patient, and (c) allow the pool of potential candidates to be broadened to include those unable or unwilling to voluntary activate the device. At this time, subjects qualifying for deglutitive pacing are those presenting with (a) a continuation or worsening of aspiration for at least 6 months to 1 year after the neurological insult, (b) the need for a tracheotomy for pulmonary toilet, and (c) appropriate hand-motor coordination to manipulate the external controller.

Practically, the receiver-stimulator portion of the implanted pacemaker, placed in a pocket on the anterior chest wall under the clavicle, is subcutaneously connected over the bone to the electrode passed around the RLN. When the patient wishes to swallow a bolus, the order for glottic closure is given at the end of the oral phase by pushing the switch of the programmable external controller. This coil then generates a transcutaneous magnetic field for the receiver-stimulator (Fig. 12.1).

Preliminary experience in two subjects has demonstrated that a tight glottis seal could be effectively secured by vocal fold adduction limited to one side, using charges as low as 42 Hz, 1 mA, 56–132 µs for a period of 1 year. Statistically significant results from an appropriate number of fluoroscopies (modified barium swallows) confirmed the safe passage of ingested contrast materials of various consistencies during paced glottic closure exclusively, while aspiration resumed during non-stimulated swallows (Fig. 12.2). Pharyngeal residuals remaining at completion of the stimulation were easily cleared by coughing, as post-supraglottic laryngectomies are taught to do routinely after surgery. Longer-term follow-up was interrupted in one case from attrition due to an unrelated problem. The vocal fold of the other patient ceased to respond to stimulation for no apparent reason. Interestingly in this case, subsequent fluoroscopies continued to show improved deglutition. This was attributed to muscle strengthening "on the job" comparable to deliberate muscle exercise applied to the latissimus dorsi [34]. Ongoing clinical trials will determine whether effective pacing for vocal fold adduction will be validated for the long term in larger numbers of subjects, and allow graduation to a second generation of miniaturized stimulators.

Dynamic Restoration of Laryngeal Patency After Bilateral Vocal Fold Paralysis

While bilateral vocal fold paralyses with airway compromise due to head and neck, chest trauma, and thyroid surgeries are now less frequently encountered than in the past, it is important to keep other causes in mind, such as invasive tumors along the RLN, endotracheal intubation, and a wide variety of neurological insults.

Early authors seem to have been fascinated with PCA reinnervation, at least in part because reinstating the lone abductory function of the larynx offered a challenge in targeted intervention. Unfortunately, plain PCA reinnervation has not been universally shown to provide dynamic abduction on its own. Hössly must be credited for being the first author to have unwittingly achieved laryngeal pacing (in 1916) as he injected "faradic" (induced) currents into nerves implanted into canine PCAs as a mean

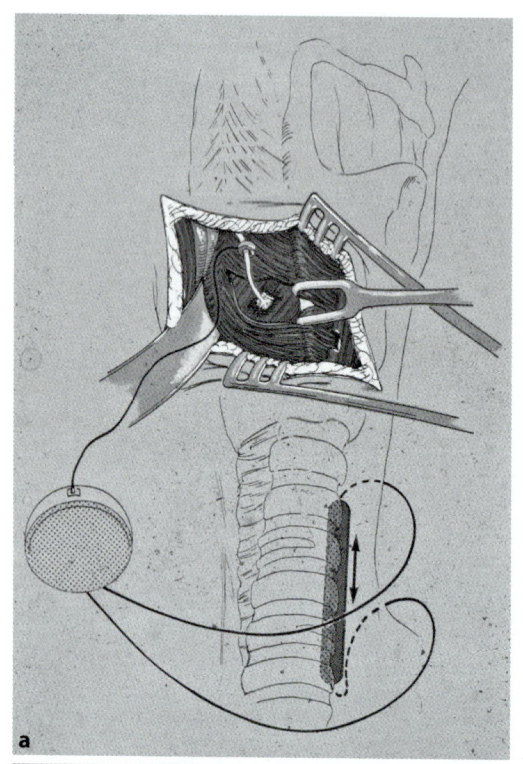

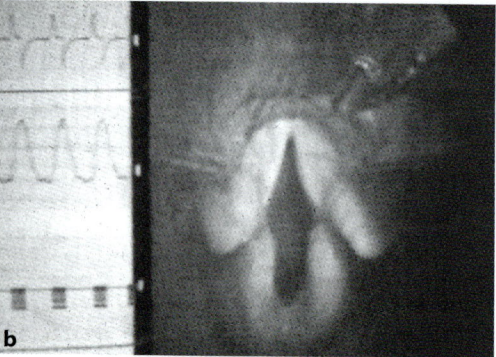

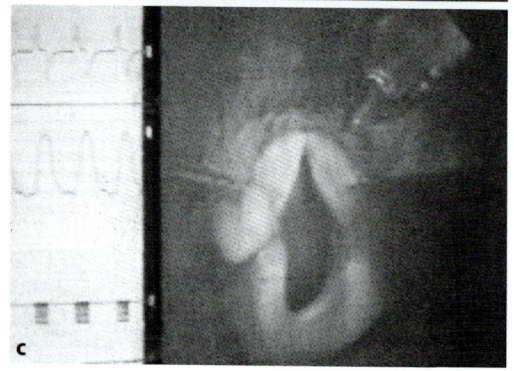

Fig. 12.3. Block diagram (upper) of an early automated experimental device for paced glottic opening after vocal fold paralysis. The afferent limb of the system transmits signals cued on inspiration (tracheal strain gauge) to the stimulator (left) which, in turn, activates as efferent limb the ipsilateral posterior cricoarytenoideus via a perineural electrode. The reinnervated vocal fold at rest (middle) abducts (lower) as the circuit fires (top) based on sensor activation (middle) synchronized with the respiratory phases (bottom tracing) (From [23, 34])

of verifying that reinnervation had actually occurred [35]. The importance of this observation was unfortunately ignored, because common wisdom taught that plain reinnervation would suffice to drive the muscle on its own, and also because, even assuming an interest in rehabilitative stimulation, medical electronics were not sufficiently developed at the time to encourage any further efforts. More recently, however, and with the progress of FES of other territories in mind, neuromuscular stimulation emerged as an added benefit to clinically established implantation techniques (e.g., Tucker's nerve-muscle pedicle) [36]. Shortcomings of plain nerve-muscle implantation include (a) the inappropriate substitution of a less effective cranial nerve power center in lieu of the incapacitated nucleus ambiguus, (b) an ensuing lack of synchronization between the borrowed command structure and the reinnervated PCA, and, importantly, (c) a lack of return of proprioceptive feedback, as was demonstrated by Grundfest-Broniatowski et al. on cross-over rabbit ansa-strap muscle preparations [37].

The first successful attempt at driving reinnervated laryngeal nerve-muscles focused, not surprisingly, on coordinated abduction, and used a fairly bulky circuit picking up inspiratory signals originating either from tracheal descent or changes in chest wall impedance. Once afferent signals reached a predetermined threshold, the system was set to fire charges as low as 50 Hz, 1.8 V, 2 ms into reinnervating pedicles, sufficient to produce exclusive and robust vocal fold abduction on the stimulated side. The abducted vocal fold returned to its original position as soon as when the circuit had ceased firing (Fig. 12.3) [23]. These experiments were modeled on an earlier pilot study examining cross-over nerve-muscle pedicle from one sternohyoid muscle to its pair using even lower charges (60 Hz, 0.5 V, 2.5 ms), possibly in line with larger sizes of more excitable nerve implants [12].

We have seen that one criticism of the reinnervation process lies in its inability to fully restore contraction patterns similar to those observed before the paralysis, since neither normal histology (the reinnervated tissue assumes an embryonal "checkerboard" distribution of myofiber types), ILM-specific aerobic and anaerobic metabolism, nor fatigability and delays of response can yet be dependably reproduced under the current conditions of practice. Nonetheless, workable short- and long-term contraction capabilities (up to 8 months) [11] have been reliably verified with charges roughly comparable to the low levels used when normal nerve-muscles are stimulated in animals paced with the implanted Itrel II (Medtronic) stimulator traditionally used for dorsal column stimulation of the spinal cord. As previously emphasized, these charges stand about 1 to 2 orders of magnitude below those necessary to stimulate the muscle directly, as further indicated by chronaxies (the shortest duration of an effective electrical stimulus having a strength equal to twice the minimum strength required for excitation), following implantation of laryngeal nerve-muscle pedicles [38]. The transformation in nerve-muscle distribution after grafting has been illustrated by retrograde tracers all the way up to the donor nucleus [39], and reinnervated muscle activities were confirmed through glycogen depletion after electrical stimulation of the pedicles [40]. Nerve pedicle vitality and satisfactory results obtained with paced adduction for aspiration should offer promise for human applications of the original canine nerve-muscle pedicle pacing experiments currently underway.

Zealear and his group have recently implanted non-reinnervated PCAs with promising results; 3 of 7 patients were decannulated after 6, 7, and 18 months, respectively. The device used was the time-honored Itrel II stimulator adjusted to deliver 30–40 Hz, 2–7 V, and 1–2 s trains of 1-ms, which were not synchronized with pa-

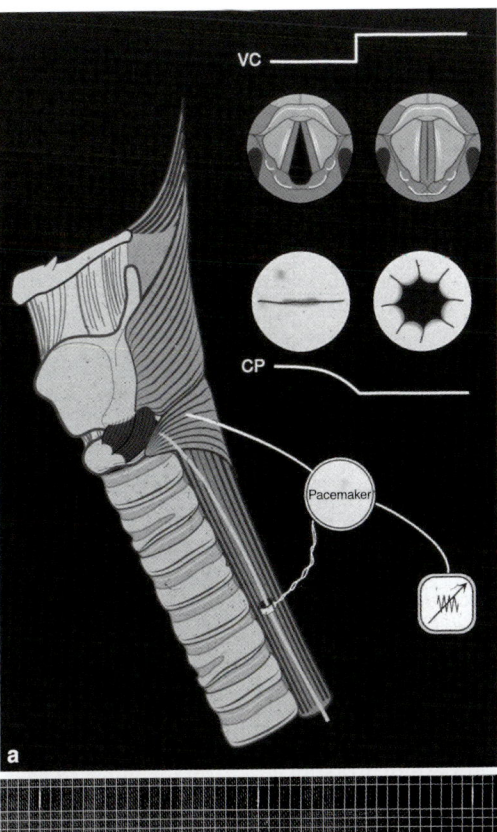

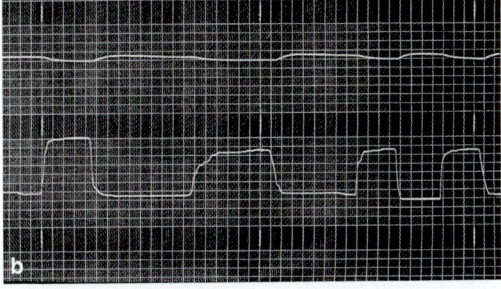

Fig. 12.4. Block diagram of an experimental system of reciprocal coupling designed to combine vocal fold and esophageal sphincter participations in the control of deglutition [45]. The glottic adductors and the cricopharyngeus muscle are put under baseline tension (*Pacemaker*) by injection of current into the RLN and the muscle. Input information from the rheostat (lower right) allows gradual increase in vocal fold tension (VC) to close the glottis as the cricopharyngeus reciprocally relaxes (CP) Recorded tracings (below) show downward deflection from cricopharyngeal relaxation (top) coordinated with RLN stimulation bursts (bottom) Baseline cricopharyngeal tone returns with cessation of electronic stimulation. (From [63])

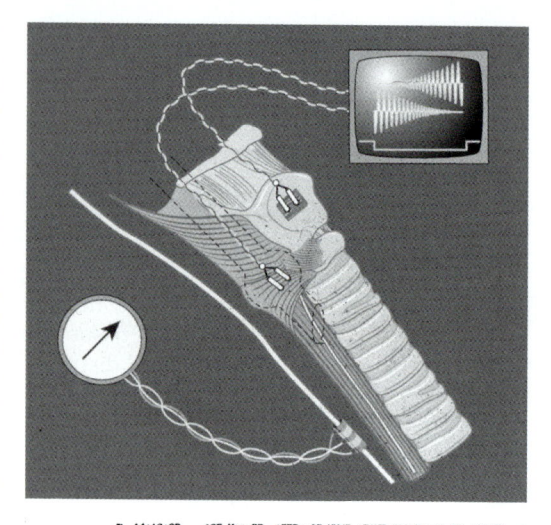

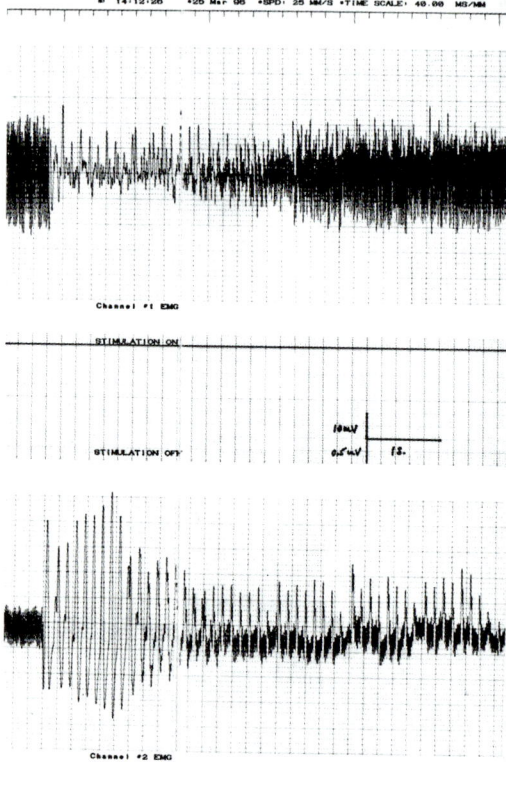

Fig. 12.5. Upper: block diagram of vagal stimulation for reciprocal coupling between glottic and upper esophageal sphincter activities [47]. A cuffed tripolar perineural electrode is passed around the vagus low in the neck (bottom) to avoid any close contact with the larynx. The RLN (running closer to the trachea and esophagus) is also exposed for further stimulation. The electrode is linked to a dual stimulating/blocking device (arrow) capable of producing orderly recruitment of the neural fibers traveling within the nerve. Pairs of spherical contact EMG electrodes placed on the surfaces of the TA through a window in the thyroid cartilage (right side) and the cricopharyngeus (left side) pick up compound motor unit action potentials (CMAPs) illustrating muscle activities. As the blocking current is progressively lifted within the stimulator, sequential activation of small to large axons allows TA and CP CMAPs to be expressed on the screen of the oscilloscope. Pressure changes within the upper esophageal sphincter are recorded via the inflated cuff of an endoluminal endotracheal tube. Lower: CP CMAP amplitudes (lower tracings) decrease as they increase for the TA (upper tracing). (From [47])

tients inspiratory effort, however. In their clinical report, the authors impute some difficulties with mildly breathy and asthenic voice to electrochemical corrosion possibly related to relatively long pulse durations administered [41] as suggested in past work [12, 23]. Direct muscle stimulation remains consistent with prior work of these authors who pioneered rehabilitative laryngeal stimulation by using the detached canine cricothyroideus as a slave muscle from activities originating on the healthy side [42].

Potential Future Human Applications

The progress of clinically implanted devices depends on popular acceptance, subsequent support for ongoing refinements of first generation units, and the application of hypotheses previously verified in the laboratory. The encouraging results so far obtained in clinical practice with fully implantable stimulators may eventually allow low cost alternatives to onerous rehabilitation processes. In an age of therapies still traditionally based on palliative surgeries and medications (e.g., for sedation, hypersecretion, infection, pain control, etc.), advantages offered by well-tolerated artificial organs may help control a wide array of neuromuscular deficits, including those affecting the larynx. Such benefits may arguably well outweigh adverse reactions of traditional approaches such as prescription drugs [43]. A short list of potential FES applications currently under consideration include integrated swallowing rehabilitation, the powering of laryngeal transplants, and artificial voice control.

Integrated Swallowing Rehabilitation

While sphincteric glottic function remains instrumental in securing separation between the airway and the foodway, a no less important end point of the swallowing cascade pertains to coordinated relaxation of the normally tonically occluded upper esophageal sphincter (UES) [28]. The normal reciprocal relationship between the two opposing neuromuscular systems has been artificially reproduced in animals by fully bypassing the brain stem by means of an experimental agonist/antagonist coupling approach [44]. This method requires that reciprocal tone adjustment between laryngeal adductors and the cricopharyngeus (CP) muscle occur over a restored baseline corresponding to levels normally controlled by proprioceptive feedback pathways. This approach offers potential advantages in situations where laryngeal afferents are impaired, especially considering that neural conduits leading to the CP are not always sufficiently well defined (i.e., plexiform) to support an electrode (Fig. 12.4) [45].

Retaining the full benefits of nerve stimulation implies clinical situations where aspiration has not necessarily resulted from a complete breakdown in neural conduction such as would necessitate a complete bypass of the brain stem described above. Since all neurofibers innervating both sphincters travel within the vagus, it is logical to use the nerve for interactive coupling activities, especially in light of the good tolerance of vagal stimulation in the human [46]. This goal may be achieved by using the tripolar blocking circuit in a canine model to activate the faster glottic adductors and relax the smaller axons to the CP along a negative feedback loop and to manipulate force (Fig. 12.5) [47].

Glottal and UES control may be further supplemented with programmed laryngeal elevation, placing electrodes directly into the strap muscles or preferably around their motor nerves [48]. It is not certain, however, that axial aerodigestive pull will not promote glottic opening under given circumstances [49]. At this time, however, it is probably safe to consider that artificial protection of the lungs should eventually combine timely glottic control with some degree of deglutitive aerodigestive ascension.

Laryngeal Transplantation

It is obviously not the purpose of this focused presentation to discuss controversies about true needs and moral issues pertaining to laryngeal transplantation addressed elsewhere in the literature [50, 51]; these notwithstanding, the clinical future of this surgery requires that at least key laryngeal functions be promptly reinstated after their obligatory loss from organ harvest. Canine experiments have clearly demonstrated that the missing sphincteric and respiratory functions could be reanimated by stimulating their supporting ILMs following reinnervation. Laryngeal transplantation would certainly constitute a case study in cybercontrol for neuromuscular integration via glottic electrodynamics [52].

Artificial Control of Voice and Spasm

From a strict perspective of laryngeal pacing, there is probably no conceptual difference between artificial control of voice and the dynamic rehabilitation of the less phylogenetically advanced functions of breathing and swallowing; however, due to its social function, voice production necessitates more attention to fine tuning [53] when compared with those fundamental mechanisms of survival.

Similar to rehabilitation of respiration and deglutition, traditional approaches to voice rehabilitation offer nondynamic solutions. Vocal fold injection and medialization thyroplasty for air escape, denervation for spasmodic dysphonia, and other "static" procedures may be credited with some degrees of success, particularly when breathing and swallowing have remained intact. It is not certain, however, how much fur-

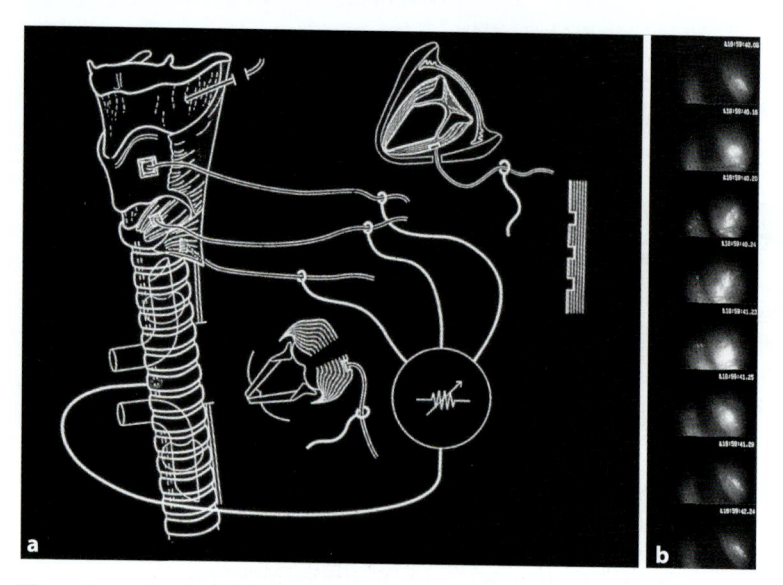

Fig. 12.6. Application of the principle of reciprocal coupling to the artificial production of voice (voice modulation) [53]. The larynx (left side) is completely denervated on one side and the ipsilateral thyroarytenoideus (TA, top), cricothyroideus (CT, middle) and posterior cricoarytenoideus (PCA, bottom) fitted with nerve-muscle pedicles harvested from the ipsilateral sternothyroid muscle. After obtaining baseline tension, amplitudes of currents injected via perineural electrodes into the reinnervated glottic sphincter (TA and CT) and the intact contralateral RLN are reciprocally modulated against PCA tone with a rheostat. Humidified air injected subglottically via the upper cannula interacts with variably paced vocal fold motion (right side) to result in higher pitched sound as the glottis progressively tightens and relaxes. (From [55])

ther progress can be achieved if a dynamic approach continues to be ignored.

Early attempts at voice modeling have used direct RLN stimulation in canine models over a background of transglottic tracheal air flow blown upstream [54]. When the nerve is missing, and compensation has not occurred, voice may be artificially restored with low balancing charges (e.g., 40–45 Hz, 12 mA, 0.02 ms) [55] between normal and reinnervated ILMs over a given level of baseline tone. In this paradigm, variable electronic charges elicit corresponding levels of glottal tension and tightness producing matching fundamental frequencies (Fig. 12.6) [56].

Determining respective excitability patterns of key ILMs involved in voice production (CT, TA, PCA) is a prerequisite to voice manipulation in the non-deafferented larynx. To this end, it has been established that the muscles' recruitment patterns may be correlated with fundamental frequencies (Fo) and intensities (I) of sounds produced under typical conditions of subglottic air pressure. Specifically, the TA was found instrumental in Fo modeling at low intensity levels when balanced with the PCA under vagal control. The CT contractions were found to enhance both Fo and I through TA/PCA coupling, a quality further observed in fine tuning at lower intensities [57]. While this method using blockage by anodal hyperpolarization [19] remains satisfactory for analysis, it does not produce immediate responses of the neuromuscular system to any projected circumstance. Rather, and in order to avoid focused breaks in the stimulating sequence, we have used another algorithm [20], proposing simultaneous stimulation of some ILMs and blockage of others. It was possible to find a statistical correlation between current amplitudes and resulting Fo and I changes along this approach, suggesting that reproducibility in contraction patterns was possible [58].

Fig. 12.7. Block diagram of an experimental closed-loop system for the control of laryngeal spasm. Supramaximal currents (lower circuit) injected into the RLN via a standard bipolar electrode produce forced adductory muscle contraction picked up by an implanted sensor (sonomicrometer crystals within the TA, inset). This afferent information is fed to a second (top) blocking circuit which relaxes (lower right) forced vocal fold adduction (lower left). (From [61])

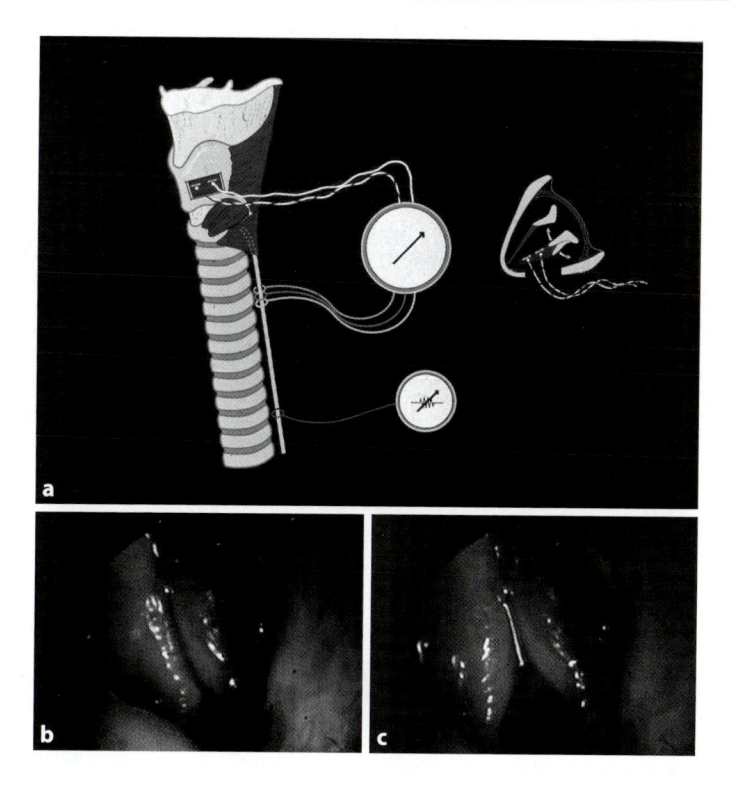

Restoration or boosting of ILM tone for paralysis represents one of the challenging aspects of voice control. Another issue pertains to restricting increasing or untimely changes in muscle tension as may be present in the inappropriate vocal fold adduction and/or abduction typical of spasmodic dysphonia (SD). Whatever its etiology, which remains largely unknown, SD often results in a "fried," "strangled," or weak voice, depending on the neuromuscle(s) involved. In order to suppress the symptoms, Friedman proposed FES with an implantable Medtronic model 3522 stimulator injecting the RLN of a patient with abductor spastic dysphonia with non-blocking 100-Hz, 2–10 mA, and 0.5 ms currents via a bipolar cuff electrode [59]. Improvement in phonation was impressive and there was no reported complication. With the possible failure of regulatory CNS commands to the larynx in mind, however, a more appropriate approach to curbing excessive muscular force may arrest responsible action potentials above a predetermined level of muscular tone judged compatible with normal function [60]. To such effect, neural arrest was produced by hyperpolarizing the RLN based on information picked up over the TA rendered "spastic" by a separate circuit (Fig. 12.7) [61]. In the future, the control of spasm should probably graduate from clipping strength "across the board" to a more specific targeted control of individual ILMs as based on clinical needs.

Conclusion

The practice of surgery has historically evolved through chronological stages of diseased tissue excision, infection control, reconstruction, grafting, and rehabilitation as driven by scientific developments often outside the specialty. Some of the more recent advances use implanted devices specifically designed for the purposes of restoring missing dynamic functions throughout the body; however, and in proportion with their originality, experimental procedures must always test clear-cut hypotheses and once a conclusion is reached, a period of development may begin [62]. While technical advances offered by FES are bountiful, they should be only applied to well-defined laryngeal deficits unable to benefit from more traditional methods. First-generation devices for the control of absent human vocal fold excursion offer promise, but further trials are necessary for confirmation prior to proceeding with improved designs. Meanwhile, while animal experimentation may not always directly apply to the human, founding hypotheses remain generally true. In all cases, the laboratory remains a necessary passage for verification and future applications in research and development in the more sophisticated aspects of laryngology.

References

1. Stedman's Medical Dictionary, 27th edn (1999) Lippincott, Williams and Wilkins, Philadelphia, p 1311
2. Taber's Cyclopedic Medical Dictionary, 19th edn (2001) F.A. Davies, Philadelphia, p 1575
3. Crumley RL (1982) Experiments in laryngeal reinnervation. Laryngoscope (Suppl 30) 92:1–27
4. Van Lith-Bijl JT et al. (1996) Laryngeal abductor function after recurrent laryngeal nerve injury in cats. Arch Otolaryngol Head Neck Surg 122:393–396
5. Sasaki CT, Buchwalter J (1984) Laryngeal function. Am J Otolaryngol 5:281–291
6. Gilman S, Winans S (1982) Spinal reflexes and muscle tone. In: Gatz AJ (ed) Manter and Gatz' s essentials of clinical neuroanatomy and neurophysiology, 6th edn. F.A. Davis, Philadelphia, pp 19–24
7. Wyke BD, Kirchner JA (1976) Neurology of the larynx. In: Harrison DFN, Hichcliffe R (eds) Scientific foundations of otolaryngology. Year-Book, Chicago, pp 546–576
8. Lazorthes Y et al. (1985) Neurostimulation, an overview. Biotechnological basis of biostimulation. Futura, Mt. Kisco, N.Y., pp 11–17
9. Crumley RL (1985) Update of laryngeal reinnervation concepts and options. In: Bailey BJ, Biller HF (eds) Surgery of the larynx. Saunders, Philadelphia, pp 135–147
10. Malmgren LT, Gacek RR (1981) Histochemical characteristics of muscle fiber types in the posterior cricoarytenoid muscle. Ann Otol Rhinol Laryngol 90:423–429
11. Broniatowski M et al. (1998) Long-term stimulation of nerve pedicles implanted in strap muscles in the canine. Ann Otol Rhinol Laryngol 107:301–311
12. Broniatowski M et al. (1986) Laryngeal pacemaker. Part I: Electronic pacing of reinnervated strap muscles in the dog. Otolaryngol Head Neck Surg 94:41–44
13. Blair E, Erlanger J (1934) A comparison of the characteristics of axons through their individual electrical response. Am J Physiol 6:524–564
14. Henneman E et al. (1965) Functional significance of cell size in spinal motor neurons . J Neurophysiol 28:560–580
15. Eisele DW (1996) Intraoperative electrophysiologic monitoring of the recurrent laryngeal nerve. Laryngoscope 106:443–449
16. Sweeney JD, Mortimer JT (1986) An Asymmetric two electrode cuff generation of unidirectional propagated action potentials. IEEE Trans Biomed Eng 33:541–549
17. Van den Honert C, Mortimer JT (1981) A technique for collision block of peripheral nerve. Frequency dependence. IEEE Trans Biomed Eng 28:373–378
18. Broniatowski M et al. (1996) Contraction patterns in intrinsic laryngeal muscles in the canine. Laryngoscope 106:1510–1515
19. Barratta R et al. (1989) Orderly stimulation of skeletal motor units with tripolar cuff electrodes. IEEE Trans Biomed Eng 36:836–843
20. Fang ZP, Mortimer JT (1991) Selective activation of small motor axons by quasitrapezoidal current pulses. IEEE Trans Biomed Eng 38:168–174
21. Schachter SC, Wheless JW (2002) Vagus nerve stimulation therapy 5 years after approval: a comprehensive update. Neurology 59 (Suppl 4):S1–S61
22. Broniatowski M et al. (2001) Dynamic laryngeal closure for aspiration: a preliminary report. Laryngoscope 111:2032–2040
23. Broniatowski M et al. (1985) Laryngeal pacemaker II. Electronic pacing of reinnervated posterior cricoarytenoid muscles in the canine. Laryngoscope 95:11941–198
24. Broderick J et al. (1998) The Greater Cincinnati/Kentucky Stroke Study: preliminary first ever and total incidence rate of strokes among blacks. Stroke:29:415–421
25. Agency for Health Policy and Research (AHCPR) (1999) Diagnosis and treatment of swallowing disorders (Dysphagia) in acute car stroke patients. Evidence Report/Technology Assessment no. 8. AHCPR publication no. 99-E024, Rockville, Maryland

26. Schmidt et al. (1994) Videofluoroscopic evidence of aspiration predicts pneumonia and death but not dehydration following stroke. Dysphagia 9:7–11
27. Hughes TAT, Wiles CM (2000) The neurologists' perspective of the patient with dysphagia. In: Rubin JS, Broniatowski M, Kelly JH (eds) The swallowing manual. Singular Publishing Group, Thomson Learning, San Diego, California, pp 119–136
28. Broniatowski M et al. (1999) Current evaluation and treatment of patients with swallowing disorders. Otolaryngol Head Neck Surg 120:464–473
29. Broniatowski M et al. (1987) A potential solution for chronic aspiration. I. Cutaneous biologic sensors in the neck triggering strap muscle contractions in the canine. Laryngoscope 97:331–333
30. Broniatowski M et al. (1988) Artificial reflex arc: II. A potential solution for chronic aspiration. A canine study based on a laryngeal prosthesis. Laryngoscope 98:235–237
31. Broniatowski M et al. (1994) Artificial reflex arc: III. A potential solution for chronic aspiration. Stimulation of implanted cervical skin triggering glottic closure in the canine. Laryngoscope 104:1259–1263
32. Rijkhoff NMJ et al. (1997) Urinary bladder control by electrical stimulation: review of electrical stimulation techniques in spinal cord injury. Neurourol Urodyn 16:39–53
33. Tarver WB et al. (1992) Clinical experiments with a helical stimulating electrode. PACE 15:1545–1546
34. Furnary A et al. (1991) Perineural leads and burst stimulation optimize contraction of skeletal muscle. ASAIO Trans 37:M164–M166
35. Hössly H (1916) Ueber Nervenimplantation bei Recurrentlahmungen, Eine Experimentale Studie. Beitrage zur Klinischen Chirurgie 99:186–192
36. Tucker HM et al. (1976) Human laryngeal reinnervation. Laryngoscope 86:769–779
37. Grundfest-Broniatowski S et al. (1989) Artificial myotatic reflex: a potential avenue to fine motor control. Otolaryngol Head Neck Surg 101:621–628
38. Broniatowski M et al. (1990) Excitation thresholds for nerves reinnervating the paralysed canine larynx. Trans Am Soc Artif Inter Organs 36:M432–M434
39. Anonsen CK et al. (1985) Reinnervation of skeletal muscles with a neuromuscular pedicle. Otolaryngol Head Neck Surg 93:48–57
40. Fata JJ et al. (1987) Histochemical evidence of posterior ricoarytenoid reinnervation by a nerve muscle pedicle in the cat. Ann Otol Rhinol Laryngol 96:479–487
41. Zealar DI et al. (2003) Reanimation of the paralysed human larynx with an implantable electric stimulating device. Laryngoscope 113:11491–156
42. Zealar DI, Dedo HH (1977) Control of paralyzed axial muscles by electrical stimulation. Acta Otolaryngol (Stockh) 83:514–527
43. Nose Y (1998) Please stop killing so many patients by drugs: artificial organs will not kill so many patients (Editorial). Artif Organs 22:7–23
44. Broniatowski M et al. (1989) Artificial agonist/antagonist coupling in the paralysed face. I: Electronic balance of reinnervated strap muscles from facial activity in the rabbit. Laryngoscope 99:647–650
45. Broniatowski M et al. (1995) Electronic integration of glottic closure and cricopharyngeal relaxation for the control of aspiration. A canine study. Otolaryngol Head Neck Surg 424–429
46. Lambert et al. (2000) Vagus nerve stimulation. Quality control in thyroid and parathyroid surgery. J Laryngol Otol 114:125–127
47. Broniatowski M et al. (1999) Vagal stimulation for reciprocal coupling between glottic and upper esophageal sphincter activities in the canine. Dysphagia 14:196–203
48. Ludlow C et al. (1999) Three dimensional changes in the upper airway during neuromuscular stimulation of laryngeal muscles. Artif Organs 23:463–465
49. Fink B (1974) Folding mechanisms of the human larynx. Acta Oto-Laryngol (Stockh) 78:124–128
50. Daly JF (1970) Is laryngeal transplantation justifiable? Laryngoscope 80 1251–1255
51. Strome M et al. (2001) Laryngeal transplantation and 40-month follow-up. N Engl J Med. 344:1676–1679
52. Broniatowski M (1988) Bionic larynx: electronic control of the reimplanted organ in the dog. Laryngoscope 98:1107–1115
53. Gould WB, Okamura H (1974) Interrelationship between laryngeal mucosal reflexes. In: Wyke BD (ed) Voluntary and phonatory control systems. An international symposium. Oxford University Press, London, pp 347–369
54. Berke GS et al. (1987) Laryngeal modeling: theoretical, in vitro, in vivo. Laryngoscope 97:871–881
55. Broniatowski M et al. (1990) Artificial restoration of voice. I: Experiments in phonatory control of the reinnervated larynx. Laryngoscope 100:1219–1224
56. Wyke BD (1974) Laryngeal muscular control systems in singing. A review of current concepts. Folia Phoniatr (Basel) 26:295–306
57. Broniatowski M et al. (2002) Electronic analysis of intrinsic laryngeal muscle contributions to canine sound production. Ann Otol Rhinol Laryngol 111:542–552
58. Broniatowski M et al. (2004) Artificial manipulation of voice in a canine model. Abstract, 9th Int

Workshop on Laser Voice Surgery and Voice Care, Paris, France
59. Friedman M et al. (1989) Implantation of a recurrent laryngeal nerve stimulator for the treatment of spastic dysphonia. Ann Otol Rhinol Laryngol 98:130–134
60. Broniatowski M et al. (1990) Electronic control of laryngeal spasm. I: Blockage of orthodromically induced action potentials in intact canine recurrent laryngeal nerves. Laryngoscope 100:892–895
61. Broniatowski M et al. (1993) Electronic control of laryngeal spasm. II: Selective blockage of glottic adduction by a closed loop in the canine. Laryngoscope 103:734–740
62. Nose Y (1998) Do you know what you are doing? Editorial. Artif Organs 22:625–626
63. Broniatowski M et al. (1995) Electronic integration of glottic closure and cricopharyngeal relaxation for the control of aspiration: a canine study. Otolaryngol Head Neck Surg 112:424–429
64. Villiers R de, Nose Y, Meier W, Kantrowitz A (1964) Long-term electrostimulation of a peripheral nerve. Trans Am Soc Artif Int Organs 10:357–365
65. Bergman K, Warzel H, Echardt U, Hopstock U, Gerhardt HJ (1984) Respiratory rhythmically regulated electrical stimulation of paralysed laryngeal muscles. Laryngoscope 94:1376–1380
66. Obert PM, Young KA, Tobey DN (1984) Use of direct posterior cricoarytenoid stimulation in laryngeal paralysis. Arch Otolaryngol 110:88–92
67. Otto RA, Templer J, Davis W, Homeyer D, Stroble M (1985) Coordinated electrical pacing of vocal cord abductors in recurrent laryngeal nerve paralysis. Otolaryngol Head Neck Surg 93:634–638
68. Kojima H, Omori K, Shoji K et al. (1990) Laryngeal pacing in unilateral vocal cord paralysis. Arch Otolaryngol Head Neck Surg 116:74–78
69. Kano S, Sasaki CT (1991) Pacing parameters of the canine posterior cricoarytenoid muscle. Ann Otol Rhinol Laryngol 100:584–588
70. Sanders I (1991) Electrical stimulation of laryngeal muscle. Otolaryngol Clin Norh Am 93:634–638
71. Zealear DL, Rainey CL, Jerles ML, Tanabe T, Herzon GD (1994) Technical approach for reanimation of the chronically denervated larynx by means of functional electrical stimulation. Ann Otol Rhinol Laryngol 103:705–712
72. Zealear DL, Rainey CL, Netterville JL, Herzon GD, Ossoff RH (1996) Electrical pacing of the paralysed human larynx. Ann Otol Rhinol Laryngol 105:689–693
73. Broniatowski M, Dessoffy R, Strome M (1998) Long-term excitability and fine tuning of nerve pedicles reinnervating strap muscles in the dog. Ann Otol Rhinol Laryngol 107:301–311

Chapter 13

Bilateral Medialization Laryngoplasty

Gregory N. Postma, Peter C. Belafsky

Introduction

Bilateral medialization laryngoplasty (BML) is an innovative procedure for voice and swallowing rehabilitation. It is an excellent surgical option for many patients with symptomatic glottal insufficiency. The glottal insufficiency may be secondary to any combination of vocal fold atrophy (presbylaryngis), vocal fold paresis and paralysis, and abductor spasmodic dysphonia. The purpose of this chapter is to discuss the indications, technique, patient selection, complications, and expected results of BML.

Unlike unilateral medialization laryngoplasty (ML), which has become widely accepted for the treatment of paralytic dysphonia [1–4], the indications and techniques used for *bilateral* ML have not been well described and are still being refined [5–8].

Initially, the surgical treatment of vocal fold bowing attempted to increase vocal fold tension [9–13]. In 1974, Isshiki et al. [9, 10] reported cricothyroid approximation in which mattress sutures were placed between the thyroid and the cricoid cartilages. Usually, the procedures were done in an attempt to elevate the pitch of the patient's voice, but in two cases, the procedure was performed to treat vocal fold bowing due to superior laryngeal neuropathy. LeJeune et al. [11] reported another technique for increasing vocal fold tension, in which an inferiorly based rectangular flap of the thyroid cartilage was pulled anteriorly and secured by a tantalum shim. Two years later, Tucker [12] reported a variation of LeJeune's method, using a superiorly based cartilage flap. In a subsequent report by Tucker [13], ten of ten patients with vocal fold bowing experienced immediate voice improvement with his procedure. Only three, however, maintained the improvement 6 months after surgery.

In 1986, Koufman [2] combined an anterior laryngoplastic approach (anterior commissure advancement) with a unilateral ML in two patients who had unilateral paralysis with bilateral vocal fold atrophy. In 1989, Koufman [5] first reported the BML procedure specifically for the treatment of vocal fold bowing. Postma et al. presented a series of 39 BML patients in 1998 with 90% of them obtaining successful outcomes [8].

Surgical Indications

Bilateral ML may be used to correct mild to severe degrees of glottal insufficiency, even if the vocal folds are normally mobile. The postoperative improvement in closure is achieved by the placement of permanent space-occupying material (Gore-Tex or Silastic in our practice) adjacent to the vocal folds. This improves glottal closure by straightening the vocal folds.

Our current indications for BML include: (a) presbylaryngis; (b) bilateral vocal fold paresis; (c) unilateral vocal fold paralysis with contralateral bowing; and (d) some neurological conditions such as Parkinson's disease and abductor-type SD.

Surgical Technique

We emphasize that the technique of BML that we use for the treatment of bowed (but mobile) vocal folds is *not* the same as the standard ML for unilateral vocal fold paralysis [8, 14, 15].

The technique differs in three principal ways:

1. Overcorrection anteriorly must be carefully avoided, since excessive anterior medialization will cause a harsh, strained voice. This error can easily occur during the performance of a BML.
2. The posterior portion of the implant must not contact the vocal process of the arytenoid cartilage. Since the vocal folds are mobile, an implant projecting far posteriorly could impinge on the arytenoid, and thus restrict arytenoid motion. In active individuals this can result in dyspnea upon exertion.
3. The implants should be fixed in place, because the vocal folds are still mobile, and therefore, displacement or extrusion may be more likely than in ML for paralysis.

A number of different implant materials have been used for ML including Silastic shims, preformed thyroplasty implants [16], hydroxylapatite implants [17], and Gore-Tex [18, 19]. We prefer Gore-Tex for BML for a variety of reasons. In our hands it is faster than using Silastic, creates less edema, decreases the chance of overcorrecting the anterior commissure, and allows placement of the implants closer to the vocal process without limiting its movement.

Bilateral medialization laryngoplasty is always performed under local anesthesia with intravenous sedation. Preoperatively, each patient is given intravenous betamethasone and antibiotics. The neck is prepared and draped with the head in a neutral position, and a fiberoptic laryngoscope is placed through one nostril after topical anesthesia and decongestion and suspended from a flexible laryngoscope holder [3]. The laryngoscope is coupled to a video monitor to allow intraoperative real-time visualization of the larynx.(Fig. 13.1). Local anesthesia is infiltrated along the anticipated 5- to 8-cm incision, which is usually made over the inferior third of the thyroid cartilage in a skin crease. Then, small subplatysmal flaps are elevated, and the strap muscles are divided at the midline raphe and reflected laterally to expose the thyroid alae.

When using Gore-Tex, an inferiorly based outer perichondrial flap is elevated off of the thyroid ala (Fig. 13.2). This is followed by removal of a small window of cartilage overlying the vocal fold. The laryngoplasty window location is determined by needle localization under direct visualization with the transnasal flexible laryngoscope. An 18-G needle is used to gently bore through the cartilage and then a 27-G needle is passed through the hole in the

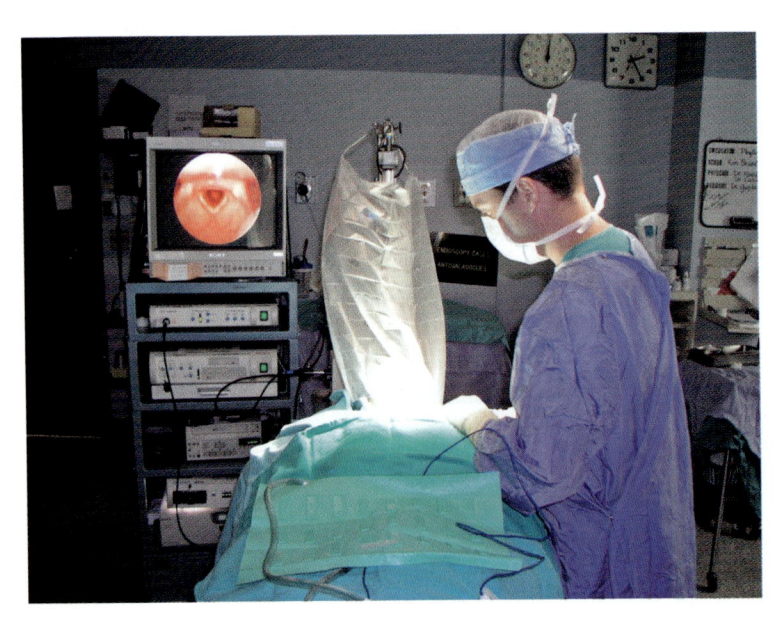

Fig. 13.1. The general setup of the operating suite. The flexible laryngoscope is in place and sterilely draped giving the surgeon a "real-time" view of the larynx

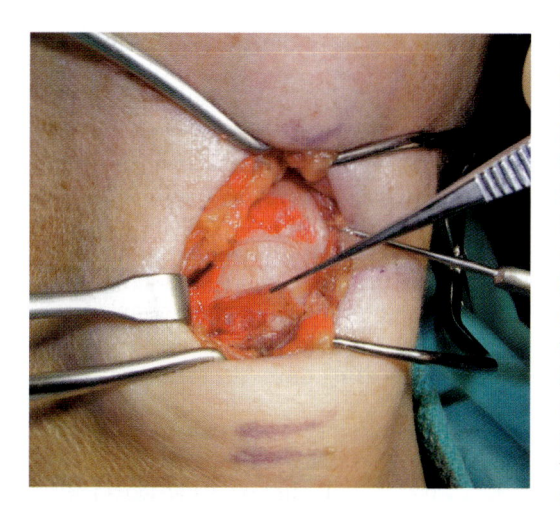

Fig. 13.2 The outer perichondrium is elevated off of the right thyroid ala and will be sutured over the implant at the conclusion of the procedure.

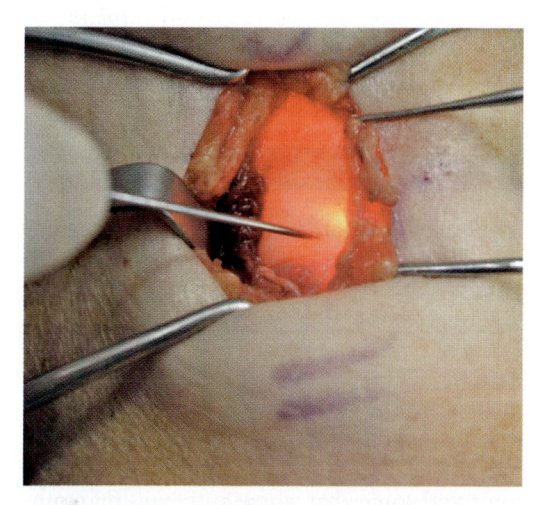

Fig. 13.3. A needle is gently passed through the cartilage determining vocal fold position prior to making the laryngoplasty window

cartilage to precisely localize the level of the vocal fold.(Fig. 13.3). Using that as a guide, small rectangular windows are then marked on the thyroid cartilage approximately 4–6 mm posterior to the midline of the thyroid cartilage and usually 2–3 mm superior to the inferior border of each thyroid ala; these are usually approximately 3–4 x 8–12 mm in size. The long axis is placed parallel to the lower border of the thyroid alae. These windows are made using a scalpel or a drill with a 3- or 4-mm cutting burr. A small Kerrison rongeur is also often helpful in removing cartilage. After removal of the cartilage window, the inner perichondrium is incised with a no. 15 or no. 11 scalpel blade. We believe that incising the perichondrium allows a much more precise control of medialization (particularly adjacent to the vocal process) with less chance for medialization of ventricular mucosa. In addition, an increased implant extrusion rate has never been reported in those patients. If there is any difference between the vocal folds, we correct the paralyzed fold, or the more bowed, or paretic, side first. After the inner perichondrium is incised, a small pocket is formed using the Woodson elevator and the vocal folds are medialized with a Woodson or Freer elevator. The effect is observed on the video monitor and using vocal feedback from the patient. Gore-Tex, which has been previously soaked in an antibiotic solution, is cut in a 3- to 4-mm-wide strip and layered in the window. The implant is placed as a stacked strip and its shape can be easily adjusted to medialize the vocal fold optimally [8, 14]. Once the preferred voice is obtained, the vocal folds are overcorrected to compensate for intraoperative edema and implant compression (Fig. 13.4). The implant is stabilized by suturing the outer perichondrial flap in its original position with 4–0 nylon sutures.

If Silastic is used, the implants are carved out of firm block Silastic (Dow Corning Corporation, Medical Products, Midland, Mich.). One or both implants may be removed to be reshaped in order to improve the vocal result. The implants, regardless of how firmly they are seated in the windows, are then secured to the cartilage itself or the surrounding perichondrium with three to four 4–0 nylon sutures. A small suction drain is rarely employed and the wound is then closed in layers. Patients are observed overnight and discharged the following morning. Patients are given oral antibiotics for 1 week. Figure 13.5 shows the appearance of a completed BML procedure.

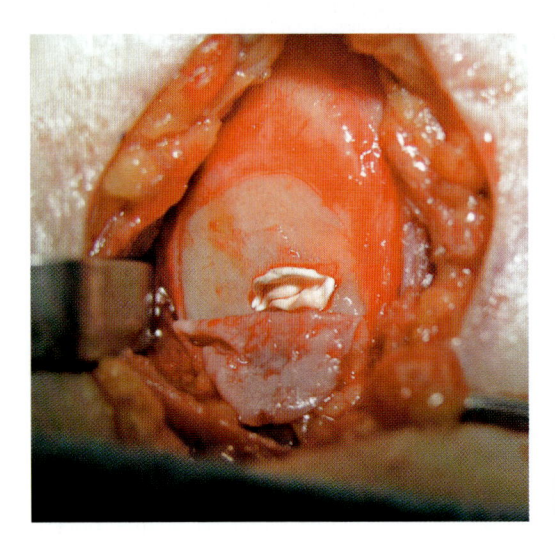

Fig. 13.4. The Gore-Tex implant layered into the window

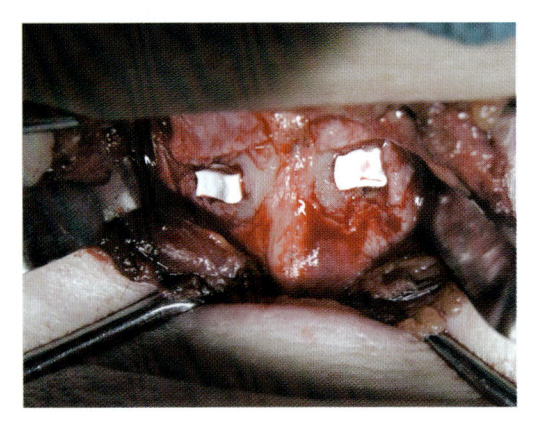

Fig. 13.5. A completed bilateral medialization laryngoplasty

Results

In our institution's initial series of 39 BML patients using Silastic implants [8], 90% (35 of 39) of the patients experienced subjective improvement in voice and/or swallowing function. Patients with aspiration and/or dysphagia appeared to benefit significantly from BML. Of the 20 individuals with dysphagia and/or aspiration in this cohort, 14 had improved swallowing function, 4 were unchanged, and 2 had worsened dysphagia but no aspiration. All 6 patients with frank aspiration preoperatively stopped aspirating after surgery. This included 2 patients in the vocal fold paralysis group, 2 with degenerative neuromuscular disorders, 1 with bilateral paresis, and 1 with presbylaryngis. One gastrostomy-dependent patient in our study (myotonic dystrophy) was able to have his gastrostomy tube removed after BML. Some of these individuals underwent adjunctive lipoinjection. Our more recent series of 89 BML patients using Gore-Tex showed a similar success rate [14].

Complications

Complications are rare. Our combined series of 128 patients yielded a total of four complications (3%). There were two extrusions in the Silastic group and two displaced implants in the Gore-Tex group; all underwent successful revision surgery.

Discussion

Incomplete glottal closure can cause dysphonia, vocal fatigue, effortful phonation, diplophonia, aphonia, dysphagia, and aspiration. The degree of glottal insufficiency and the severity of symptoms may be interrelated, or they may be a function of the specific underlying medical condition. This point is reinforced by the observation that patients with degenerative neurological diseases have more severe symptoms and somewhat worse outcomes than other groups of patients. Conversely, patients with unilateral paralysis and pre-existing presbylaryngis who underwent ipsilateral medialization (with or without arytenoid adduction), as well as a contralateral medialization procedure, had uniformly excellent results. The postoperative voices in this group were superior to the voice of the patients prior to the onset of the paralysis.

Approach to Surgical Treatment

The majority of patients with glottal insufficiency do not require (or desire) surgery. In general, surgery is indicated for patients with life-altering symptoms, and the decision to perform surgery is multifactorial, with the severity of the patient's symptoms and the patient's needs being key variables. For most individuals with mild glottal insufficiency, their symptoms do not alter their lifestyles or professions and surgery is not indicated.

In our hands, BML provides the best option for surgical treatment of symptomatic patients with moderate to severe vocal fold atrophy/bowing or paresis. For mild glottal insufficiency, when the glottal gap is 1 mm or less, we recommend autologous fat or calcium hydroxylapatite (CaHA) injection [20].

Some patients require more than one procedure to correct vocal fold bowing, particularly those with glottal gaps of 4 mm or more. In some cases closure can also be improved when needed by staged, adjunctive injection augmentation with CaHA or fat. Adjunctive injection augmentation is especially worthwhile in patients with a persistent gap just anterior to the vocal processes. This area is difficult to correct by BML, because of the need to avoid using large posterior implants that might impact the vocal processes. In practice, we counsel patients preoperatively that injection may be employed as a secondary procedure and that the two procedures are complimentary. Our revision rate is just under 10%.

It is important to emphasize that BML helps facilitate glottal closure, but it does *not* improve neuromuscular function. In addition, BML does not improve pulmonary function, breath support for speech, or other illnesses. Patients who have very poor pulmonary function do not respond particularly well to BML, because they lack sufficient subglottal pressure to drive the vocal folds. We cannot overemphasize the importance of careful patient selection for BML.

Conclusion

Bilateral medialization laryngoplasty appears to be a safe and effective treatment for patients with glottal incompetence due to a wide array of causes. Patients with degenerative neuromuscular diseases and/or poor pulmonary function appear to have inferior results when compared with those with paralysis, paresis, or presbylaryngis. Appropriate patient selection is essential.

References

1. Isshiki N, Okamura H, Ishikawa T (1975) Thyroplasty type I (lateral compression) for dysphonia due to vocal cord paralysis or atrophy. Acta Otolaryngol (Stockh) 80:465–473
2. Koufman JA (1986) Laryngoplasty for vocal cord medialization: an alternative to Teflon. Laryngoscope 96:726–731
3. Wanamaker JR, Netterville JL, Ossoff RH (1993) Phonosurgery. Silastic medialization for unilateral vocal fold paralysis. Oper Techniques Otolaryngol Head Neck Surg 4:207–217
4. Maves MD, McCabe BF, Gray S (1989) Phonosugery: indications and pitfalls. Ann Otol Rhinol Laryngol 98:577–580
5. Koufman JA (1989) Surgical correction of dysphonia due to bowing of the vocal cords. Ann Otol Rhinol Laryngol 98:41–45
6. Koufman JA, Isaacson G (1991) Laryngoplastic phonosurgery. Otolaryngol Clin N Am 24:1151–1177
7. Isshiki N, Shoji K, Kojima H, Hirano S (1996) Vocal fold atrophy and its surgical treatment. Ann Otol Rhinol Laryngol 105:182–188
8. Postma GN, Blalock PD, Koufman JA (1998) Bilateral medialization laryngoplasty. Laryngoscope 108:1429–1434
9. Isshiki N, Morita H, Okamura H, Hiramoto M (1974) Thyroplasty as a new phonosurgical technique. Acta Otolaryngol 78:451–457
10. Isshiki N, Taira T, Tanube M (1983) Surgical alternation of the vocal pitch. J Otolaryngol 12:335–340
11. LeJeune FE, Guice CE, Samuels PM (1983) Early experiences with vocal ligament tightening. Ann Otol Rhinol Laryngol 92:475–477
12. Tucker HM (1985) Anterior commissure laryngoplasty for adjustment of vocal fold tension. Ann Otol Rhinol Laryngol 94:547–549
13. Tucker HM (1988) Laryngeal framework surgery and the management of the aged larynx. Ann Otol Rhinol Laryngol 97:534–536

14. Cohen JT, Bates DD, Postma GN (2004) Revision Gore-Tex medialization laryngoplasty. Otol Head Neck Surg 131:236–240
15. Koufman JA, Postma GN (1999) Bilateral medialization laryngoplasty. Oper Techniques Otolaryngol Head Neck Surg 10:321–324
16. Montgomery WM, Blaugrund SM, Varvares MA (1993) Thyroplasty: a new approach. Acta Otol Rhinol Laryngol 102:571–579
17. Cummings CW, Purcell LL, Flint PW (1993) Hydroxylapatite laryngeal implants for medialization. Preliminary report. Ann Otol Rhinol Laryngol 102:843–851
18. Hoffman HT, McCulloch TM (1996) Anatomic considerations in the surgical treatment of unilateral laryngeal paralysis. Head Neck 18:174–187
19. Zeitels SM, Mauri M, Dailey SH (2003) Medialization laryngoplasty with Gore-Tex for voice restoration secondary to glottal incompetence: indications and observations. Ann Otol Rhinol Laryngol 112:180–184
20. Belafsky PC, Postma GN (2004) Vocal fold augmentation using calcium hydroxylapatite. Otol Head Neck Surg 131:351–354

Chapter 14

Vocal Fold Paralysis in Children

Marshall E. Smith

Introduction

Stridor and hoarseness are frequently encountered by otolaryngologists who care for children, so vocal fold paralysis is usually on their mind. It is generally a straightforward diagnosis to make, especially in the past 20 years with the use of the flexible fiberoptic laryngoscope. Once vocal fold paralysis is identified, the otolaryngologist has two tasks: to identify the etiology of the condition and to decide among options for treatment. In children, there are a variety of causes of vocal fold paralysis that are not usually considered in adults. The age of the children influences treatment decisions, with special attention to airway considerations in infants.

This chapter reviews the presentations of vocal fold paralysis, with focus on age-related differences. The causes of vocal fold paralysis are reviewed, and other tests in evaluation of the problem are discussed. The options for treatment, as in adults, depend on whether the deficit is unilateral or bilateral, and address the attendant airway, feeding, and voice problems. These options are outlined with attention to some new choices in management.

Spectrum of Presentation

Over 500 cases of pediatric vocal fold paralysis have been tabulated in many case series and case reports [1–14]. Several patterns emerge from these cases. Bilateral vocal fold paralysis (BVFP) is more commonly seen in neonates, whereas unilateral vocal fold paralysis (UVFP) is seen more commonly in older children. There is significant overlap, however. Although the distinction between unilateral and bilateral is commonly made, patients are not always so easily compartmentalized. The entity may even be descriptively termed "impaired vocal fold mobility" [15]. There is a spectrum of vocal fold movement impairment. The term "paralysis" implies a complete lower motor neuron dysfunction, but in practice there is often motion impairment without complete flaccidity or denervation [16]. Some adductor movement may be seen even though abductor movement is impaired. Dysfunctional innervation of the "paralyzed" vocal fold, rather than complete denervation, is likely responsible for the spectrum of observations regarding laryngeal movement in vocal fold paralysis [17]. Other causes of impaired vocal fold mobility include cricoarytenoid joint fixation and interarytenoid scar; these may only be able to be distinguished by microlaryngoscopy under general anesthesia.

Table 14.1 is a modification of Dedo and Dedo [18] which includes an extensive list of the causes of vocal fold paralysis in children. This list can be somewhat intimidating; however, most causes of laryngeal paralysis are evident from the history, physical examination, and imaging studies of the patient. The categorization of these into central neurological conditions, cardiac anomalies, post-surgical or neck trauma, infectious and inflammatory causes, and idiopathic is similar to that in adults. As children get older, unilateral vocal fold paralysis becomes more common, with similar etiologies as are seen in adults. Other reported causes of laryngeal paralysis are mentioned, including vincristine neurotoxicity [19, 20], vagal nerve stimulator implant [21], esophageal foreign body ingestion [22], and cricopharyngeal stenosis [23].

Table 14.1. Etiologies of laryngeal paralysis in infants and children

Congenital
    Central nervous system
    Cerebral agenesis
    Hydrocephalus
    Encephalocele
    Meningomyelocele
    Meningocele
    Arnold-Chiari malformation
    Nucleus ambiguous dysgenesis
    Peripheral nervous system
    Congenital myasthenia gravis
    Skull base platybasia
    Cardiovascular anomalies
    Cardiomegaly
    Interventricular septal defect
    Tetralogy of Fallot
    Abnormal great vessels
    Vascular ring
    Dilated aorta
    Double aortic arch
    Patent ductus arteriosus
    Transposition of the great vessels
    Associated with other congenital anomalies
    Bronchogenic cyst
    Esophageal cyst, duplication, atresia
    Cricopharyngeal stenosis
Inherited
    Genetic
    Autosomal dominant
    Autosomal recessive
    X-linked
    Isolated mutation
    Associated neurologic disease
    Charcot-Marie-Tooth disease
Acquired
    Trauma
    Birth injury
    Postsurgical correction of cardiovascular or esophageal abnormalities
    Vagal nerve stimulator
    Foreign body ingestion
    Infections
    Pertussis encephalitis
    Polyneuritis
    Polioencephalitis
    Diphtheria
    Rabies
    Syphilis
    Tetanus
    Botulism
    Tuberculosis
    Guillain-Barré syndrome
    Neurotoxicity
    Vincristine

The Newborn and Infant: Airway and Swallowing Assessment and Management

The neonate or infant with stridor demands urgent attention. This situation may arise at or shortly after birth, after extubation, or spontaneously. The pediatrician or neonatologist relies on the otolaryngologist to evaluate the problem and direct treatment. Although vocal fold paralysis is only one of the causes of stridor, it is an important one and is generally regarded as the second most common congenital laryngeal anomaly (next to laryngomalacia), accounting for 10% of all cases [7].

The airway is intimately tied to swallowing in infants, due to the high position of the larynx in the neck and their physiology as preferential nasal breathers. There is a spectrum of findings in infants with respect to nasal breathing [24]. Airway obstruction anywhere from the nasal valve through the upper aerodigestive tract often affects the infant's ability to swallow. Because the swallowing reflex is still developing, the infant can be at increased risk for aspiration from laryngeal problems such as unilateral vocal fold paralysis, as compared with the adult.

Table 14.2 summarizes various published series that focus on newborns and infants. An interesting finding is that BFVP is generally more commonly seen than UVFP. An exception is the report by Zbar and Smith [6], in which they acknowledge a high number of PDA ligations at their institution. The volume of pediatric cardiothoracic surgery will affect the frequency of UVFP that is seen at an individual center, whereas the occurrence of BFVP should be fairly consistent. A few case reports exist of congenital cardiac anomalies that cause left UVFP, an infant form of Ortner's cardiovocal syndrome [25–27].

The first examination of the infant with stridor is flexible laryngoscopy. This examination is not always straightforward in infants and small children. Assessment of vocal fold movement may be affected by the rapid respiratory rate, vigorous breathing, and movement of the larynx, swallowing, overlying supraglottic tissues, and arytenoid cartilages which are large relative to the length of the membranous folds

Table 14.2. Vocal fold paralysis series in neonates and infants

Reference	Age	Bilateral	Unilateral
[6]	0–12 months	4	13
[7]	Birth	56	28
[3]	0–12 months	11	8
[9]	Congenital	13	6
[11]	Congenital	52	61
[12]	0–12 months	42	18
[1]	0–12 months	12	10
[96]	Neonatal	28	8

when compared with adults. Flexible laryngoscopes may not pass easily through the nose; thus, the exam can be done via the peroral route, if needed [96]. The author prefers videotaping these examinations so that they can be reviewed frame by frame should the "real-time" examination be ambiguous. If vocal fold paralysis is suspected but cannot be confirmed, follow-up examinations are needed. Another option to assess vocal fold mobility in infants and children is laryngeal ultrasound. Friedman studied 15 normal patients (ages 1 month to 14 years) and 12 patients with vocal fold paralysis (ages 1 day to 8 years) with laryngeal ultrasound and found that blinded raters of the recorded examinations could reliably distinguish between the groups with an accuracy of 87–94% [28]. The question of when to perform laryngoscopy under anesthesia in these cases is reasonable. The advantages of general anesthesia allow a more systematic examination of the entire upper airway. This is helpful in looking for concomitant airway obstructive lesions, and palpating the arytenoid cartilages to rule out arytenoid fixation. If laryngeal EMG is done, general anesthesia is usually required for infants and small children. It should be recognized that the sedation from general anesthesia affects vocal fold mobility assessment. An immobile vocal fold seen under general anesthesia should be confirmed with the child awake using the flexible laryngoscope in the recovery room, or later. In the practice of the present author, an uncomplicated (no serious airway obstruction symptoms) case of clearly diagnosed UVFP by flexible laryngoscopy does not require a subsequent examination under general anesthesia. Bilateral vocal fold paralysis, or complicated cases when other airway pathology is suspected, requires an evaluation of the airway in the operating room. This includes palpation of the arytenoid to rule out cricoarytenoid fixation.

When a vocal fold paralysis is identified (unilateral or bilateral), the cause should be investigated if it is not evident from the history and examination. In infants this usually means obtaining an MRI of the brain to look for a central neurological abnormality.

Management of Airway, Voice, and Swallowing in Vocal Fold Paralysis in Infants

The airway of the infant with vocal fold paralysis is of pre-eminent concern. The main issue involves the need for tracheostomy. In most cases of unilateral vocal fold paralysis presented tracheostomy is not needed, as substantiated by the findings in Table 14.3. In 32 cases of UVFP diagnosed at birth or infancy at our institution from 1997–2002, none required a tracheotomy (personal observation). In bilateral vocal fold paralysis, this issue is more complicated. Table 14.3 reveals that in most older studies the practice was to perform a tracheostomy in most cases of bilateral vocal fold paralysis. However, there are also a substantial percentage of infants with bilateral vocal fold

Table 14.3. Frequency of tracheostomy in several published case series of infant vocal fold paralysis

Reference	Bilateral	Unilateral
[7]	36 of 56 Birth	3 of 28
[8]	45 of 62	0 of 38
[3]	7 of 13	
[10]	19 of 29	8 of 22
[5]	0 of 11	
[6]	0 of 4	0 of 13
[11]	10 of 52	0 of 61
[12]	28 of 49	7 of 53
Average	145 of 276 (53%)	18 of 215 (8%)

paralysis that have been managed without a tracheostomy. This includes an astounding 11 of 11 patients reported by Murty et al. [5]. In their study, all patients had eventual recovery of vocal fold movement at 5–26 months. Improvements in neonatal care, the assessment and monitoring of apnea, and use of nasal CPAP to "buy time" may be responsible for this. In order to make the decision regarding tracheostomy, the otolaryngologist needs to fully evaluate the cause of the vocal fold paralysis, and assess the infant for sleep apnea, lung disease of prematurity, gastroesophageal reflux, neurological status, and swallowing function, as well as the severity of airway obstruction and work of breathing. All these factors influence airway management decisions. For example, the BVFP patient found to have hydrocephalus and Chiari malformation who receives a ventriculoperitoneal shunt may be observed to see if the relief of brainstem compression improves laryngeal nerve function and vocal fold mobility [29]. The BVFP patient who had a traumatic birth from forceps delivery with neck stretching may also be observed as this neuropraxic injury often recovers. Infants with more profound central neurological injury may be less likely to recover quickly. However, long-term recovery can be seen in these patients, even up to 11 years after diagnosis [12].

The evaluation of these cases usually involves sleep apnea studies, neurological assessment and imaging studies, tests for gastroesophageal reflux, and swallowing studies (by radiography or videoendoscopy). Swallowing studies are especially important in the assessment of the infant with BVFP. The act of swallowing becomes an additional stress on the airway in infants who share the pharynx for both functions. For some infants, oxygen desaturation and obstruction may become symptomatic with oral feedings, and gavage tube feedings are required for an interval while observing for clinical improvement in vocal fold mobility and stridor symptoms.

Bilateral Vocal Fold Paralysis: Long-Term Management Options

Children with BVFP and a tracheotomy have several options for surgical procedures for decannulation. There is no consensus regarding the age at which to pursue these options. Because of reports of long-term (greater than 3 years) recovery of vocal fold movement in some patients [12], the argument to wait is compelling, especially if the etiology of the vocal fold paralysis is central neurological injury. This would not be the case for unrecovered peripheral nerve injuries from trauma or surgery. Daya et al. reported that iatrogenic VFP had the lowest rate of spontaneous recovery (46%) [12]. The child with a tracheotomy from BVFP can usually acquire speech by means of a speaking valve or by covering the tracheotomy tube with his or her chin. Removal of the tracheotomy is often desirable before children start attending school. Some parents, however, may choose to keep the tracheotomy because of the effects of airway augmentation procedures to facilitate decannulation on the voice. These include posterior cricoidotomy and cartilage grafting [15, 30], posterior cordotomy [31], suture lateralization [32], and arytenoidectomy or arytenoidopexy [13]. The posterior cricoidotomy and cartilage graft can even be done endoscopically [33]. The posterior cricoidotomy is felt to be preferable when there is some adductor vocal fold movement observed but no abductor movement, and the child has no aspiration symptoms [15]. Brigger and Hartnick reviewed the results of several studies, including 55 children treated with various procedures for BVFP, and concluded that a combination of external arytenoidopexy and vocal fold suture lateralization was the most reliably successful [34]. All these studies use tracheotomy decannulation as a standard outcome measure. No reports have specifically addressed the effects of these procedures on the voice. However, they all have a predictable effect on vocal function: creating a larger glottal airway necessarily creates a degree of glottal insufficiency for phonation, with consequent reduction in volume and a breathy voice quality.

Another procedure reported for BVFP is laryngeal reinnervation by ansa cervicalis nerve–muscle pedicle (NMP) transfer to the posterior cricoarytenoid muscle. Tucker reported a 50% decannulation rate in children following this procedure in 9 of 18 tracheotomized children under 5 years of age [35]. A recent study at another institution of six children with BVFP treated with this procedure also reported a 50% decannulation rate [36]. Two of the three failures were felt in retrospect to have impaired cricoarytenoid mobility that should have been a contraindication for the procedure. The procedure has theoretical appeal because it does not impair voice at the expense of the airway. In the future, laryngeal pacing may add to the options for these patients [37].

We have treated ten BVFP pediatric patients at our institution over the past 10 years with vocal fold botulinum toxin injections to avoid tracheotomy, facilitate tracheotomy decannulation, or maintain tracheotomy decannulation (unpublished observations). Although four of the ten patients required a tracheotomy or could not be decannulated, the procedure had clinical benefit in the others. Five of the patients continue to receive injections every 6–12 months as stridor recurs. This idea is not new; Cohen et al. in the late 1980s reported canine experiments on augmentation of the airway through chemodenervation, targeting the cricothyroid muscles [38, 39]. Our experience has shown thyroarytenoid muscle injections to be more effective than cricothyroid for airway augmentation. Other authors have also reported use of thyroarytenoid botulinum toxin injections for laryngeal breathing problems in adults [40, 41].

Voice Concerns in the Older Child and Adolescent

The approach to evaluation of a child with a voice problem differs from that of the adult in several respects [42]. Voice disorders in children often co-occur with speech, language, and developmental delays. Children have limited ability to cooperate, so that any procedures or assessment techniques must be performed in the least invasive and non-threatening manner. Parents, family members, and other caregivers are also included in the acquisition of historical information and involved with therapy.

Laryngeal examination is a crucial aspect of the voice evaluation. The flexible fiberoptic laryngoscope has become the tool of choice for the evaluation of voice problems in children [43]. Even young children can tolerate this examination well with proper preparation of the child and parent, use of topical nasal anesthesia, and an engaging, non-threatening atmosphere. These methods have been well described [44–46]. The use of video equipment has advantages of engaging the child's attention, providing visual feedback for the parent, and facilitating communication between the physician and speech pathologist and others. Several points may be emphasized in the course of this examination. After the fiberscope is passed beyond the turbinates, the velopharynx is examined for velopharyngeal insufficiency. The adenoid pad and tonsils are seen as the fiberscope passes beyond the nose into the pharynx. In the hypopharynx, the laryngopharyngeal mucosa is inspected for erythema and mucosal thickening, especially the arytenoid mucosa, posterior glottis, and true vocal fold mucosa. Edema of the vocal folds or subglottic mucosa, termed "pseudosulcus," may be present [47]. These are signs of extraesophageal reflux. Diffuse edema of the laryngeal mucosa, "cobblestoning" of the posterior pharynx, and edematous nasal mucosa may be a sign of allergy. Vocal fold mobility is inspected, including observation during coughing and sniffing maneuvers. The larynx is observed during connected speech, such as counting to ten, or repetition of phrases. These tasks are helpful for observing supraglottal hyperfunction seen both in functional dysphonias and as compensatory behavior in organic lesions [43]. The vocal folds themselves are examined for irregularities, swelling, or lesions. Such abnormalities of the vocal fold, when seen unilaterally, may represent congenital cysts [48, 49]. During sustained vowel /i/ phonation, the glottal closure is assessed. Incomplete posterior glottal closure (posterior "chink") is common in children as it is in many adult women [50, 51]. During endoscopic visualization, a determination may be made regarding whether stroboscopic examination would help elucidate the problem (e.g., suspicion of abnormal mucosal wave vibration due to scar or sulcus in the absence of nodules; unilateral cord lesion). Laryngostroboscopy has limitations in young children, who may not be able to vocalize a sufficient length of time (4–5 s) for a useful examination to be obtained. Average maximum phonation time increases from 6 to 8 s in normal 3-year-olds up to 10 s in children under 7 years [52]. This can be even more difficult for the child with UVFP and glottal incompetence. Older children can sometimes tolerate a rigid oral telescopic examination of the larynx. A 70° rod lens telescope is usually used. This yields a more detailed view of the vocal fold and laryngeal mucosa, which is helpful for examining vocal fold mass lesions, inflammation, and obtaining a stroboscopic exam. Only sustained vowel phonation is possible, usually by having the patient say the vowel /i/ with the mouth open and tongue extended. Rigid peroral laryngoscopy has the disadvantage of not being able to examine the larynx during connected speech and sometimes yields a less adequate view of vocal fold movement. A sensitive gag reflex precludes the performance of transoral laryngeal examination of some patients.

The voice assessment by the speech/language pathologist is ideally conducted during the same visit to the otolaryngologist. The child's voice is rated perceptually during a variety of speech tasks and sustained vowels. The voice is recorded for acoustic measures. Aerodynamic and glottographic measurements may also contribute information to the problem. These are easily conducted with current instrumentation. They have certain advantages: documentation of the problem; corroboration of findings with the laryngeal imaging examination; documentation of treatment efficacy; and use as biofeedback during therapy.

Unilateral Laryngeal Paralysis: Management Options

Several large reviews have reported that the natural history of laryngeal paralysis in children tends toward spontaneous "recovery." Cohen et al. described 38 children with UVFP: although 14 were lost to follow-up, 13 recovered completely [8]. Emery and Fearon reported 30 cases of UVFP in children [53]. Peripheral nerve injuries usually recovered (60% of cases). In laryngeal paralysis it is important to distinguish between neuromotor (return of vocal fold movement) and phonatory (improvement in voice) recovery, since they are not always the same [54]. This is demonstrated in the series of Emery and Fearon [53]: in eight patients observed for an average of 6 years vocal fold mobility did not return, yet in six of them, the voice recovered. Only one patient had a surgical procedure (Teflon injection). The infrequent reports of surgical management of dysphonia in children from laryngeal paralysis attest to the trend toward natural improvement in voice through compensatory means, with or without recovery of vocal fold movement. It can also reflect a social accommodation to the child with mild or moderate degrees of dysphonia.

Surgical management of glottal insufficiency and laryngeal paralysis has received much attention. Beginning in the early 1960s, Teflon paste injection of the vocal fold was commonly performed in adults until other techniques superseded it in the 1980s. There are reports of Teflon injection in three children [53, 55]. It has several disadvantages in children, including irreversibility and unpredictable long-term effects [35]. However, the principle of vocal fold injection for medialization to treat glottal incompetence has merit. Other materials for injection, including Gelfoam and collagen, are available as a temporary treatment of glottal incompetence, and have been successfully used in a few children [35, 55, 56]. We have had favorable results with Cymetra collagen injection for temporary medialization in a series of adolescents with UVFP [57]. Autologous fat is also an option. It also yields temporary medialization but has not had long-lasting results in children (personal observation).

A variety of phonosurgical techniques have been popularized as alternatives to vocal fold injection [58, 59]. These laryngeal framework procedures have had some limited application in children [60-62]. Link et al. reported on eight patients with UVFP treated with type-I medialization thyroplasty for dysphonia or aspiration symptoms [61]. The arytenoid adduction procedure [63], while appropriate in theory for closure of posterior glottic defects, has technical problems that preclude its use in young children [60]. The arytenoid muscular process is not as well defined and easily palpable in the pediatric larynx as it is in adults. The arytenoid and thyroid ala cartilage is softer and does not hold the suture as well. Even with adduction of the arytenoid, the larger posterior pediatric glottis (relative to the anterior half of the glottis) still remains partially open during phonation, resulting in a more breathy voice.

Development of exertional dyspnea may also be a concern with arytenoid adduction, although it has not been a problem in our limited experience. This procedure may be appropriate in adolescents with UVFP and large glottal gap and concomitant aspiration symptoms. Although our experience has been positive, a recent review of three studies on the topic found that arytenoid adduction yielded no benefit over medialization laryngoplasty alone [64]. These laryngoplasty procedures can be done under local anesthesia in adults. This is not possible in most children. The use of laryngeal mask airway and intraoperative fiberoptic laryngoscopy to adjust implant location has been reported in two children [62].

Reinnervation of the paralyzed larynx is another surgical option for dysphonia from UVFP. Two variations of this approach have been investigated: ansa hypoglossi to recurrent laryngeal nerve anastomosis [65], and NMP implantation into adductor laryngeal muscles (lateral cricoarytenoid or thyroarytenoid) [66]. Both of these techniques aim to reinnervate laryngeal muscle to prevent atrophy, increase tone, and improve glottal adduction and voice. A recent experimental study in canines that compared these techniques found direct suture neurorrhaphy to be superior to NMP in amplitude of EMG and strength of muscle contraction [67]. In the series reported by Tucker of eight children with UVFP, three underwent the nerve–muscle pedicle procedure, in addition to voice therapy, with "good" voice results [35]. In older pre-teens and adolescents with UVFP we have utilized the technique of combining arytenoid adduction with ansa hypoglossi reinnervation [57, 68]. This combines the benefits of framework surgery to close the posterior glottis and reinnervation.

Laryngeal EMG in Children

Electromyography (EMG) measures the electrical activity of muscle and is used to study paralysis in a variety of clinical situations. In the larynx it has been used to make prognostic determinations regarding recovery from laryngeal paralysis. There are many theoretical and technical issues regarding laryngeal EMG [69] which likely account for the variable results in numerous papers detailing clinical experiences. There are several reports of its use in children [70-75]. It is usually done under general anesthesia, which can itself affect EMG results depending on agents used and depth of anesthesia. Monopolar electrode insertion into the posterior cricoarytenoid or thyroarytenoid muscle is done while the patient is breathing spontaneously [70, 73–75]. Bipolar hooked wire electrodes have also been used [71, 72]. Laryngeal EMG does not appear to have much utility in prognostic assessment of congenital vocal fold paralysis [73, 74], but it has been helpful in selected cases of pediatric new-onset paralysis, tumors affecting laryngeal nerves, or decannulation decisions [74]. It has also been used to monitor the left vocal fold and recurrent laryngeal nerve during video thoracoscopic patent ductus arteriosus ligation [76].

Familial Vocal Fold Paralysis

Although rare, vocal fold paralysis can run in families. In the seminal paper by Plott in 1964 congenital laryngeal abductor paralysis was found in three brothers, who also had mental retardation [77]. Inheritance was determined to be X-linked recessive. Subsequent reports have substantiated this observation, but with different variations. An article by Raza et al. summarized 21 reports of familial vocal fold paralysis [78]. Although there is a spectrum of associated findings, several themes are present. It usually presents with stridor or respiratory distress after birth or in childhood and is usually described as an abductor paralysis, although it has also been reported as adductor paralysis [79], or to have onset in adulthood [80]. There may be associated neurological delays [77, 81–84]. The inheritance of this condition has most frequently been determined to be autosomal dominant [79, 85–87]. Gene linkage analysis of one family with this disorder localized to chromosome 6q16 [88]. Autosomal-dominant mode of inheritance in three generations was observed in the family of a patient cared for by the author (personal observation). In the 21 reports summarized by Raza et al., nine were autosomal dominant, two were X-linked recessive [77, 81], three were X-linked or autosomal dominant [86, 89, 90], three were autosomal recessive [78, 89, 91], one was a single mutant gene, and four were unknown. Although the condition is unusual, study of these cases may further elucidate the neural development of the larynx [82]. These cases are managed along the same lines as patients with vocal fold paralysis due to other causes. Because there is a tendency toward spontaneous improvement in laryngeal function, a conservative approach is advised [78].

Other inherited neurological diseases may be associated with vocal fold paresis or paralysis in children. Charcot-Marie-Tooth (CMT) disease (or hereditary motor and sensory neuropathy) is the most commonly described disorder [92–95]. Its onset can occur in infancy or later childhood. Although CMT type 2, especially CMT-2C, is particularly associated with laryngeal paralysis, it is also seen in type 1 [92]. This condition persists into adulthood.

Conclusion

The following points are made in conclusion:
- Bilateral vocal fold paralysis is generally a problem of neonates and infants. Unilateral vocal fold paralysis is seen in infants and older children.
- Pediatric vocal fold paralysis is diagnosed by fiberoptic laryngoscopy, and supplemented by direct microlaryngoscopy.
- Airway and swallowing are of pre-eminent concern in the infant with vocal fold paralysis. In reported series of bilateral vocal fold paralysis, tracheotomy is performed in half the cases. In unilateral vocal fold paralysis, tracheotomy is uncommonly required.
- Voice becomes an increasing concern in the older child and adolescent with vocal fold paralysis. There is a reported trend toward spontaneous recovery of voice, although long-term studies are lacking.
- Laryngeal EMG has a limited role in management of vocal fold paralysis in children.
- Familial vocal fold paralysis is uncommon but occurs with several series, and with several forms of genotypic and phenotypic expression.

References

1. Gentile RD (1986) Vocal cord paralysis in children 1 year of age and younger. Ann Otol Rhinol Laryngol 95:622–625
2. Dedo DD (1979) Pediatric vocal cord paralysis. Laryngoscope 89:1378–1384
3. Swift AC, Rogers J (1987) Vocal cord paralysis in children. J Laryngol Otol 101:169–171
4. Holinger LD, Holinger P, Holinger P (1976) Etiology of bilateral abductor vocal cord paralysis. Ann Otol Rhinol Laryngol 85:428–436
5. Murty GE, Shinkwin C, Gibbin KP (1994) Bilateral vocal fold paralysis in infants: tracheostomy or not? J Laryngol Otol 108:329–331
6. Zbar RI, Smith RJ (1996) Vocal fold paralysis in infants twelve months of age and younger. Otolaryngol Head Neck Surg 114:18–21
7. Holinger PH, Brown WT (1967) Congenital webs, cysts, laryngoceles, and other anomalies of the larynx. Ann Otol Rhinol Laryngol 76:744–752
8. Cohen SR, Geller KA, Birns JW, Thompson JW (1982) Laryngeal paralysis in children: a long-term retrospective study. Ann Otol Rhinol Laryngol 91:417
9. Goff WF (1970) Vocal cord paralysis analysis of 229 cases. J Am Med Assoc 212:1378–1379
10. Rosin DF, Handler SD, Potsic WP, Wetmore RF, Tom WC (1990) Vocal cord paralysis in children. Laryngoscope 100:1174–1179
11. de Gaudemar I, Roudaire M, Francois M, Narcy P (1996) Outcome of laryngeal paralysis in neonates: a long-term retropective study of 113 cases. Int J Pediatr Otorhinolaryngol 34:101–110
12. Daya H, Hosni A, Bejar-Solar I, Evans JN, Bailey M (2000) Pediatric vocal fold paralysis. Arch Otolaryngol Head Neck Surg 126:21–25
13. Narcy P, Contencin P, Viala P (1990) Surgical treatment for laryngeal paralysis in infants and children. Ann Otol Rhinol Laryngol 99:124–128
14. Cavanaugh F (1955) Vocal palsies in children. J Laryngol Otol 69:399–418
15. Gray SD, Kelly SM, Dove H (1994) Arytenoid separation for impaired pediatric vocal fold mobility. Ann Otol Rhinol Laryngol 103:510
16. Crumley RL (1989) Laryngeal synkinesis: its significance to the laryngologist. Ann Otol Rhinol Laryngol 98:87–92
17. Maronian NC, Robinson L, Waugh P, Hillel AD (2004) A new electromyographic definition of laryngeal synkinesis. Ann Otol Rhinol Laryngol 113:877–886
18. Dedo DD, Dedo HH (2003) Neurogenic diseases of the larynx. In: Bluestone CD, Stool SE et al. (eds) Pediatric otolaryngology, 4th edn. Saunders, Philadelphia, pp 1505–1510
19. Tobias JD, Bozeman PM (1991) Vincristine-induced recurrent laryngeal nerve paralysis in children. Intensive Care Med 17:304–305
20. Annino DJ, MacArthur CJ, Friedman EM (1992) Vincristine-induced recurrent laryngeal nerve paralysis. Laryngoscope 102:1260
21. Zalvan C, Sulica L, Wolf S, Cohen J, Gonzalez-Yanes O, Blitzer A (2003) Laryngopharyngeal dysfunction from the implant vagal nerve stimulator. Laryngoscope 113:221–225
22. Virgilis D, Weinberger JM, Fisher D, Goldberg S, Picard E, Kerem E (2001) Vocal cord paralysis secondary to impacted esophageal foreign bodies in young children. Pediatrics 107:E101
23. Johnson DG, Gray S, Smith M, Kelly S (2004) Vocal fold paralysis and progressive cricopharyngeal stenosis reversed by cricopharyngeal myotomy. J Pediatr Surg 39:1715–1718
24. Bergeson PS, Shaw JC (2001) Are infants really obligatory nasal breathers? Clin Pediatr (Phila) 40:567–569
25. Robida A, Povhe B (1988) Cardiovocal syndrome in an infant with a double outlet of the right ventricle. Eur J Pediatr 148:15–16
26. Polaner DM, Billet AL, Richardson MA (1986) Cardiovocal syndrome. Pediatrics 78:380
27. Condon LM, Katkov H, Singh A, Helseth HK (1985) Cardiovocal syndrome in infancy. Pediatrics 76:22–25
28. Friedman EM (1997) Role of ultrasound in the assessment of vocal cord function in infants and children. Ann Otol Rhinol Laryngol 106:199–209
29. Bluestone CD, Delerme A, Samuelson G (1972) Airway obstruction due to vocal cord paralysis in infants with hydrocephalus and meningomyelocele. Ann Otol Rhinol Laryngol 81:778–783
30. Cotton RT (1991) The problem of pediatric laryngotracheal stenosis: a clinical and experimental study on the efficacy of autogenous cartilaginous grafts placed between the vertically divided halves of the posterior lamina of the cricoid cartilage. Laryngoscope 101:1
31. Kashima HK (1991) Bilateral vocal fold motion impairment: pathophysiology and management by transverse cordotomy. Ann Otol Rhinol Laryngol 100:717–721
32. Mathur NN, Kumar S, Bothra R (2004) Simple method of vocal cord lateralization in bilateral abductor cord paralysis in paediatric patients. Int J Pediatr Otorhinolaryngol 68:15–20
33. Inglis AF Jr, Perkins JA, Manning SC, Mouzakes J (2003) Endoscopic posterior cricoid split and rib grafting in 10 children. Laryngoscope 113:2004–2009
34. Brigger MT, Hartnick CJ (2002) Surgery for pediatric vocal cord paralysis: a meta-analysis. Otolaryngol Head Neck Surg 126:349–355

35. Tucker HM (1986) Vocal cord paralysis in small children: principles of management. Ann Otol Rhinol Laryngol 95:618
36. Nunez DA, Hanson DR (1993) Laryngeal reinnervation in children: the Leeds experience. Ear Nose Throat J 72:542–543
37. Zealear DL, Billante CR, Courey MS, Netterville JL, Paniello RC, Sanders I, Herzon GD, Goding GS, Mann W, Ejnell H, Habets AM, Testerman R, Van de Heyning P (2003) Reanimation of the paralyzed human larynx with an implantable electrical stimulation device. Laryngoscope 113:1149–1156
38. Cohen SR, Thompson JW (1987) Use of botulinum toxin to lateralize true vocal cords: a biochemical method to relieve bilateral abductor vocal cord paralysis. Ann Otol Rhinol Laryngol 96:534–541
39. Cohen SR, Thompson JW, Camilon FS Jr (1989) Botulinum toxin for relief of bilateral abductor paralysis of the larynx: histologic study in an animal model. Ann Otol Rhinol Laryngol 98:213–216
40. Grillone GA, Blitzer A, Brin MF, Annino DJ Jr, Saint-Hilaire MH (1994) Treatment of adductor laryngeal breathing dystonia with botulinum toxin type A. Laryngoscope 104:30–32
41. Merlo IM, Occhini A, Pacchetti C, Alfonsi E (2002) Not paralysis, but dystonia causes stridor in multiple system atrophy. Neurology 58:649–652
42. Rammage L, Morrison J, Nichol H (2001) Pediatric voice disorders: special considerations. In: Morrison M, Rammage L (eds) Management of the voice and it's disorders, 2nd edn. Singular, San Diego
43. Koufman JA (1991) Approach to the patient with a voice disorder. Otolaryngol Clin North Am 24:989
44. Chait DH, Lotz WK (1991) Successful pediatric examinations using nasoendoscopy. Laryngoscope 101:1016
45. D'Antonio LL, Chait DH, Lotz WK et al. (1986) Pediatric videonasoendoscopy for speech and voice disorders. Otolaryngol Head Neck Surg 94:578
46. Lotz WK, D'Antonio LL, Chait DH, Netsell RW (1993) Successful nasoendoscopic and aerodynamic examinations of children with speech/voice disorders. Int J Pediatr Otorhinolaryngol 26:165–172
47. Hickson C, Simpson CB, Falcon R (2001) Laryngeal pseudosulcus as a predictor of laryngopharyngeal reflux. Laryngoscope 111:1742–1745
48. Monday LA, Cornut G, Bouchayer M et al. (1983) Epidermoid cysts of the vocal cords. Ann Otol Rhinol Laryngol 92:124
49. Bouchayer M, Cornut G (1992) Microsurgical treatment of benign vocal fold lesions: indications, technique, results. Folia Phoniatr (Basel) 44:155
50. Glaze LE, Bless DM, Susser RD (1990) Acoustic analysis of vowel and loudness differences in children's voice. J Voice 4:37
51. Hirano M, Bless DM (1993) Videostroboscopic examination of the larynx. Singular, San Diego
52. Baken RJ, Orlikoff RF (1999) Clinical measurement of speech and voice, 2nd edn. Singular, San Diego
53. Emery PJ, Fearon B (1984) Vocal cord palsy in pediatric practice: a review of 71 cases. Int J Pediatr Otorhinolaryngol 8:147
54. Hirano M, Nozoe I, Shin T, Maeyama T (1987) Electromyography for laryngeal paralysis. In: Hirano M, Kirchner JA, Bless DM (eds) Neurolaryngology: recent advances. College-Hill Press, Boston, pp 232–248
55. Levine BA, Jacobs IN, Wetmore RF, Handler SD (1995) Vocal cord injection in children with unilateral vocal cord paralysis. Arch Otolaryngol Head Neck Surg 121:116–119
56. Patel NJ, Kerschner JE, Merati AL (2003) The use of injectable collagen in the management of pediatric vocal unilateral fold paralysis. Int J Pediatr Otorhinolaryngol 67:1355–1360
57. Smith ME, Muntz HR (2003) Unilateral vocal fold paralysis in adolescents. American Society of Pediatric Otolaryngology, Nashville, Tennessee
58. Isshiki N (1991) Laryngeal framework surgery. In: Myers EN, Bluestone CD et al. (eds) Advances in otolaryngology–head neck surgery, vol 5. Mosby, St. Louis, pp 37–56
59. Benninger MS, Crumley RL, Ford CN, Gould WJ, Hanson DG, Ossoff RH, Sataloff RT (1994) Evaluation and treatment of the unilateral paralyzed vocal fold. Otolaryngol Head Neck Surg 111:497–508
60. Smith ME, Gray SD (1994) Laryngeal framework surgery in children. In: Myers EN, Bluestone CD et al. (eds) Advances in otolaryngology–head neck surgery, vol 5. Mosby, St. Louis, pp 91–106
61. Link DT, Rutter MJ, Liu JH, Willging JP, Myer CM, Cotton RT (1999) Pediatric type I thyroplasty: an evolving procedure. Ann Otol Rhinol Laryngol 108:1105–1110
62. Gardner GM, Altman JS, Balakrishnan G (2000) Pediatric vocal fold medialization with silastic implant: intraoperative airway management. Int J Pediatr Otorhinolaryngol 52:37–44
63. Isshiki N, Tanabe M, Sawada M (1978) Arytenoid adduction for unilateral vocal cord paralysis. Arch Otolaryngol 104:555
64. Chester MW, Stewart MG (2003) Arytenoid adduction combined with medialization thyroplasty: an evidence-based review. Otolaryngol Head Neck Surg 129:305–310
65. Crumley RL (1991) Nerve transfer technique as it relates to phonatory surgery. In: Cummings CW, Fredrickson JM et al. (eds) Otolaryngology–head and neck surgery, update II. Mosby, St. Louis, pp 100–106

66. Goding GS (1991) Nerve-muscle pedicle reinnervation of the paralyzed vocal cord. Otolaryngol Clin North Am 24:1239
67. Zheng H, Zhou S, Chen S, Li Z, Cuan Y (1998) An experimental comparison of different kinds of laryngeal muscle reinnervation. Otolaryngol Head Neck Surg 119:540–547
68. Chhetri DK, Gerratt BR, Kreiman J, Berke GS (1999) Combined arytenoid adduction and laryngeal reinnervation in the treatment of vocal fold paralysis. Laryngoscope 109:1928–1936
69. Sulica L, Blitzer A (2004) Electromyography and immobile vocal fold. Otolaryngol Clin North Am 37:59–74
70. Koch BM, Milmoe G, Grundfast KM (1987) Vocal cord paralysis in children studied by monopolar electromyography. Pediatr Neurol 3:288
71. Woo P, Arandia H (1992) Intraoperative laryngeal electromyographic assessment of patients with immobile vocal fold. Ann Otol Rhinol Laryngol 101:799–806
72. Gartlan MG, Peterson KL, Luschei ES, Hoffman HT, Smith RJ (1993) Bipolar hooked-wire electromyographic technique in the evaluation of pediatric vocal cord paralysis. Ann Otol Rhinol Laryngol 102:695–700
73. Berkowitz RG (1996) Laryngeal electromyography findings in idiopathic congenital bilateral vocal cord paralysis. Ann Otol Rhinol Laryngol 105:207–212
74. Wohl DL, Kilpatrick JK, Leshner RT, Shaia WT (2001) Intraoperative pediatric laryngeal electromyography: experience and caveats with monopolar electrodes. Ann Otol Rhinol Laryngol 110:524–531
75. Jacobs IN, Finkel RS (2002) Laryngeal electromyography in the management of vocal cord mobility problems in children. Laryngoscope 112:1243–1248
76. Odegard KC, Kirse DJ, Nido PJ del, Laussen PC, Casta A, Booke J, Kenna MA, McGowan FX Jr (2000) Intraoperative recurrent laryngeal nerve monitoring during video-assisted throracoscopic surgery for patent ductus arteriosus. J Cardiothorac Vasc Anesth 14:562–564
77. Plott D (1964) Congenital laryngeal-abductor paralysis due to nucleus ambiguus dysgenesis in three brothers. N Engl J Med 271:593–597
78. Raza SA, Mahendran S, Rahman N, Williams RG (2002) Familial vocal fold paralysis. J Laryngol Otol 116:1047–1049
79. Mace M, Williamson E, Worgan D (1978) Autosomal dominantly inherited adductor laryngeal paralysis: a new syndrome with a suggestion of linkage to HLA. Clin Genet 14:265–270
80. Barbieri F, Pellecchia MT, Esposito E, Stasio E di, Castaldo I, Santorelli F, Perretti A, Santoro L, Michele G de (2001) Adult-onset familial laryngeal abductor paralysis, cerebellar ataxia, and pure motor neuropathy. Neurology 56:1412–1414
81. Watters G, Fitch N (1973) Familial laryngeal abductor paralysis and psychomotor retardation. Clin Genet 4:429–433
82. Tucker HM (1983) Congenital bilateral recurrent nerve paralysis and ptosis: a new syndrome. Laryngoscope 93:1405–1407
83. Johnson JA, Stern LZ (1981) Bilateral vocal cord paralysis in a patient with familial hypertrophic neuropathy. Arch Neurol 38:532
84. Grundfast KM, Milmoe G (1982) Congenital hereditary bilateral abductor vocal cord paralysis. Ann Otol Rhinol Laryngol 91:564–566
85. Isaacson G, Moya F (1987) Hereditary congenital laryngeal abductor paralysis. Ann Otol Rhinol Laryngol 96:701–704
86. Gacek RR (1976) Hereditary abductor vocal cord paralysis. Ann Otol Rhinol Laryngol 85:90–93
87. Cunningham MJ, Eavey RD, Shannon DC (1985) Familial vocal cord dysfunction. Pediatrics 76:750–753
88. Manaligod JM, Skaggs J, Smith RJ (2001) Localization of the gene for familial laryngeal abductor paralysis to chromosome 6q16. Arch Otolaryngol Head Neck Surg 127:913–917
89. Schinzel A, Hof E, Dangel P, Robinson W (1990) Familial congenital laryhngeal abductor paralysis: different expression in a family with one male and three females affected. J Med Genet 27:715–716
90. Hawkins DB, Liu-Shindo M, Kahlstrom EJ, MacLaughlin EF (1990) Familial vocal cord dysfunction associated with digital anomalies. Laryngoscope 100:1001–1004
91. Koppel R, Friedman S, Fallet S (1996) Congenital vocal cord paralysis with possible autosomal recessive inheritance. Am J Med Genet 64:485–487
92. Sulica L, Blitzer A, Lovelace RE, Kaufmann P (2001) Vocal fold paresis of Charcot-Marie-Tooth disease. Ann Otol Rhinol Laryngol 110:1072–1076
93. Lacy PD, Hartley BE, Rutter MJ, Cotton RT (2001) Familial bilateral vocal cord paralysis and Charcot-Marie-Tooth disease type II-C. Arch Otolaryngol Head Neck Surg 127:322–324
94. Holinger PC, Vuckovich DM, Holinger LD, Holinger PH (1979) Bilateral abductor vocal cord paralysis in Charcot-Marie-Tooth disease. Ann Otol Rhinol Laryngol 88:205–209
95. Dyck PJ, Litchy WJ, Minnerath S, Bird TD, Chance PF, Schaid DJ, Aronson AE (1994) Hereditary motor and sensory neuropathy with diaphragm and vocal cord paresis. Ann Neurol 35:608—615
96. Schild JA, Holinger LD (1980) Peroral endoscopy in neonates. Int J Pediatr Otorhinolaryngol 2:133–138

1

Chapter 15

Bilateral Vocal Fold Immobility

George Goding

Introduction

Bilateral vocal fold immobility (BVFI) presents a significant challenge for which complete rehabilitation can be accomplished in only a minority of patients with favorable etiologies. Despite a number of significant technological advances, the principles of surgical therapy have remained the unchanged over the past few decades. Surgical intervention, however, is able to provide a majority of patients with adequate airway, voice, and swallowing function without the presence of a tracheotomy. The major points of this chapter are summarized as follows:

- BVFI can be secondary to paralysis, cricoarytenoid joint fixation, infiltrative lesions, and posterior glottic scar.
- Surgery continues to be the most common etiology of BVFI, but a significant number of patients present without laryngeal paralysis.
- Laryngeal electromyography and flow-volume loop spirometry are useful adjuncts in the evaluation of BVFI.
- Reversible etiologies should be eliminated or treated prior to destructive surgery.
- Tissue removal and vocal fold lateralization, alone or in combination, provide the mainstays of therapy.
- Direct muscle reinnervation and functional electrical stimulation provide opportunities for improved rehabilitation in patients with mobile arytenoids.

History

Vocal fold movement allows the larynx to perform multiple critical functions. When movement is lost the larynx can no longer provide airway protection, airway patency, and phonation at a peak level. Current therapy often imposes a compromise in laryngeal function that allows adequate, but not optimal, function to allow the best conditions for daily living. The ultimate goal of therapy in bilateral vocal fold immobility (BVFI) is to restore vocal fold motion and restore the divergent functions of airway protection and airway maintenance. Anastomosis of a divided nerve would appear to be an ideal solution when the paralysis is due to trauma. Such attempts were made in the 1920s [1, 2] but were soon abandoned, because the lack of specific adductor and abductor reinnervation resulted in a synkinesis with little functional vocal fold movement.

Following the failure to reestablish vocal fold movement in cases of bilateral vocal fold paralysis, procedures were designed to improve the airway while minimizing the detrimental effect on phonation and swallow. Jackson [3] experimented with simple cordectomy but changed to ventriculo-cordectomy by removing the vocal cord as well as the ventricle. The arytenoid cartilage was left undisturbed. The voice result was poor and the airway result was variable; primarily due to the amount of scarring that resulted. Multiple laryngoscopies and dilations were sometimes required. In 1936 Lore [4] recommended removing the arytenoid cartilage. He felt that cordectomy failed because of scar tissue formation between the original anterior and posterior points of attachment of the vocal fold. By removing the arytenoid cartilage, a more lateral position of the scar tissue could be obtained.

An external approach to provide a lateral position of the posterior vocal fold was recommended by King [5]. Through a lateral approach the anterior belly of the omohyoid muscle was attached to the arytenoid cartilage on the paralyzed side. Initially, the improved airway was attributed to arytenoid movement due to the action of the transferred omohyoid muscle. The arytenoid cartilage was subsequently found to be fixed in the abducted position and held in place by fibrosis [6]. Contraction resulted in lateral rotation of the vocal process and restoration of effective glottic opening. Morrison [6] presented a number of modifications on the King procedure including disarticulation of the arytenoid cartilage, division of the interarytenoid muscle, and fixation of the arytenoid in a lateralized position to allow enough time for scar tissue to form and maintain that position. Further modifications included removing the arytenoid cartilage through a window in the thyroid cartilage [7].

In 1946, Woodman [8] described removal of the body of the arytenoid cartilage via a lateral approach. Rather than placing a window in the thyroid ala, the arytenoid was approached from behind the thyroid ala after disarticulating the thyroid from the cricoid cartilage. The vocal process of the arytenoid was then lateralized by placing a traction suture between it and the inferior cornu of thyroid cartilage.

Arytenoidectomy via midline thyrotomy was established early as a technique for bilateral vocal fold paralysis. The first successful thyrotomy with cordectomy and arytenoidectomy, performed in a 9-year-old child, was reported by Baker in 1916 [9]. In the 1950s several further reports of midline thyrotomy and arytenoidectomy were published [10, 11], and in 1968, Downey and Kennon reported a 12-case series [72]. A wire lateralizing suture was used. The airway was successfully opened but the resulting voice was breathy. Arytenoidectomy in the subperichondrial plane using microsurgical technique was emphasized by Helmus in his description [12]. A stent was placed but not felt to be necessary for effective lateralization of the vocal fold. Ten patients were reported to have a good airway and a good or serviceable voice.

Removal of the arytenoid by an endoscopic approach was described by Thornell in 1948 [13]. Following a tracheotomy, the arytenoid was removed and both its bed and thyroarytenoid muscle [14] cauterized for hemostasis as well as induction of scar formation.

These techniques form the basis of the current surgical therapies used presently. A number of modifications and technical advances have been made that allow increased efficiency of the surgical procedure and improved results. Patients with BVFI, in most cases, nevertheless must still compromise between the functions of the larynx. In some difficult cases, procedures quite similar to those described above provide important therapeutic options.

Etiology

Bilateral vocal fold immobility is a clinical finding with multiple causes. Bilateral vocal fold paralysis has always been the most common cause of BVFI and has received the most attention. A noteworthy minority of patients with BVFI have an etiology other than vocal fold paralysis so that careful attention to causes other than lower motor neuron disease is important. Kashima [15] divided the causes of BVFI into four categories including vocal fold paralysis, fixation of the cricoarytenoid joint, infiltrative lesions, and cicatricial webs. Although descriptions vary in other reports, these categories are useful in considering the various etiologies of BVFI (Table 15.1).

Surgical trauma, especially at thyroidectomy, continues to be a major cause of bilateral vocal fold paralysis [16]. Cervical malignancy and the associated surgery are also prominent etiologies. Depending on the series, surgical intervention results in 26% [16] to 70% [17] of cases of BVFI. As expected, pulmonary malignancy typically results in unilateral paralysis. Prolonged intubation can result in BVFI either by direct pressure on the nerves secondary to high cuff position [18] or formation of posterior glottic scar [17, 19, 20]. Other etiologies include inflammatory disease such as tuberculosis, caustic ingestion, and inhalation of toxins [21]. With intubation, the injury is typically limited to the posterior glottis, including the posterior third of the vocal folds. The injury occurs because the endotracheal tube lies in the posterior aspect of the larynx and the

Table 15.1. Etiologies of bilateral vocal fold immobility. (From [15, 16, 23, 37, 71])

Paralysis/neurologic
  Surgical trauma
  Prolonged intubation
  Thyroid, esophageal, and tracheal malignancies
  Midbrain stroke
  Amyotrophic lateral sclerosis
  Arnold–Chiari malformation
  Diabetic neuropathy
  Post-polio syndrome
  Multiple sclerosis
  Guillain–Barré syndrome
Cricoarytenoid joint fixation
  Arytenoid dislocation
    (blunt or intubation trauma)
  Rheumatoid arthritis
  Ankylosing spondylitis
Infiltrative or inflammatory lesions of the vocal fold
  Sarcoidosis
  Amyloidosis
  Wegener's granulomatosis
  Lipoid granulomatosis
  Radiation therapy
  Laryngeal neoplasms
  Idiopathic fibrosis
Posterior glottic scar
  Prolonged intubation
  Cicatricial pemphigoid
  Endolaryngeal surgery
  Gastroesophageal reflux disease

mucosa of the posterior glottis overlies firm cartilaginous structures with little submucosal soft tissue to provide a cushion effect. Posterior glottic inflammation secondary to refluxed gastric material is a significant contributor to the development of posterior glottic scar during intubation [22]. Other risk factors predisposing to posterior glottic scar include diabetes mellitus, large endotracheal tube size, excessive endotracheal tube movement, and multiple intubations [23].

Cricoarytenoid joint fixation secondary to rheumatoid arthritis has been estimated to occur in up to 25% of affected patients [24]. By the time cricoarytenoid joint mobility is compromised enough to restrict respiration, the diagnosis of rheumatoid arthritis is typically well established. Rheumatoid arthritis and other inflammatory diseases are less common causes of BVFI accounting for only (3.4%) of cases in the series by Benninger et al. [16] and less than 1% of cases reported by Eckel et al. [17]. Although the incidence of BVFI due to inflammatory disease is low, successful therapy carries the potential for return of vocal fold motion.

Evaluation

The presentation of bilateral vocal fold immobility is relatively consistent with stridor and/or exercise intolerance being the most prominent symptoms. The clinical presentation often does little to help distinguish among the various possible etiologies. The severity of the airway obstruction determines the extent of the evaluation that can be undertaken prior to therapeutic intervention. Once the airway is stable, a more deliberate evaluation can proceed. A number of questions need to be answered by the diagnostic work-up:
1. Is this the presentation of a life-threatening or disabling condition?
2. Is this a temporary or permanent condition?
3. Is the neuromuscular function of the larynx intact and appropriate?
4. What is the status of the arytenoid cartilage mobility?
5. What is the degree of airway impairment relative to the patient's anticipated needs?

The answers to these questions determine the therapeutic options available to the patient.

In many cases the etiology of the BVFI can be established by an adequate history and a thorough physical examination. The BVFI is often a consequence of a long-term disease process or an acute complication of a surgical intervention. As in unilateral vocal fold immobility, the presence of malignant infiltration of the recurrent laryngeal nerve must be considered. Imaging of the skull base to upper mediastinum is important in patients with an unclear etiology of BVFI. The patient must also be examined for the presence of other causes of airway obstruction that might need to be addressed. Examination for the presence of subglottic and tracheal pathology in particular can be hampered by a narrow glottic opening.

Laryngeal electromyography (LEMG) provides electrophysiologic information that can be used to distinguish neurologic from structural causes of vocal fold immobility. In neuromuscular disease it can be used to localize the site of the lesion. Finally, LEMG can be used to predict the chances of neuromuscular recovery [25]. In patients with a marginal and unprotected airway, the risk of further airway compromise from the LEMG test must be taken into consideration.

Determination of the status of the cricoarytenoid joint can be inferred but not confirmed by LEMG findings. Although laryngoscopy in the clinic can demonstrate asymmetry or limitation of vocal fold motion, limited passive motion of the vocal folds can sometimes be difficult to distinguish from intrinsic muscular activity. Definitive examination of the status of the cricoarytenoid joint involves direct laryngoscopy and palpation of the arytenoid cartilage under general anesthesia. The larynx is also examined for the presence of posterior glottic scar.

The most important indicator of the severity of airway obstruction is the patient's own assessment. Patients with a longstanding glottic stenosis can tolerate a surprisingly narrow glottic aperture. Flow-volume loop spirometry can provide a quantifiable estimate of the severity and nature of the airway obstruction. The absolute value of inspiratory flow is affected by the patient's effort and the presence of lower airway or respiratory muscle dysfunction. Two flow-volume loop spirometry patterns are observed in upper airway obstruction [15]. In a variable extrathoracic obstruction pattern, the inspiratory flow rate effect is predominantly affected. The pliable vocal folds respond to the airway pressure during respiration resulting in greater restriction during inspiration (reduced intratracheal pressure) and glottic expansion during expiration (increased intratracheal pressure). This pattern is seen in laryngeal paralysis, cricoarytenoid joint fixation, and posterior glottic scarring [15]. A flow rate which is limited during both inspiration and expiration is consistent with an infiltrative lesion that reduces vocal fold pliability. This pattern is referred to as fixed. Serial examinations using flow-volume loop spirometry provide an objective assessment of an individual's airway either in response to surgical intervention or with progression of disease.

Adjunctive Measures and Nonsurgical Management

Surgical intervention is the mainstay of therapy for patients with airway compromise and BVFI. Adjuncts to surgical intervention include the topical application of mitomycin to reduce fibroblast proliferation. The application of mitomycin results in an improved post-procedure airway in animals [26]. Preliminary studies have not demonstrated mitomycin-related complications in laryngeal surgery but a definitive positive effect has yet to be shown clinically [27]. Anti-reflux therapy is frequently used in combination with laryngeal surgery involving raw mucosal surfaces or exposed subepithelial tissues [22]. Local injection of steroid and systemic administration of a perioperative antibiotic has also been employed.

In patients with BVFI secondary to systemic disease (see Table 15.1) therapy directed at the disease process can result in improvement of the airway symptoms.

When exercise limitation is the primary complaint, nonsurgical options exist. Reports of nonsurgical interventions consist primarily of single subject case reports. Improvement of the inspiratory airflow through a training program was able to reduce exercise-related dyspnea in a patient with bilateral vocal fold paralysis [28]. Patients can take advantage of passive movement of the arytenoids brought about through the aryepiglottic folds with exaggerated vertical movement of the larynx. Botulinum toxin injection into the adductor muscles of the larynx has been employed in animals [29] and humans [30, 31] to improve the glottic airway.

Application of continuous positive airway pressure (CPAP) takes advantage of the variable extrathoracic airway obstruction present in most cases of BVFI. In patients that desire an alternative to surgical correction or have primarily nocturnal hypoventilation secondary to

BVFI, application of positive airway pressure can be beneficial [32, 33].

Surgical Management

Tracheotomy continues to be the most common technique to consistently provide an airway with a high maximum inspiratory flow with out detrimental effects on the voice. The disadvantages of living with a tracheotomy have led to a number of techniques which aim to provide an adequate airway through the glottis while minimizing the detriment to vocal quality and swallowing function. In patients with a posterior glottic scar band or adhesion, remobilization of the vocal folds is possible. Direct reinnervation of the posterior cricoarytenoid muscle can be accomplished but is performed less frequently than other techniques. The two principal surgical approaches consist of lateralization of the intact vocal fold and removal of vocal fold or arytenoid tissue. In most instances, when a lateralization is performed, some tissue is removed as well. For successful lateralization, it is important that the arytenoid not be fixed. When ankylosis is present, tissue removal is usually necessary. The majority of procedures performed are endoscopic, but open techniques continue to be available for more difficult cases.

Posterior Glottic Stenosis

Posterior glottic stenosis can be divided into four levels of severity [34]. An isolated vocal process adhesion is the simplest form of posterior glottic stenosis (Fig. 15.1). In these patients the posterior commissure mucosa is intact and the interarytenoid muscle and soft tissue shows no evidence of scar formation. Excision of a simple posterior glottic scar in a neurologically intact larynx can result in the return of vocal fold mobility and normal laryngeal function. No other surgical procedure can duplicate these results. It is important, therefore, that every patient considered for a glottic opening procedure be examined for the presence of a posterior glottic scar. The diagnosis should be suspected in all BVFI patients with a history of prolonged intubation. When soft tissue stenosis of the posterior commissure is present (Fig. 15.2), the second level of severity, endoscopic incision, can be performed but recurrence is more likely. Repeat incisions with the application of mitomycin have resulted in return of vocal fold mobility in certain patients. Laryngofissure and rotation of local mucosal flaps as well as placement of endolaryngeal stents can be effective in reducing the incidence of recurrent stenosis [34]. Unilateral and bilateral involvement of the cricoarytenoid joint resulting in joint ankylosis comprise the third and fourth levels of severity. Remobilization of the scarred arytenoids can be performed by a midline thyrotomy approach and excision of local adhesions [35]. If bilateral cricoarytenoid joint fixation exists, the success rate of remobilization is minimal. There is a discrepancy, however, between the clinical impression of arytenoid fixation and the lack of joint fibrosis and obliteration of the joint space seen on histologic evaluation. Muscle atrophy and fibrosis may play a larger role than joint ankylosis in reduction of arytenoid mobility [36]. For patients with severe posterior glottic stenosis, placing a cartilage graft in a posterior cricoid split to enlarge the interarytenoid area has been performed [37]; otherwise, the airway can be enlarged by tissue removal techniques.

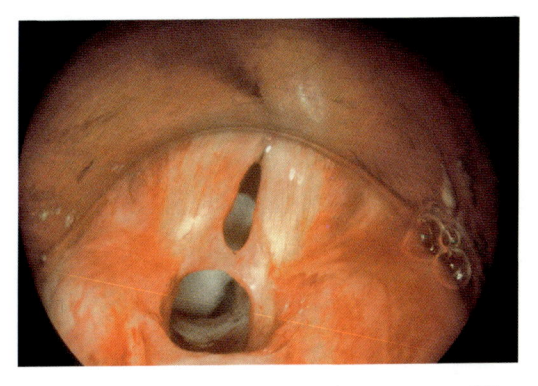

Fig. 15.1 Posterior glottic scar band. Note mucosal lining of posterior commissure

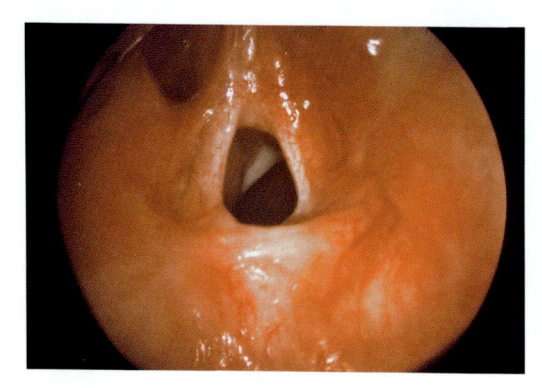

Fig. 15.2. Posterior commissure scar

Direct Muscle Reinnervation

The neuromuscular pedicle (NMP) procedure, developed in the 1970s, involves placement of the distal portion of the ansa cervicalis branch to the omohyoid muscle along with a small block of muscle into a denervated laryngeal muscle. The block of muscle is included in order to preserve and transfer intact motor units with the nerve. Depending on the success of reinnervation and the nature of the stimulus, there is a potential for recovery of vocal fold motion.

The NMP can be considered for any patient with bilateral vocal cord paralysis that has persisted for 6 months [38] to 1 year [39]. In practice, however, only half of patients are suitable candidates [40]. Fixation or limitation of the cricoarytenoid joint is the most common contraindication, and effects approximately one-third of patients [39]. The ansa cervicalis nerve and its insertion into the appropriate strap muscle must be available for this technique. The history should be carefully reviewed to identify any prior surgery or trauma that may have injured the ansa cervicalis. Central nervous system disease resulting in vocal fold paralysis is a relative contraindication. Tucker [39] has reported only a 40–50% success rate in these patients. Finally, the laryngeal muscles must be able to accept reinnervation. Although successful reinnervation has been reported after 22 and 50 years of denervation [41, 42], muscle atrophy probably plays a role in hampering the outcome. The incidence of cricoarytenoid fixation may increase with time [43], but this finding has not been confirmed histologically [36] and may be less common than previously suspected.

In 1976 Tucker reported using the NMP in humans for bilateral vocal fold paralysis [41]. All five patients studied demonstrated vocal cord abduction with inspiration within 6–8 weeks of the procedure. In two patients with a marked improvement in exercise tolerance, vocal fold motion was not seen without an increased respiratory effort. In 1978 an 88.8% (40 of 45) success rate was reported in 45 cases of NMP laryngeal reinnervation for bilateral vocal fold paralysis [38]. Follow-up ranged from 3 months to 4 years and duration of paralysis ranged from 6 months to 50 years. The time to return of function varied from 6 to 12 weeks. In approximately 40% of cases, airway improvement was accompanied by visible motion of the vocal fold with inspiratory effort [39]. Twenty percent of patients had no airway improvement. The remaining patients had airway improvement but little vocal fold motion. Most of these patients demonstrated motion or tonic abduction only with increased respiratory demand. A second NMP procedure to the opposite PCA muscle has been performed successfully in patients with an inadequate result from the first procedure [39].

A 74% long-term success rate was reported in 202 bilateral vocal fold paralysis patients treated with the NMP technique [40]. Success was defined as decannulation with improved airway that did not limit regular daily activities or exacerbate acute upper respiratory disease. Minimum follow-up was 2 years. Six-month results showed an 89% success rate (180 of 202 patients), but 31 additional patients had subsequent deterioration of their airway. In a majority of late-failure patients that were evaluated endoscopically, limited motion of the cricoarytenoid joint was identified as a cause of failure.

A few other authors have reported a variable amount of success in smaller groups of patients with the NMP technique. Of eight patients reported by May et al. [44], only three were improved. Applebaum et al. [42] reported successful results in four patients. Dyspnea and stridor were relieved in all four; vocal cord movement was seen only after physical exertion.

It is possible that the surgical approach rather than reinnervation itself results in an improved airway. Postoperative scarring which could stabilize the arytenoid and lateral tethering of the arytenoid to the thyroid cartilage is a potential explanation for vocal fold motion and a more lateral position not related to reinnervation [45].

With successful use limited to only a few authors' experience, widespread use of the NMP has not materialized. Reinnervation can occur with implantation of an NMP into denervated muscle, but the ansa cervicalis continues to be an imperfect source for neural input. Even in the absence of movement with respiration, the NMP can maintain muscular tone. The NMP can provide a mechanism to access a denervated muscle for long-term pacing [46, 47]. With electrical pacing, the options for a potential triggering source, and the stimulus for muscle contraction, are increased, providing a potentially more effective treatment of airway impairment secondary to bilateral vocal fold paralysis.

Lateralization

Lateralization of the vocal fold was described by Kirchner in 1979 [48]. The technique also involves excision of a wedge of thyroarytenoid muscle with a microcautery. The resulting defect is closed and the vocal fold is lateralized by passing a suture across it via two needles placed through the skin entering the larynx above and below the vocal fold. The suture is tightened to appropriately position the vocal fold and is secured on the skin surface. If the vocal process is not adequately lateralized, then it is removed. The sutures are removed after 2 weeks at which time the vocal fold is presumably fixed in its new position.

A pure laterofixation technique was introduced by Ejnell et al. [49]. In this technique the thyroid lamina is exposed by an external approach and two needles are placed above and below the vocal fold and just behind the tip of the vocal process. A permanent suture is passed through the needles and around the vocal fold. After the correct positioning of the vocal fold has been determined by the operating surgeon, the suture is secured on the external surface of the thyroid lamina. Of 10 patients with severe airway obstruction reported in the initial study, 9 had an improvement in airway function. Patients with only a moderate airway restriction did not substantially improve. Five patients required repeat operation. No tracheotomy is necessary for the technique.

To facilitate placement of the suture for vocal fold lateralization an endo-extralaryngeal needle carrier was developed [50]. Similar to the technique of Ejnell et al. [49], the thyroid ala is exposed by an external approach. The sutures to be used for lateralization are placed under endoscopic control from inside the larynx. The first suture is placed under the posterior third of the vocal fold and through the thyroid cartilage. A second suture is threaded through the needle carrier of the instrument and passed above the vocal fold. The suture is then secured over the external surface of the thyroid ala. The most effective direction of traction by the suture on the vocal fold appears to be perpendicular to the median line of the glottis rather than perpendicular to the thyroid lamina [51].

A combination of the suture lateralization technique with excision of the thyroarytenoid muscle or the arytenoid itself can be used to enlarge the airway. A submucous cordectomy in combination with suture lateralization using an endo-extralaryngeal needle carrier [52] is similar to the original operation described by Kirchner [48]. A modification is the use of the carbon dioxide laser. Preservation of the overlying vocal fold mucosa is emphasized. A balance exists between the extent of thyroarytenoid muscle excision and the resulting vocal and airway results. Sutures are placed submucosally using the endo-extralaryngeal needle carrier anterior to the vocal process. If needed, a second suture is placed at the middle third of the vocal fold to further enlarge the resulting airway. In this method, the sutures are secured over the skin of the neck for 3 weeks. The suture lateralization technique can also be combined with carbon dioxide laser excision of the arytenoid when arytenoid cartilage ankylosis is present.

Pure lateralization of the vocal fold provides a reversible technique to be used early in the course of bilateral vocal fold immobility [53]. The technique involves suture lateralization of the vocal folds without removal of any tissue. Reversible lateralization of the vocal folds using an endo-extralaryngeal needle carrier was performed in 63 patients over a 20-year-period [53]. Fifty-seven of the cases were a result of thyroid surgery. The procedure was successful in obviating a tracheotomy in 61 of the 63 patients. Two additional patients medialized over a 4- to 6-month period and required an additional procedure to maintain the airway. Eight of the patients had return of vocal fold movement and the lateralization suture was removed. Pain with swallowing and mild aspiration was an early complication in some of the patients. In patients with damage to the vocal fold mucosa it is possible for the suture to cut into the vocal fold resulting in a less effective medialization.

Lateralization of the arytenoid may also be aided by release of the muscular attachments of the interarytenoid and thyroarytenoid muscles to the arytenoid cartilage [54]. The muscular pull on the arytenoid cartilage is changed so that the primary tension moves it laterally. The technique involves submucosal division of the interarytenoid attachment to the arytenoid and removal of the vocal process. A mucosal flap is sutured into the defect created by removal of the vocal process. In their study Rontal and Rontal [54] were able to remove the tracheotomy in all of their eight patients with good to excellent exercise tolerance.

Tissue Removal

Excision of vocal fold tissue is an effective but irreversible method of increasing airway diameter in cases of obstructive vocal fold immobility. Ankylosis of the arytenoid cartilage is not a contraindication to these techniques.

Arytenoidectomy has long been an important part of therapy for bilateral vocal fold paralysis. The long-term results of unilateral or bilateral arytenoidectomy demonstrated relief of laryngeal obstruction in 135 of 147 patients (92%) [55]. The use of the carbon dioxide laser in conjunction with the operating microscope further advanced the technique, allowing the arytenoidectomy to be performed more easily in a narrower operative field. Instead of removing the arytenoid, the CO_2 laser was used to ablate the cartilage. In Ossoff et al.'s study [56], improved hemostasis and precision were cited as advantages of the laser technique over endoscopic arytenoidectomy described by Thornell in 1948 [13]. Less control in the placement of the vocal fold, the complications of a laser-associated fire, and the potential for submucosal thermal injury are disadvantages.

The technique [56] involves endoscopic exposure of the posterior aspect of the larynx. The arytenoid is carefully ablated along with the overlying mucosa. The lateral ligamentous attachments of the arytenoid are removed along with the vocal process. The interarytenoid space and the attachments of the interarytenoid muscle are preserved to reduce posterior glottic scar. In the original study 10 of 11 patients were able to be decannulated. In a subsequent study of 28 patients, 27 were decannulated with 2 requiring a revision procedure [57]. All patients had a reduction in vocal quality.

Complete removal of one or both arytenoids raises concern about immediate or future ability of the larynx to protect the airway. Should additional insult to pharyngeal function occur with subsequent aging or illness, swallowing function could be significantly compromised. More conservative procedures with partial arytenoid preservation should more effectively preserve swallowing function. Laser arytenoidectomy can be modified to remove only the medial portion of the arytenoid [58]. The procedure can be repeated on the opposite side after healing is complete if additional airway is needed. Eight patients comprised the original report. In the 2 patients without tracheotomy, the airway was improved. Only 2 of the 6 patients presenting with a tracheotomy were able to be decannulated.

An attempt to improve airway with better voice preservation using the CO_2 laser was presented by Dennis and Kashima [59]. A 6- to 7-

mm transverse incision is made fully dividing the vocal ligament and thyroarytenoid muscle attachment just anterior to the vocal process (Fig. 15.3). Excision of the false vocal fold on the same side improves visualization to complete the incision. Healing at the surgical site dramatically reduces the surgically created opening and revision or contralateral procedures are often needed.

In the original study [59], six patients were decannulated with four of them requiring revision or contralateral procedures. All patients had voice judged to be good and no laryngeal incompetence. The posterior cordotomy technique along with a temporary tracheotomy was successful in improving the airway in 18 of 20 patients [60]. Laccourreye et al. [61] were able to restore the airway in 23 of 25 patients (92%) with the CO_2 laser posterior cordotomy technique. Revision surgery was required in 6 patients and bilateral procedures in 10 patients.

The improvement in airway is directly related to the amount of tissue removed and the subsequent healing of the surgical defect. Attempts to increase the size of the residual defect include application of mitomycin, enlargement of the lateral aspect of the cordotomy defect, and rotation of mucosal flaps to cover the exposed submucosal tissue. Posterior cordotomy appears to be more effective when the airway restriction is modest.

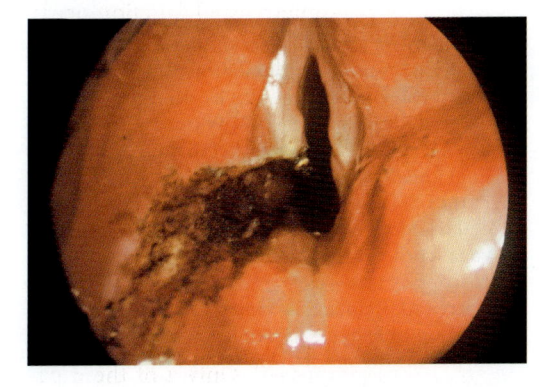

Fig. 15.3. Posterior cordotomy. Note extensive lateral dissection

Research

Investigation of alternate therapies has been driven by the persistent need to compromise between voice and airway results when attempting to avoid tracheotomy in patients with bilateral vocal fold immobility. Most experimental techniques that attempt to adjust or remobilize the vocal fold require that ankylosis of the cricoarytenoid joint is not present.

The possibility of implanting a double-helix screw into the soft tissues of the vocal fold that could retract the vocal fold to varying degrees was examined in the sheep model [62]. In the four animals studied, lateralization of the paralyzed vocal fold was accomplished without endolaryngeal complications. A major advantage of the device is that it can be adjusted relative to voice and airway symptoms. A report of human use is pending.

Reinnervation procedures designed to generate muscle movement must bypass the main trunk of the recurrent laryngeal nerve and address its distal branches or individual muscles directly. Selective innervation of individual laryngeal muscles, in particular the posterior cricoarytenoid muscle, can be accomplished by neuromuscular transfer technique [63], selective anastomosis [64, 65], or direct nerve implantation [66, 67].

As an alternative to reinnervation, electrical pacing of the paralyzed laryngeal muscles has been investigated. Functional electrical stimulation of the posterior cricoarytenoid muscle is applied during the inspiratory phase of respiration. Stimulation is turned off during the expiratory phase of respiration to allow for phonation and deglutition. In animal studies, electrical stimulation of the posterior cricoarytenoid muscle has been able to produce abduction in denervated larynges [68–70]. The result of efforts at vocal fold pacing in humans is discussed elsewhere in this book. With improvements in device hardware, functional electrical stimulation carries promise of improved airway function without additional impairment in voice or swallowing function.

Conclusion

Bilateral vocal fold immobility continues to be a challenge to treating physician and patient. When evaluating BVFI, it is important to look for and treat reversible pathology as well as significant extra-laryngeal disease. Surgical intervention is often able to establish a static glottic opening that allows a compromise between airway and voice in the absence of a tracheotomy. Because this compromise is not always satisfactory, efforts to remobilize at least one vocal fold continue, and provide the greatest promise in improving patient outcomes.

References

1. Frazier CH, Mosser WB (1926) Treatment of recurrent laryngeal nerve paralysis by nerve anastomosis. Surg Gynecol Obstet 43:134–139
2. Lahey FH (1928) Successful suture of recurrent laryngeal nerve for bilateral abductor paralysis, with restoration of function. Ann Surg 87:481–484
3. Jackson C (1922) A new operation for the cure of goitrous paralytic stenosis. Arch Surg 4:257–274
4. Lore JM (1936) A suggested operative procedure for relief of stenosis in double abductor paralysis: an anatomic study. Ann Otol 45:679–686
5. King BT (1939) A new and function-restoring operation for bilateral abductor cord paralysis: preliminary report. J Am Med Assoc 112:814–823
6. Morrison LF (1945) Further observations on the King operation for bilateral abductor paralysis. Ann Otol Rhinol Laryngol 54:390–408
7. Kelley JD (1941) Surgical treatment of bilateral paralysis of the abductor muscles. Arch Otolaryngol 33:293–304
8. Woodman DG (1946) A modification of the extralaryngeal approach to arytenoidectomy for bilateral abductor paralysis. Arch Otolaryngol 43:63–65
9. Baker CH (1916) Report of a case of abductor paralysis with removal of one vocal cord. J Mich Med Soc 15:485
10. DeBord B (1951) Bilaateral abductor paralysis complicated by fractured ribs. Arch Otolaryngol 54:308
11. Pearlman SG, Killian EW (1953) Thyrotomy approach for arytenoidectomy and bilateral abductor paralysis of the vocal cords. Ann Otol Rhinol Laryngol 52:207–212
12. Helmus C (1972) Microsurgical thyrotomy and arytenoidectomy for bilateral recurrent laryngeal nerve paralysis. Laryngoscope 82:491–503
13. Thornell WC (1948) Intralaryngeal approach for arytenoidectomy in bilateral abductor paralysis of the vocal cords, a preliminary report. Arch Otolaryngol 47:505–508
14. Thornell WC (1950) A new intralaryngeal approach for arytenoidectomy in the treatment of bilateral abductor vocal cord paralysis. J Clin Endocrinol Metab 10:1118–1125
15. Kashima HK (1991) Bilateral vocal fold motion impairment: pathophysiology and management by transverse cordotomy. Ann Otol Rhinol Laryngol 100:717–721
16. Benninger MS, Gillen JB, Altman JS (1998) Changing etiology of vocal fold immobility. Laryngoscope 108:1346–1350
17. Eckel HE, Wittekindt C, Klussmann JP et al. (2003) Management of bilateral arytenoid cartilage fixation versus recurrent laryngeal nerve paralysis. Ann Otol Rhinol Laryngol 112:103–108
18. Cavo JW Jr (1985) True vocal cord paralysis following intubation. Laryngoscope 95:1352–1359
19. Weymuller EA Jr, Bishop MJ, Fink BR et al. (1983) Quantification of intralaryngeal pressure exerted by endotracheal tubes. Ann Otol Rhinol Laryngol 92:444–447
20. Whited RE (1983) Posterior commissure stenosis post long-term intubation. Laryngoscope 93:1314–1318
21. Montgomery WW (1973) Posterior and complete laryngeal (glottic) stenosis. Arch Otolaryngol 98:170–175
22. Koufman JA (1991) The otolaryngologic manifestations of gastroesophageal reflux disease (GERD): a clinical investigation of 225 patients using ambulatory 24-hour pH monitoring and an experimental investigation of the role of acid and pepsin in the development of laryngeal injury. Laryngoscope 101:1–78
23. Gardner GM (2000) Posterior glottic stenosis and bilateral vocal fold immobility: diagnosis and treatment. Otolaryngol Clin North Am 33:855–878
24. Lofgren RH, Montgomery WW (1962) Incidence of laryngeal involvement in rheumatoid arthritis. N Engl J Med 267:193–195
25. Parnes SM, Satya-Murti S (1985) Predictive value of laryngeal electromyography in patients with vocal cord paralysis of neurogenic origin. Laryngoscope 95:1323–1326
26. Correa AJ, Reinisch L, Sanders DL et al. (1999) Inhibition of subglottic stenosis with mitomycin-C in the canine model. Ann Otol Rhinol Laryngol 108:1053–1060
27. Rahbar R, Valdez TA, Shapshay SM (2000) Preliminary results of intraoperative mitomycin-C in the treatment and prevention of glottic and subglottic stenosis. J Voice 14:282–286

28. Baker SE, Sapienza CM, Martin D et al. (2003) Inspiratory pressure threshold training for upper airway limitation: a case of bilateral abductor vocal fold paralysis. J Voice 17:384–394
29. Cohen SR, Thompson JW, Camilon FS Jr (1989) Botulinum toxin for relief of bilateral abductor paralysis of the larynx: histologic study in an animal model. Ann Otol Rhinol Laryngol 98:213–216
30. Ptok M, Schonweiler R (2001) Botulinum toxin type A-induced "rebalancing" in bilateral vocal cord paralysis? HNO 49:548–552 [in German]
31. Zealear DL, Billante CR, Courey MS et al. (2002) Electrically stimulated glottal opening combined with adductor muscle botox blockade restores both ventilation and voice in a patient with bilateral laryngeal paralysis. Ann Otol Rhinol Laryngol 111:500–506
32. Chetty KG, McDonald RL, Berry RB et al. (1993) Chronic respiratory failure due to bilateral vocal cord paralysis managed with nocturnal nasal positive pressure ventilation. Chest 103:1270–1271
33. Zitsch RP III (1992) Continuous positive airway pressure. Use in bilateral vocal cord paralysis. Arch Otolaryngol Head Neck Surg 118:875–876
34. Bogdasarian RS, Olson NR (1980) Posterior glottic laryngeal stenosis. Otolaryngol Head Neck Surg 88:765–772
35. Schaefer SD, Close LG, Brown OE (1986) Mobilization of the fixated arytenoid in the stenotic posterior laryngeal commissure. Laryngoscope 96:656–659
36. Gacek M, Gacek RR (1996) Cricoarytenoid joint mobility after chronic vocal cord paralysis. Laryngoscope 106:1528–1530
37. Hillel AD, Benninger M, Blitzer A et al. (1999) Evaluation and management of bilateral vocal cord immobility. Otolaryngol Head Neck Surg 121:760–765
38. Tucker HM (1978) Human laryngeal reinnervation: long-term experience with the nerve-muscle pedicle technique. Laryngoscope 88:598–604
39. Tucker HM (1982) Nerve–muscle pedicle reinnervation of the larynx: avoiding pitfalls and complications. Ann Otol Rhinol Laryngol 91:440–444
40. Tucker HM (1989) Long-term results of nerve-muscle pedicle reinnervation for laryngeal paralysis. Ann Otol Rhinol Laryngol 98:674–676
41. Tucker HM (1976) Human laryngeal reinnervation. Laryngoscope 86:769–779
42. Applebaum EL, Allen GW, Sisson GA (1979) Human laryngeal reinnervation: the Northwestern experience. Laryngoscope 89:1784–1787
43. Tucker HM (1979) Reinnervation of the paralyzed larynx: a review. Head Neck Surg 1:235–242
44. May M, Lavorato AS, Bleyaert AL (1980) Rehabilitation of the crippled larynx: application of the Tucker technique for muscle–nerve reinnervation. Laryngoscope 90:1–18
45. Crumley RL (1985) Update of laryngeal reinnervation concepts and options. In: Bailey BJ, Biller HF (eds) Surgery of the larynx. Saunders, Philadelphia, pp 135–147
46. Broniatowski M, Kaneko S, Jacobs G et al. (1985) Laryngeal pacemaker. II. Electronic pacing of reinnervated posterior cricoarytenoid muscles in the canine. Laryngoscope 95:1194–1198
47. Broniatowski M, Tucker HM, Kaneko S et al. (1986) Laryngeal pacemaker. Part I. Electronic pacing of reinnervated strap muscles in the dog. Otolaryngol Head Neck Surg 94:41–44
48. Kirchner FR (1979) Endoscopic lateralization of the vocal cord in abductor paralysis of the larynx. Laryngoscope 89:1779–1783
49. Ejnell H, Mansson I, Hallen O et al. (1984) A simple operation for bilateral vocal cord paralysis. Laryngoscope 94:954–958
50. Lichtenberger G (1983) Endo-extralaryngeal needle carrier instrument. Laryngoscope 93:1348–1350
51. Tamura E, Kitahara S, Ogura M et al. (2002) Direction of lateral traction in Ejnell's technique: an experimental study and case report of bilateral vocal cord paralysis. Acta Otolaryngol 122:420–423
52. Lichtenberger G, Toohill RJ (1997) Technique of endo-extralaryngeal suture lateralization for bilateral abductor vocal cord paralysis. Laryngoscope 107:1281–1283
53. Lichtenberger G (2002) Reversible lateralization of the paralyzed vocal cord without tracheostomy. Ann Otol Rhinol Laryngol 111:21–26
54. Rontal M, Rontal E (1994) Use of laryngeal muscular tenotomy for bilateral midline vocal cord fixation. Ann Otol Rhinol Laryngol 103:583–589
55. Whicker JH, Devine KD (1972) Long-term results of Thornell arytenoidectomy in the surgical treatment of bilateral vocal cord paralysis. Laryngoscope 82:1331–1336
56. Ossoff RH, Sisson GA, Duncavage JA et al. (1984) Endoscopic laser arytenoidectomy for the treatment of bilateral vocal cord paralysis. Laryngoscope 94:1293–1297
57. Ossoff RH, Duncavage JA, Shapshay SM et al. (1990) Endoscopic laser arytenoidectomy revisited. Ann Otol Rhinol Laryngol 99:764–771
58. Crumley RL (1993) Endoscopic laser medical arytenoidectomy for airway management in bilateral laryngeal paralysis. Ann Otol Rhinol Laryngol 102:81–84
59. Dennis DP, Kashima H (1989) Carbon dioxide laser posterior cordectomy for treatment of bilateral vocal cord paralysis. Ann Otol Rhinol Laryngol 98:930–934

60. Segas J, Stavroulakis P, Manolopoulos L et al. (2001) Management of bilateral vocal fold paralysis: experience at the University of Athens. Otolaryngol Head Neck Surg 124:68–71
61. Laccourreye O, Paz Escovar MI, Gerhardt J et al. (1999) CO2 laser endoscopic posterior partial transverse cordotomy for bilateral paralysis of the vocal fold. Laryngoscope 109:415–418
62. Cummings CW, Redd EE, Westra WH et al. (1999) Minimally invasive device to effect vocal fold lateralization. Ann Otol Rhinol Laryngol 108:833–836
63. Chang SY (1985) Studies of early laryngeal reinnervation. Laryngoscope 95:455–457
64. Sercarz JA, Nguyen L, Nasri S et al. (1997) Physiologic motion after laryngeal nerve reinnervation: a new method. Otolaryngol Head Neck Surg 116:466–474
65. van Lith-Bijl JT, Mahieu HF (1998) Reinnervation aspects of laryngeal transplantation. Eur Arch Otorhinolaryngol 255:515–520
66. Brondbo K, Hall C, Teig E et al. (1987) Experimental laryngeal reinnervation by phrenic nerve implantation into the posterior cricoarytenoid muscle. Acta Otolaryngol 103:339–344
67. Jacobs IN, Sanders I, Wu BL et al. (1990) Reinnervation of the canine posterior cricoarytenoid muscle with sympathetic preganglionic neurons. Ann Otol Rhinol Laryngol 99:167–174
68. Obert PM, Young KA, Tobey DN (1984) Use of direct posterior cricoarytenoid stimulation in laryngeal paralysis. Arch Otolaryngol 110:88–92
69. Otto RA, Templer J, Davis W et al. (1985) Coordinated electrical pacing of vocal cord abductors in recurrent laryngeal nerve paralysis. Otolaryngol Head Neck Surg 93:634–638
70. Sanders I (1991) Electrical stimulation of laryngeal muscle. Otolaryngol Clin North Am 24:1253–1274
71. Holinger LD, Holinger PC, Holinger PH (1976) Etiology of bilateral abductor vocal cord paralysis: a review of 389 cases. Ann Otol Rhinol Laryngol 85:428–436
72. Downey WL, Kennon WG Jr (1968) Laryngofissure approach for bilateral abductor paralysis. Arch Otolaryngol 88:513–517

Subject Index

A

ACD, see anterior approach to the cervical spine
adduction arytenoidopexy 17, 180, 181
airway obstruction 240
Alloderm (acellular human dermis) 117
amplification 93
amyotrophic lateral sclerosis 208
ansa cervicalis 192
anterior
- approach to the cervical spine 38, 42
- cervical diskectomy, see anterior approach to the cervical spine
anti-reflux therapy 240
aorta 7
aortic
- aneurysm 38
- dissection 47
Arnold-Chiari malformation, see Chiari malformation
artery
- common carotid 6, 7
- inferior thyroid 8
- internal carotid 5, 6
- subclavian 6, 7
- superior laryngeal 5
arytenoid
- adduction, see arytenoid repositioning procedure
- cartilage 57, 178
- dislocation, see cricoarytenoid dislocation
- repositioning procedure (arytenoid adduction) 58, 78, 83, 137, 170, 174, 177, 179, 181
- - in children 231
arytenoidectomy 24, 198, 229, 237, 238, 244
arytenoidopexy 229
aspiration 24, 44, 55, 59, 77, 78, 83, 98, 136, 203, 208, 222, 226
atrophy 22, 23, 24, 97, 219
autologous fat, see also injection augmentation, autologous fat 105
axonotmesis 21, 33

B

barium swallow 59
behavioral rehabilitation, see voice therapy
bioplastique 98
botulinum toxin injection 229
bowing 219, 223
Brünings syringe, see syringe, Brünings
Buffalo voice profile 87

C

calcium hydroxylapatite (Radiesse, Radiance) 81, 83, 123
- allergic reaction 123
- implant (VoCoM), see hydroxylapatite implant
- injected percutaneously 124
- paste 137
- technique 124
cardiac valve repair 45
carotid endarterectomy 38, 43, 44, 78, 79
central venous catheterization 45
cepstrum analysis 88
cervical spine, anterior approach 38, 42, 79
Charcot-Marie-Tooth disease 47, 63, 232
chest radiography 59
Chiari malformation 228
cisplatin 46, 56
collagen 113, 114
- autologous 98, 112
- bovine 98, 102, 111, 118
- homologous 112
- human 112
- in children 231
compensation 89, 91
complex repetitive discharge 66
computed tomography (CT) 21, 38, 59, 61
continuous positive airway pressure 240
cordectomy 198, 237, 243
cordotomy 24
coronary artery bypass 45
cricoarytenoid
- dislocation (arytenoid dislocation) 45, 56–58, 59, 66
- joint 180, 182, 241
- - arthritis, see cricoarytenoid joint fixation
- - fixation (cricoarytenoid ankylosis) 59, 225, 237, 239, 241
- muscle, see muscle, posterior cricoarytenoid
cricoarytenoid ankylosis, see cricoarytenoid joint fixation
cricoid cartilage 178
cricopharyngeal myotomy 44, 78, 182
cricopharyngeus muscle 181
cricothyroid
- approximation 219
- joint 180
CT, see computed tomography or cricothyroid
Cymetra, see micronized acellular dermis
cytomegalovirus 47

D

DiHA (Deflux) 130
diphtheria 38
dysfunctional reinnervation, see synkinetic reinnervation
dysphagia 42, 55, 56, 77, 83
dysphonia plica ventricularis 55, 58, 77, 136, 203
dyspnea 24, 56, 136

E

electrical pacing, *see* functional electrial stimulation
electrical stimulation, *see* functional electrical stimulation
electromyography (EMG) 23, 59, 61, 63, 64, 66, 70, 71, 77, 80, 81, 83, 138, 189, 190, 195, 227, 237, 240
- in children 231
EMG, *see* electromyography
endotracheal intubation, *see* intubation
Epstein-Barr virus 47
esophageal cancer 46
esophagectomy 45
examination, laryngeal 57

F

fascia 98, 102
fat 102
- harvest 105, 106
FEES, *see* fiberoptic endoscopic evaluation of swallowing
fiberoptic endoscopic evaluation of swallowing (FEES) 59, 61
fibrillation 64
flu, *see* influenza
forceps delivery 228
framework surgery, *see* medialization laryngoplasty
functional electrical stimulation (pacing) 24, 28, 203, 237, 245
- aspiration 208
- deglutitive 209
- for abduction 209
- for laryngeal transplantation 213
- for swallowing 213
- for voice 213
- in spasmodic dysphonia 215
- pattern 207
- recurrent laryngeal nerve 205, 207, 209, 214

G

ganglion, inferior cervical (nodose) 5
gelfoam in children 231
gene therapy 28
Gore-tex, *see* polytetrafluoroethylene, expanded
Graves disease 41
GRBAS 87
groove, tracheoesophageal (TE) 7
Guillain-Barré syndrome 208

H

HA, *see* hyaluronic acid
hematoma 184
Henneman's size principle 20, 205
herpes
- simplex 47
- zoster 47
hIGF-1, *see* human insulin-like growth factor
hoarseness 56
Horner's syndrome 43, 47
human insulin-like growth factor (hIGF) 28
hyaluronan, *see* hyaluronic acid (HA)
hyaluronic acid (HA) 98, 127, 128, 130
- complications 131
- injection 131
- resorption 127, 131
- allergy 130
hydrocephalus 228
hydroxylapatite implant (VoCoM) 159
- airway compromise 163
- complications 163
- hematoma 163
- revision 163
- thyroplasty 159
hyperfunction, supraglottic 55, 58
hyperfunctional compensation 89, 90
hyperthyroidism 41
hypoglossal nerve, *see* nerve, hypoglossal

I

idiopathic vocal fold paralysis, *see* vocal fold paralysis, idiopathic
inferior cervical (nodose) ganglion 5
influenza (flu) 47
injection augmentation 81, 97, 101, 102, 105, 111, 119, 123, 135, 137, 177
- direct microlaryngoscopy 99
- indirect laryngoscopy 99
- autologous fat 105, 108, 109
- - complications 109
- - contraindication 106
- percutaneous 114
- techniques 99
- transcutaneous 99
- transoral 99
interarytenoid muscle, *see* muscle, interarytenoid
intubation 45
- endotracheal 45
- injury 238
Isshiki type I thyroplasty, *see* medialization laryngoplasty
Itrel II neural stimulator 211

J

jostle sign 58

L

large-amplitude motor unit 66
laryngeal
- dystonia, *see* spasmodic dysphonia
- electromyography, *see* electromyography
- pacing, *see* functional electrical stimulation
- transplantation 199
- ultrasound 227
laryngoscopy
- fiberoptic 57
- indirect 57
- rigid 57
laryngostroboscopy, *see* stroboscopy
laser, carbon dioxide 244
lateralization
- arytenoid 244
- vocal fold 229, 243
laterofixation 243
LEMG, *see* electromyography
ligament
- inferior cricothyroid 11
- of Berry 10
ligamentum arteriosum 7
ligation of a patent ductus arteriosus 45
lipoinjection, *see* injection, autologous fat
liposuction 106
lobectomy 44
lung cancer 34

Subject Index

Lyme borreliosis 47
lymphoma 46

M

magnetic resonance imaging (MRI) 38, 59, 61
malignancy 34, 46, 59
maximum phonation time (MPT) 58, 87, 88, 102
medialization laryngoplasty 83, 136, 145, 177, 180, 195, 197
– bilateral 105, 219
– cartilage 135
– complications 140
– Gore-tex 169
– hydroxylapatite 159
– implant extrusion 140
– implant malposition 141
– over-medialization 141
– perforation 140
– persistent glottic gap 141
– postoperative airway obstruction 140
– revision 142
– silastic 145
– technique 138–140
– timing 138
– titanium 165
– undercorrection 141
– unsatisfactory voice result 141
– in children 231
mediastinal
– metastases 46
– procedure 44
MHC, see myosin heavy chain
micronized acellular dermis (Cymetra) 98, 102, 114, 117
– allergic reactions 117
– complications 119
– in children 231
– preparation 118, 120
– viral transmission 117
– Alloderm 114
– homologous dermis 98
mitomycin 240
modified barium swallow 59, 61, 77
Montgomery thyroplasty implant system 153
– complications 157
– results 157
Morrison procedure 179
motor
– innervation 4

– unit 20, 66
– – action potential 64
MPT, see maximum phonation time
MRI, see magnetic resonance imaging
multiple sclerosis 208
muscle
– cricoarytenoid 178
– cricopharyngeus 6, 7, 181, 213
– cricothyroid (CT) 4, 7, 20, 17, 197
– fast-twitch type-II fibers 19
– Galen's anastomosis 21
– inferior pharyngeal constrictor 6
– interarytenoid (IA) 11, 17, 20, 178, 190
– lateral cricoarytenoid (LCA) 11, 17, 190
– posterior cricoarytenoid (PCA) 10, 11, 17, 19, 20–22, 178, 189, 190
– slow contracting type-I fibers 20
– slow-twitch type-I fibers 19
– thyroarytenoid (TA) 4, 5, 11, 17, 19, 22, 23, 190
– type-I (slow-twitch) fibers 27
– type-II (fast-twitch) fibers 20, 27
– vocalis 19, 20
myasthenia gravis 63, 64
myokymia 66
myosin heavy chain (MHC) 27, 28

N

nasogastric tube insertion 45
nerve
– anastomosis of Galen 3, 12, 13
– ansa cervicalis 242
– communicating 13
– cricoid anastomosis 13
– for laryngeal reinnervation, hypoglossal 194
– glossopharyngeal 43
– hypoglossal 43, 192–194
– interarytenoid plexus 13
– recurrent laryngeal 3, 4, 7-10, 13, 14, 17, 20, 21, 33, 189, 190, 192–194
– – adductor division 11
– – cervical segment 6
– – primary 197
– – reanastomosis 191, 196

– – repair of 197
– spinal accessory 43
– stimulator, see neuroprosthesis
– superior laryngeal, 3, 4, 13, 14, 17, 197
– – descending division 5
– – external branch 5, 20
– – Galen's anastomosis 5, 17
– – injury 78
– – internal branch 5, 17, 21
– – middle division 5
– – superior division 5
– vagus 6, 7, 43
neurapraxia 21
neuromuscular
– junction 12
– pedicle 199, 242, 243
– plasticity 27
neuroprosthesis 207
– problems 207
neuroprosthetic device, see neuroprosthesis
neurorrhaphy 25, 190, 193
– recurrent laryngeal nerve 21, 24
neurotmesis 21, 33
NMP 199, 243
nodose ganglion, see ganglion, inferior cervical
nucleus
– ambiguous 4
– retrofacial 4
– tractus solitarius 4

O

organophosphate 46
Ortner's cardiovocal syndrome 38, 226
outcome scale 88

P

pacing, see functional electrica stimulation
palatal paralysis 57
paraffin 98, 135
paraganglioma 45
paralytic falsetto 55
paresis 63, 79, 114, 119, 219
Parkinson's disease 208
patent ductus arteriosus 45
– ligation 45
pericardial effusion 38
pleuritis 38

pneumonectomy 44, 79
polyphasic potential 66, 69
Polytef, see polytetrafluoroethylene polymer
polytetrafluoroethylene 98, 135
- expanded (gore-tex) 169, 220
- - complications 174
- - edema 174
- - extrusion 174
- - hematoma 174
- - medialization 169
- - thyroplasty 170
- polymer (teflon, polytef) 81, 98, 100, 101, 135
- - granuloma 102, 179
- - injection, in children 231
positive sharp wave 64
posterior
- cordotomy 229, 245
- cricoarytenoid muscle (PCA) 178, 209
- cricoidotomy 229
- gap 178
- glottic scar 237, 241
- glottic stenosis (posterior glottic scar) 241
presbylaryngis 98
presbyphonia 114
puerperal fever 38

R

Radiance, see calcium hydroxylapatite
radiation 46
Radiesse, see calcium hydroxylapatite
radioactive iodine 46
recruitment 64, 66, 69, 71
regeneration, nerve 26
reinnervation 21, 57, 79, 80, 138, 190, 200, 231, 237, 242, 243, 245
- abductor 198, 199
- ansa cervicalis 191, 194, 199, 229
- - to recurrent laryngeal nerve 192, 195
- dysfunctional, see synkinetic reinnervation
- hypoglossal nerve 191
- - to recurrent laryngeal nerve 25, 193, 196
- inappropriate, see synkinetic reinnervation
- lateral cricoarytenoid 189

- of the CT muscle 197
- PCA (posterior cricoarytenoid muscle) 209
- phrenic nerve 24, 198
- posterior cricoarytenoid muscle 241
- selective 25, 27
- thyroarytenoid 189
repair of thoracic aortic aneurysm 45
resonance 93
Restylane, see hyalouronic acid (HA)
rheumatoid arthritis 239
RLN, see nerve, recurrent laryngeal

S

s/z ratio 87, 88
sarcoidosis 46
scar 97, 113, 114, 127, 129.130, 136, 225
Semon's law 8
serology 59
silicone elastomer, see silastic
silastic 98, 145, 221
- implant, carving 147
- laryngoplasty 145
silicosis 47
skull base surgery 45, 78, 80
SLN, see nerve, superior laryngeal
spasmodic dysphonia (laryngeal dystonia) 63, 64, 219
spirometry 237, 240
stimulator, implantable 24
stridor 24, 239
- in infants 226
stroboscopy (videostroboscopy) 58, 63, 137, 230
stroke 47, 56, 78, 208
sulcus vocalis 127, 129, 130, 136
synkinesis, see synkinetic reinnervation
synkinetic reinnervation (synkinesis) 21–24, 28, 33, 57, 64, 69, 80, 190, 194, 195, 204, 225, 237
syringe, Brünings 100, 108, 124

T

Teflon, see polytetrafluoroethylene polymer
therapy, voice, see voice therapy
thoracic aortic aneurysm, repair 45
thyroid
- carcinoma 42, 46
- disease 42
- gland 6, 10
- scan 59
- surgery, see thyroidectomy
thyroidectomy 33, 38, 41, 42, 79, 238
thyroplasty, see medialization laryngoplasty
titanium vocal medialization implant 165
- complications 167
- granulation tissue 168
- hematoma 168
- outcome 167
tracheoesophageal (TE) groove 7, 10
tracheotomy 24
- for aspiration 208
- in BVFP 241
- in children 227, 228
transplantation of the larynx 199
tubercle of Zuckerkandl 10
tuberculosis 46, 238
tuberculous lymphadenopathy 38
TVFMI, see titanium vocal fold medialization implant
thyphoid fever 38
typhus 38

U

upper esophageal sphincter 213

V

vagal nerve stimulator 44, 225
valsalva maneuver 56, 136
velopharyngeal insufficiency 56
ventriculoperitoneal shunt failure 47
videostroboscopy, see stroboscopy
vinblastine 46, 56
vincristine 46, 56, 225
vocal fold paralysis
- bilateral 225, 226, 229
- evaluation 60
- familial 232
- iatrogenic 38, 39, 56
- idiopathic 47, 80
- left 36
- natural history 79
- prognosis 77–80

- recovery 79, 80, 138
- right 37
- treatment 82

VoCoM implant, *see* hydroxylapatite implant

voice handicap index 88

voice related quality-of-life instrument 88

voice therapy (behavioral rehabilitation) 87–93
- direct therapy 91
- head position 91
- indirect therapy 90

W

Wagner-Grossmann hypothesis 8
Wallenberg syndrome 47
Wallerian degeneration 33
West Nile virus 47

Z

Zyderm, *see* collagen, bovine
Zyplast, *see* collagen bovine

Printing: Krips bv, Meppel
Binding: Stürtz, Würzburg